# Changes | An Insider's View

# *cpt*®

current procedural
terminology

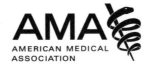

AMA
AMERICAN MEDICAL
ASSOCIATION

# Contents

# Contents

# Foreword

The American Medical Association (AMA) is pleased to offer *CPT® Changes 2022: An Insider's View* (CPT Changes). Since this book was first published in 2000, it has served as the definitive text on additions, revisions, and deletions to the CPT code set.

In developing this book, our intention was to provide CPT users with a glimpse of the logic, rationale, and proposed function of the changes in the CPT code set that resulted from the decisions of the CPT Editorial Panel and the yearly update process. The AMA staff members have the unique perspective of being both participants in the CPT editorial process and users of the CPT code set.

*CPT Changes* is intended to bridge understanding between clinical decisions made by the CPT Editorial Panel regarding appropriate service or procedure descriptions with functional interpretations of coding guidelines, code intent, and code combinations, which are necessary for users of the CPT code set. A new edition of this book, like the codebook, is published annually.

To assist CPT users in applying the new and revised CPT codes, this book includes clinical examples that describe the typical patient who might undergo the procedure and detailed descriptions of the procedure. Both of these are required as a part of the CPT code change proposal process, which are used by the CPT Editorial Panel in crafting language, guidelines, and parenthetical notes associated with the new or revised codes. In addition, many of the clinical examples and descriptions of the procedures are used in the AMA/Specialty Society Relative Value Scale (RVS) Update (RUC) process to conduct surveys on physician work and to develop work relative value recommendations to the Centers for Medicare & Medicaid Services (CMS) as part of the Medicare physician fee schedule (MPFS).

We are confident that the information provided in *CPT Changes* will prove to be a valuable resource to CPT users, not only as they apply changes for the year of publication, but also as a resource for frequent reference as they continue their education in CPT coding. The AMA makes every effort to be a voice of clarity and consistency in an otherwise confusing system of health care claims and payment, and *CPT Changes 2022: An Insider's View* demonstrates our continued commitment to assist users of the CPT code set.

# Using This Book

This book is designed to serve as a reference guide to understanding the changes contained in the Current Procedural Terminology (CPT®) 2022 code set and is not intended to replace the CPT codebook. Every effort is made to ensure accuracy; however, if differences exist, you should always defer to the information in the *CPT® 2022* codebook.

## The Symbols

This book uses the same coding conventions as those used in the CPT nomenclature.

● Indicates a new procedure number was added to the CPT nomenclature

▲ Indicates a code revision has resulted in a substantially altered procedure descriptor

+ Indicates a CPT add-on code

⊘ Indicates a code that is exempt from the use of modifier 51 but is not designated as a CPT add-on procedure or service

►◄ Indicates revised guidelines, cross-references, and/or explanatory text

⁄ Indicates a code for a vaccine that is pending FDA approval

\# Indicates a resequenced code. Note that rather than deleting and renumbering, resequencing allows existing codes to be relocated to an appropriate location for the code concept, regardless of the numeric sequence. Numerically placed references (ie, Code is out of numerical sequence. See...) are used as navigational alerts in the CPT codebook to direct the user to the location of an out-of-sequence code. Therefore, remember to refer to the CPT codebook for these references.

★ Indicates a telemedicine code

⌘ Indicates a duplicate PLA test

⇅ Indicates a Category I PLA

Whenever possible, complete segments of text from the CPT codebook are provided; however, in some instances, only pertinent text is included.

## The Rationale

After listing each change or series of changes from the CPT codebook, a rationale is provided. The rationale is intended to provide a brief clarification and explanation of the changes. Nevertheless, it is important to note that they may not address every question that may arise as a result of the changes.

## Reading the Clinical Examples

The clinical examples and their procedural descriptions, which reflect typical clinical situations found in the health-care setting, are included in this text with many of the codes to provide practical situations for which the new and/or revised codes in the CPT 2022 code set would be appropriately reported. It is important to note that these examples do not suggest limiting the use of a code; instead, they are meant to represent the typical patient and service or procedure, as previously stated. In addition, they do not describe the universe of patients for whom the service or procedure would be appropriate. It is important to also note that third-party payer reporting policies may differ.

## Summary of Additions, Deletions, and Revisions and Indexes

A **summary of additions, deletions, and revisions** for the section is presented in a tabular format at the beginning of each section. This table provides readers with the ability to quickly search and have an overview of all of the new, revised, and deleted codes for 2022. In addition to the tabular review of changes, the coding index individually lists all of the new, revised, and deleted codes with each code's status (new, revised, deleted) in parentheses. For more information about these indexes, please read the **Instructions for the Use of the Changes Indexes** on page 287.

## CPT Codebook Conventions and Styles

Similar to the CPT codebook, the guidelines and revised and new CPT code descriptors and parenthetical notes in *CPT Changes 2022* are set in green type. Any revised text, guidelines, and/or headings are indicated with the ▶ ◀ symbols. To match the style used in the codebook, the revised or new text symbol is placed at the beginning and end of a paragraph or section that contains revisions, and the use of green text visually indicates new and/or revised content. Similarly, each section's and subsections' (Surgery) complete code range are listed in the tabs, regardless if these codes are discussed in this book. In addition, all of the different level of headings in the codebook are also picked up, as appropriate, and set in the same style and color. Besides matching the convention and style used in the CPT codebook, the Rationales are placed within a shaded box to distinguish them from the rest of the content for quick and easy reference.

# Evaluation and Management

## Summary of Additions, Deletions, and Revisions

The summary of changes shows the actual changes that have been made to the code descriptors.

New codes appear with a bullet (●) and are indicated as "Code added." Revised codes are preceded with a triangle (▲). Within revised codes, or if a code symbol has been deleted, the deleted language and code symbol appear with a ~~strikethrough~~, while new text appears underlined.

The ✔ symbol is used to identify codes for vaccines that are pending FDA approval. The # symbol is used to identify codes that have been resequenced. CPT add-on codes are annotated by the ✚ symbol. The ⊘ symbol is used to identify codes that are exempt from the use of modifier 51. The ★ symbol is used to identify codes that may be used for reporting telemedicine services. The ✣ symbol is used to identify a proprietary laboratory analyses (PLA) test that has an identical descriptor as another PLA test. A PLA code that satisfies Category I code criteria and has been accepted by the CPT Editorial Panel is annotated with the ↕ symbol.

| Code | Description |
|---|---|
| ★▲99211 | **Office or other outpatient visit** for the evaluation and management of an established patient~~,~~ that may not require the presence of a physician or other qualified health care professional. ~~Usually, the presenting problem(s) are minimal.~~ |
| ▲99483 | Assessment of and care planning for a patient with cognitive impairment, requiring an independent historian, in the office or other outpatient, home or domiciliary or rest home, with all of the following required elements: |
| | ■ Cognition-focused evaluation including a pertinent history and examination; |
| | ■ Medical decision making of moderate or high complexity; |
| | ■ Functional assessment (eg, basic and instrumental activities of daily living), including decision-making capacity; |
| | ■ Use of standardized instruments for staging of dementia (eg, functional assessment staging test [FAST], clinical dementia rating [CDR]); |
| | ■ Medication reconciliation and review for high-risk medications; |
| | ■ Evaluation for neuropsychiatric and behavioral symptoms, including depression, including use of standardized screening instrument(s); |
| | ■ Evaluation of safety (eg, home), including motor vehicle operation; |
| | ■ Identification of caregiver(s), caregiver knowledge, caregiver needs, social supports, and the willingness of caregiver to take on caregiving tasks; |
| | ■ Development, updating or revision, or review of an Advance Care Plan; |
| | ■ Creation of a written care plan, including initial plans to address any neuropsychiatric symptoms, neuro-cognitive symptoms, functional limitations, and referral to community resources as needed (eg, rehabilitation services, adult day programs, support groups) shared with the patient and/or caregiver with initial education and support. |
| | Typically, 50 minutes are spent face-to-face with the patient and/or family or caregiver. |

| Code | Description |
|---|---|
| #▲99490 | Chronic care management services with the following required elements: |
| | ■ multiple (two or more) chronic conditions expected to last at least 12 months, or until the death of the patient, |
| | ■ chronic conditions that place the patient at significant risk of death, acute exacerbation/decompensation, or functional decline, |
| | ■ comprehensive care plan established, implemented, revised, or monitored; |
| | first 20 minutes of clinical staff time directed by a physician or other qualified health care professional, per calendar month. |
| #+▲99439 | each additional 20 minutes of clinical staff time directed by a physician or other qualified health care professional, per calendar month (List separately in addition to code for primary procedure) |
| #▲99491 | Chronic care management services, provided personally by a physician or other qualified health care professional, at least 30 minutes of physician or other qualified health care professional time, per calendar month, with the following required elements: |
| | ■ multiple (two or more) chronic conditions expected to last at least 12 months, or until the death of the patient,; |
| | ■ chronic conditions that place the patient at significant risk of death, acute exacerbation/decompensation, or functional decline,; |
| | ■ comprehensive care plan established, implemented, revised, or monitored;: |
| | first 30 minutes provided personally by a physician or other qualified health care professional, per calendar month. |
| #+●99437 | Code added |
| ▲99487 | Complex chronic care management services with the following required elements: |
| | ■ multiple (two or more) chronic conditions expected to last at least 12 months, or until the death of the patient, |
| | ■ chronic conditions that place the patient at significant risk of death, acute exacerbation/decompensation, or functional decline, |
| | ■ comprehensive care plan established, implemented, revised, or monitored, |
| | ■ moderate or high complexity medical decision making; |
| | first 60 minutes of clinical staff time directed by a physician or other qualified health care professional, per calendar month. |
| +▲99489 | each additional 30 minutes of clinical staff time directed by a physician or other qualified health care professional, per calendar month (List separately in addition to code for primary procedure) |
| #●99424 | Code added |
| #+●99425 | Code added |
| #●99426 | Code added |
| #+●99427 | Code added |

★ = Telemedicine   ✚ = Add-on code   𝒩 = FDA approval pending   # = Resequenced code   ⊘ = Modifier 51 exempt

| Code | Description |
|---|---|
| ▲99492 | **Initial psychiatric collaborative care management,** first 70 minutes in the first calendar month of behavioral health care manager activities, in consultation with a psychiatric consultant, and directed by the treating physician or other qualified health care professional, with the following required elements: <br><br>■ outreach to and engagement in treatment of a patient directed by the treating physician or other qualified health care professional; <br><br>■ initial assessment of the patient, including administration of validated rating scales, with the development of an individualized treatment plan; <br><br>■ review by the psychiatric consultant with modifications of the plan if recommended; <br><br>■ entering patient in a registry and tracking patient follow-up and progress using the registry, with appropriate documentation, and participation in weekly caseload consultation with the psychiatric consultant; and <br><br>■ provision of brief interventions using evidence-based techniques such as behavioral activation, motivational interviewing, and other focused treatment strategies. |
| ▲99493 | **Subsequent psychiatric collaborative care management,** first 60 minutes in a subsequent month of behavioral health care manager activities, in consultation with a psychiatric consultant, and directed by the treating physician or other qualified health care professional, with the following required elements: <br><br>■ tracking patient follow-up and progress using the registry, with appropriate documentation; <br><br>■ participation in weekly caseload consultation with the psychiatric consultant; <br><br>■ ongoing collaboration with and coordination of the patient's mental health care with the treating physician or other qualified health care professional and any other treating mental health providers; <br><br>■ additional review of progress and recommendations for changes in treatment, as indicated, including medications, based on recommendations provided by the psychiatric consultant; <br><br>■ provision of brief interventions using evidence-based techniques such as behavioral activation, motivational interviewing, and other focused treatment strategies; <br><br>■ monitoring of patient outcomes using validated rating scales; and <br><br>■ relapse prevention planning with patients as they achieve remission of symptoms and/or other treatment goals and are prepared for discharge from active treatment. |
| #▲99484 | Care management services for behavioral health conditions, at least 20 minutes of clinical staff time, directed by a physician or other qualified health care professional, per calendar month, with the following required elements: <br><br>■ initial assessment or follow-up monitoring, including the use of applicable validated rating scales; <br><br>■ behavioral health care planning in relation to behavioral/psychiatric health problems, including revision for patients who are not progressing or whose status changes; <br><br>■ facilitating and coordinating treatment such as psychotherapy, pharmacotherapy, counseling and/or psychiatric consultation; and <br><br>■ continuity of care with a designated member of the care team. |

Evaluation / Management 99202-99499

# Evaluation and Management

## Office or Other Outpatient Services

### Established Patient

★ ▲ **99211**    **Office or other outpatient visit** for the evaluation and management of an established patient that may not require the presence of a physician or other qualified health care professional

### Rationale

Code 99211 has been editorially revised with the removal of the phrase, "usually the presenting problems are minimal." Prior to 2021, the descriptors of the office or other outpatient services codes (99202-99215) included a description of the patient's presenting problem(s). Effective 2021, many revisions were made to the office or other outpatient services codes including the removal of the description of the patient's presenting problem(s). The description was inadvertently left in the descriptor of code 99211 and, therefore, has been removed for consistency. This revision does not change the way code 99211 is reported.

# Critical Care Services

Critical care is the direct delivery by a physician(s) or other qualified health care professional of medical care for a critically ill or critically injured patient. A critical illness or injury acutely impairs one or more vital organ systems such that there is a high probability of imminent or life threatening deterioration in the patient's condition. Critical care involves high complexity decision making to assess, manipulate, and support vital system function(s) to treat single or multiple vital organ system failure and/or to prevent further life threatening deterioration of the patient's condition. Examples of vital organ system failure include, but are not limited to: central nervous system failure, circulatory failure, shock, renal, hepatic, metabolic, and/or respiratory failure. Although critical care typically requires interpretation of multiple physiologic parameters and/or application of advanced technology(s), critical care may be provided in life threatening situations when these elements are not present. Critical care may be provided on multiple days, even if no changes are made in the treatment rendered to the patient, provided that the patient's condition continues to require the level of attention described above.

Providing medical care to a critically ill, injured, or post-operative patient qualifies as a critical care service only if both the illness or injury and the treatment being provided meet the above requirements. Critical care is usually, but not always, given in a critical care area, such as the coronary care unit, intensive care unit, pediatric intensive care unit, respiratory care unit, or the emergency care facility.

Inpatient critical care services provided to infants 29 days through 71 months of age are reported with pediatric critical care codes 99471-99476. The pediatric critical care codes are reported as long as the infant/young child qualifies for critical care services during the hospital stay through 71 months of age. Inpatient critical care services provided to neonates (28 days of age or younger) are reported with the neonatal critical care codes 99468 and 99469. The neonatal critical care codes are reported as long as the neonate qualifies for critical care services during the hospital stay through the 28th postnatal day. The reporting of the pediatric and neonatal critical care services is not based on time or the type of unit (eg, pediatric or neonatal critical care unit) and it is not dependent upon the type of physician or other qualified health care professional delivering the care. To report critical care services provided in the outpatient setting (eg, emergency department or office), for neonates and pediatric patients up through 71 months of age, see the critical care codes 99291, 99292. If the same individual provides critical care services for a neonatal or pediatric patient in both the outpatient and inpatient settings on the same day, report only the appropriate neonatal or pediatric critical care code 99468-99472 for all critical care services provided on that day. Also report 99291-99292 for neonatal or pediatric critical care services provided by the individual providing critical care at one facility but transferring the patient to another facility. Critical care services provided by a second individual of a different specialty not reporting a per day neonatal or pediatric critical care code can be reported with codes 99291, 99292. For additional instructions on reporting these services, see the Neonatal and Pediatric Critical Care section and codes 99468-99476.

Services for a patient who is not critically ill but happens to be in a critical care unit are reported using other appropriate E/M codes.

Critical care and other E/M services may be provided to the same patient on the same date by the same individual.

▶For reporting by professionals, the following services are included in critical care when performed during the critical period by the physician(s) providing critical care: the interpretation of cardiac output measurements

★ = Telemedicine    ✚ = Add-on code    ◢ = FDA approval pending    # = Resequenced code    ⊘ = Modifier 51 exempt

(93598), chest X rays (71045, 71046), pulse oximetry (94760, 94761, 94762), blood gases, and collection and interpretation of physiologic data (eg, ECGs, blood pressures, hematologic data); gastric intubation (43752, 43753); temporary transcutaneous pacing (92953); ventilatory management (94002-94004, 94660, 94662); and vascular access procedures (36000, 36410, 36415, 36591, 36600). Any services performed that are not included in this listing should be reported separately. Facilities may report the above services separately. ◄

Codes 99291, 99292 should be reported for the attendance during the transport of critically ill or critically injured patients older than 24 months of age to or from a facility or hospital. For transport services of critically ill or critically injured pediatric patients 24 months of age or younger, see 99466, 99467.

**99291** **Critical care, evaluation and management** of the critically ill or critically injured patient; first 30-74 minutes

**+ 99292** each additional 30 minutes (List separately in addition to code for primary service)

(Use 99292 in conjunction with 99291)

—— *Coding Tip* ——

**Services Included in Critical Care Services**

For reporting by professionals, the following services are included in critical care when performed during the critical period by the physician(s) providing critical care: the interpretation of cardiac output measurements (93598), chest X rays (71045, 71046), pulse oximetry (94760, 94761, 94762), blood gases, and collection and interpretation of physiologic data (eg, ECGs, blood pressures, hematologic data); gastric intubation (43752, 43753); temporary transcutaneous pacing (92953); ventilatory management (94002-94004, 94660, 94662); and vascular access procedures (36000, 36410, 36415, 36591, 36600). Any services performed that are not listed above should be reported separately. Facilities may report the above services separately.

*CPT Coding Guideline, Critical Care*

# Domiciliary, Rest Home (eg, Assisted Living Facility), or Home Care Plan Oversight Services

**99339** Individual physician supervision of a patient (patient not present) in home, domiciliary or rest home (eg, assisted living facility) requiring complex and multidisciplinary care modalities involving regular physician development and/or revision of care plans, review of subsequent reports of patient status, review of related laboratory and other studies, communication (including telephone calls) for purposes of assessment or care decisions with health care professional(s), family member(s), surrogate decision maker(s) (eg, legal guardian) and/or key caregiver(s) involved in patient's care, integration of new information into the medical treatment plan and/or adjustment of medical therapy, within a calendar month; 15-29 minutes

**99340** 30 minutes or more

(Do not report 99339, 99340 for patients under the care of a home health agency, enrolled in a hospice program, or for nursing facility residents)

▶(Do not report 99339, 99340 during the same month with 99424, 99425, 99426, 99427, 99437, 99439, 99487, 99489, 99490, 99491)◄

### Rationale

To accommodate the addition of the new principal care management services codes and other changes made to clarify the reporting of these services, the parenthetical note following code 99340 has been revised.

Refer to the codebook and the Rationale for codes 99424-99427 for a full discussion of these changes.

# Prolonged Services

## Prolonged Service Without Direct Patient Contact

Codes 99358 and 99359 are used when a prolonged service is provided that is neither face-to-face time in the outpatient, inpatient, or observation setting, nor additional unit/floor time in the hospital or nursing facility setting. Codes 99358, 99359 may be used during the same session of an evaluation and management service, except office or other outpatient services (99202, 99203, 99204, 99205, 99212, 99213, 99214, 99215). For prolonged total time in addition to office or other outpatient services (ie, 99205, 99215) on the same date of service without direct patient contact, use 99417. Codes 99358, 99359 may also be used for prolonged services on a date other than the date of a face-to-face encounter.

This service is to be reported in relation to other physician or other qualified health care professional services, including evaluation and management services at any level. This prolonged service may be reported on a different date than the primary service to which it is related. For example, extensive record review may relate to a previous evaluation and management service performed at an earlier date. However, it must relate to a service or patient where (face-to-face) patient care has occurred or will occur and relate to ongoing patient management.

Codes 99358 and 99359 are used to report the total duration of non-face-to-face time spent by a physician or other qualified health care professional on a given date providing prolonged service, even if the time spent by the physician or other qualified health care professional on that date is not continuous. Code 99358 is used to report the first hour of prolonged service on a given date regardless of the place of service. It should be used only once per date.

Prolonged service of less than 30 minutes total duration on a given date is not separately reported.

Code 99359 is used to report each additional 30 minutes beyond the first hour. It may also be used to report the final 15 to 30 minutes of prolonged service on a given date.

Prolonged service of less than 15 minutes beyond the first hour or less than 15 minutes beyond the final 30 minutes is not reported separately.

►Do not report 99358, 99359 for time without direct patient contact reported in other services, such as care plan oversight services (99339, 99340, 99374-99380), chronic care management by a physician or other qualified health care professional (99491), home and outpatient INR monitoring (93792, 93793), medical team conferences (99366-99368), interprofessional telephone/Internet/electronic health record consultations (99446, 99447, 99448, 99449, 99451, 99452), online digital evaluation and management services (99421, 99422, 99423), or principal care management services (99424).◄

**99358**  **Prolonged evaluation and management service** before and/or after direct patient care; first hour

**+ 99359**  each additional 30 minutes (List separately in addition to code for prolonged service)

---

### Rationale

To accommodate the addition of the new principal care management services codes and other changes made to clarify the reporting of these services, guidelines within the Prolonged Service Without Direct Patient Contact subsection have been revised.

Refer to the codebook and the Rationale for codes 99424-99427 for a full discussion of these changes.

---

# Case Management Services

## Medical Team Conferences

### Medical Team Conference, Direct (Face-to-Face) Contact With Patient and/or Family

**99366**  **Medical team conference** with interdisciplinary team of health care professionals, face-to-face with patient and/or family, 30 minutes or more, participation by nonphysician qualified health care professional

(Team conference services of less than 30 minutes duration are not reported separately)

(For team conference services by a physician with patient and/or family present, see Evaluation and Management services)

►(Do not report 99366 for the same time reported for 99424, 99425, 99426, 99427, 99437, 99439, 99487, 99489, 99490, 99491)◄

### Medical Team Conference, Without Direct (Face-to-Face) Contact With Patient and/or Family

**99367**  **Medical team conference** with interdisciplinary team of health care professionals, patient and/or family not present, 30 minutes or more; participation by physician

**99368**  participation by nonphysician qualified health care professional

(Team conference services of less than 30 minutes duration are not reported separately)

►(Do not report 99367, 99368 during the same month with 99424, 99425, 99426, 99427, 99437, 99439, 99487, 99489, 99490, 99491)◄

---

## Rationale

To accommodate the addition of the new principal care management services codes and other changes made to clarify the reporting of these services, the parenthetical notes following codes 99366 and 99368 have been revised.

Refer to the codebook and the Rationale for codes 99424-99427 for a full discussion of these changes.

# Care Plan Oversight Services

Care plan oversight services are reported separately from codes for office/outpatient, hospital, home, nursing facility or domiciliary, or non-face-to-face services. The complexity and approximate time of the care plan oversight services provided within a 30-day period determine code selection. Only one individual may report services for a given period of time, to reflect the sole or predominant supervisory role with a particular patient. These codes should not be reported for supervision of patients in nursing facilities or under the care of home health agencies unless they require recurrent supervision of therapy.

The work involved in providing very low intensity or infrequent supervision services is included in the pre- and post-encounter work for home, office/outpatient and nursing facility or domiciliary visit codes.

> (For care plan oversight services of patients in the home, domiciliary, or rest home [eg, assisted living facility], see 99339, 99340, and for hospice agency, see 99377, 99378)

> (Do not report 99374-99380 for time reported with 98966, 98967, 98968, 99421, 99422, 99423, 99441, 99442, 99443)

> ▶(Do not report 99374-99378 during the same month with 99487, 99489)◀

## Rationale

The parenthetical note for codes 99374-99378 that follows the care plan oversight services guidelines has been revised to reflect that only two codes are included for Complex Chronic Care Management Services (99487, 99489) by replacing the hyphen between codes 99487 and 99489 with a comma.

Refer to the codebook and the Rationale for codes 99424-99427 for a full discussion of these changes.

# Preventive Medicine Services

The following codes are used to report the preventive medicine evaluation and management of infants, children, adolescents, and adults.

The extent and focus of the services will largely depend on the age of the patient.

If an abnormality is encountered or a preexisting problem is addressed in the process of performing this preventive medicine evaluation and management service, and if the problem or abnormality is significant enough to require additional work to perform the key components of a problem-oriented evaluation and management service, then the appropriate office/outpatient code 99202, 99203, 99204, 99205, 99211, 99212, 99213, 99214, 99215 should also be reported. Modifier 25 should be added to the office/outpatient code to indicate that a significant, separately identifiable evaluation and management service was provided on the same day as the preventive medicine service. The appropriate preventive medicine service is additionally reported.

An insignificant or trivial problem/abnormality that is encountered in the process of performing the preventive medicine evaluation and management service and which does not require additional work and the performance of the key components of a problem-oriented E/M service should not be reported.

The "comprehensive" nature of the preventive medicine services codes 99381-99397 reflects an age- and gender-appropriate history/exam and is **not** synonymous with the "comprehensive" examination required in evaluation and management codes 99202-99350.

Codes 99381-99397 include counseling/anticipatory guidance/risk factor reduction interventions which are provided at the time of the initial or periodic comprehensive preventive medicine examination. (Refer to 99401, 99402, 99403, 99404, 99411, and 99412 for reporting those counseling/anticipatory guidance/risk factor reduction interventions that are provided at an encounter separate from the preventive medicine examination.)

(For behavior change intervention, see 99406, 99407, 99408, 99409)

▶Vaccine/toxoid products, immunization administrations, ancillary studies involving laboratory, radiology, other procedures, or screening tests (eg, vision, hearing, developmental) identified with a specific CPT code are reported separately. For immunization administration and vaccine risk/benefit counseling, see 90460, 90461, 90471-90474, 0001A, 0002A, 0011A, 0012A, 0021A, 0022A, 0031A, 0041A, 0042A. For vaccine/toxoid products, see 90476-90759, 91300, 91301, 91302, 91303, 91304.◀

## Rationale

In support of the changes made to accommodate the addition of new codes for reporting the severe acute respiratory syndrome coronavirus 2 (SARS-CoV-2) (coronavirus disease [COVID-19]) vaccines, the preventive medicine services guidelines have been revised.

Refer to the codebook and the Rationale for codes 0001A-0042A for a full discussion of these changes.

# Counseling Risk Factor Reduction and Behavior Change Intervention

## Other Preventive Medicine Services

**99424** Code is out of numerical sequence. See 99487-99493

**99425** Code is out of numerical sequence. See 99487-99493

**99426** Code is out of numerical sequence. See 99487-99493

**99427** Code is out of numerical sequence. See 99487-99493

# Non-Face-to-Face Services

## Telephone Services

**99437** Code is out of numerical sequence. See 99480-99489

## Online Digital Evaluation and Management Services

# **99421** Online digital evaluation and management service, for an established patient, for up to 7 days, cumulative time during the 7 days; 5-10 minutes

# **99422** 11-20 minutes

# **99423** 21 or more minutes

(Report 99421, 99422, 99423 once per 7-day period)

(Clinical staff time is not calculated as part of cumulative time for 99421, 99422, 99423)

(Do not report online digital E/M services for cumulative service time less than 5 minutes)

(Do not count 99421, 99422, 99423 time otherwise reported with other services)

(Do not report 99421, 99422, 99423 on a day when the physician or other qualified health care professional reports E/M services [99202, 99203, 99204, 99205, 99212, 99213, 99214, 99215, 99241, 99242, 99243, 99244, 99245])

▶(Do not report 99421, 99422, 99423 when using 99091 99339, 99340, 99374, 99375, 99377, 99378, 99379, 99380, 99424, 99425, 99426, 99427, 99437, 99487, 99489, 99491, 99495, 99496, for the same communication[s])◀

(Do not report 99421, 99422, 99423 for home and outpatient INR monitoring when reporting 93792, 93793)

## Rationale

To accommodate the addition of the new principal care management services codes and other changes made to clarify the reporting of these services, a parenthetical note following code 99423 has been revised.

Refer to the codebook and the Rationale for codes 99424-99427 for a full discussion of these changes.

# Digitally Stored Data Services/ Remote Physiologic Monitoring

Codes 99453 and 99454 are used to report remote physiologic monitoring services (eg, weight, blood pressure pulse oximetry) during a 30-day period. To report 99453, 99454, the device used must be a medical device as defined by the FDA, and the service must be ordered by a physician or other qualified health care professional. Code 99453 may be used to report the set-up and patient education on use of the device(s). Code 99454 may be used to report supply of the device for daily recording or programmed alert transmissions. Codes 99453, 99454 are not reported i monitoring is less than 16 days. Do not report 99453, 99454 when these services are included in other codes for the duration of time of the physiologic monitoring service (eg, 95250 for continuous glucose monitoring requires a minimum of 72 hours of monitoring).

Code 99091 should be reported no more than once in a 30-day period to include the physician or other qualified health care professional time involved with data accession review and interpretation, modification of care plan as necessary (including communication to patient and/or caregiver), and associated documentation.

If the services described by 99091 or 99474 are provided on the same day the patient presents for an evaluation and management (E/M) service to the same provider, these services should be considered part of the E/M service and not reported separately.

▶Do not report 99091 for time in the same calendar month when used to meet the criteria for care plan oversight services (99374, 99375, 99377, 99378, 99379, 99380), home, domiciliary, or rest home care plan oversight services (99339, 99340), remote physiologic monitoring services (99457, 99458), or personally performed chronic or principal care management (99424, 99425, 99426, 99427, 99437, 99491). Do not report 99091 if other more specific codes exist (eg, 93227, 93272 for cardiographic services; 95250 for continuous glucose monitoring). Do not report 99091 for transfer and interpretation of data from hospital or clinical laboratory computers.◄

## Rationale

To accommodate the addition of the new principal care management services codes and other changes made to clarify the reporting of these services, guidelines within the Digitally Stored Data Services/Remote Physiologic Monitoring subsection have been revised.

Refer to the codebook and the Rationale for codes 99424-99427 for a full discussion of these changes.

---

Code 99453 is reported for each episode of care. For coding remote monitoring of physiologic parameters, an episode of care is defined as beginning when the remote monitoring physiologic service is initiated, and ends with attainment of targeted treatment goals.

\# **99453**  Remote monitoring of physiologic parameter(s) (eg, weight, blood pressure, pulse oximetry, respiratory flow rate), initial; set-up and patient education on use of equipment

(Do not report 99453 more than once per episode of care)

(Do not report 99453 for monitoring of less than 16 days)

\# **99454**  device(s) supply with daily recording(s) or programmed alert(s) transmission, each 30 days

(For physiologic monitoring treatment management services, use 99457)

(Do not report 99454 for monitoring of less than 16 days)

(Do not report 99453, 99454 in conjunction with codes for more specific physiologic parameters [eg, 93296, 94760])

▶(For remote therapeutic monitoring, see 98975, 98976, 98977)◄

(For self-measured blood pressure monitoring, see 99473, 99474)

## Rationale

An instructional parenthetical note has been added following code 99454 to direct users to codes 98975, 98976, and 98977 for remote therapeutic monitoring services.

Refer to the codebook and the Rationale for codes 98975, 98976, and 98977 for a full discussion of these changes.

\# **99091**  Collection and interpretation of physiologic data (eg, ECG, blood pressure, glucose monitoring) digitally stored and/or transmitted by the patient and/or caregiver to the physician or other qualified health care professional, qualified by education, training, licensure/regulation (when applicable) requiring a minimum of 30 minutes of time, each 30 days

▶(Do not report 99091 in conjunction with 99457, 99458)◄

▶(Do not report 99091 for time in a calendar month when used to meet the criteria for 99339, 99340, 99374, 99375, 99377, 99378, 99379, 99380, 99424, 99425, 99426, 99427, 99437, 99457, 99487, 99491)◄

## Rationale

The two parenthetical notes following code 99091 have been revised. To accommodate the addition of the new remote therapeutic monitoring services codes and remote therapeutic monitoring treatment management services codes and other changes made to clarify the reporting of these services, the first parenthetical note following code 99091 has been revised with the addition of code 99458.

To accommodate the addition of the new principal care management services codes and other changes made to clarify the reporting of these services, the second parenthetical note following code 99091 has been revised.

Refer to the codebook and the Rationale for codes 98975-98981 and 99424-99427 for a full discussion of these changes.

---

\# **99473**  Self-measured blood pressure using a device validated for clinical accuracy; patient education/training and device calibration

(Do not report 99473 more than once per device)

(For ambulatory blood pressure monitoring, see 93784, 93786, 93788, 93790)

\# **99474**  separate self-measurements of two readings one minute apart, twice daily over a 30-day period (minimum of 12 readings), collection of data reported by the patient and/or caregiver to the physician or other qualified health care professional, with report of average systolic and diastolic pressures and subsequent communication of a treatment plan to the patient

▶(Do not report 99473, 99474 in the same calendar month as 93784, 93786, 93788, 93790, 99091, 99424, 99425, 99426, 99427, 99437, 99439, 99453, 99454, 99457, 99487, 99489, 99490, 99491)◄

(Do not report 99474 more than once per calendar month)

## Rationale

To accommodate the addition of the new principal care management services codes and other changes made to clarify the reporting of these services, a parenthetical note following code 99474 has been revised.

Refer to the codebook and the Rationale for codes 99424-99427 for a full discussion of these changes.

# Remote Physiologic Monitoring Treatment Management Services

▶Remote physiologic monitoring treatment management services are provided when clinical staff/physician/other qualified health care professional use the results of remote physiological monitoring to manage a patient under a specific treatment plan. To report remote physiological monitoring, the device used must be a medical device as defined by the FDA, and the service must be ordered by a physician or other qualified health care professional. Do not use 99457, 99458 for time that can be reported using codes for more specific monitoring services. Codes 99457, 99458 may be reported during the same service period as chronic care management services (99437, 99439, 99487, 99489, 99490, 99491), principal care management services (99424, 99425, 99426, 99427), transitional care management services (99495, 99496), and behavioral health integration services (99484, 99492, 99493, 99494).  However, time spent performing these services should remain separate and no time should be counted twice toward the required time for any services in a single month. Codes 99457, 99458 require a live, interactive communication with the patient/caregiver. The interactive communication contributes to the total time, but it does not need to represent the entire cumulative reported time of the treatment management service. For the first completed 20 minutes of clinical staff/physician/other qualified health care professional time in a calendar month report 99457, and report 99458 for each additional completed 20 minutes. Do not report 99457, 99458 for services of less than 20 minutes. Report 99457 one time regardless of the number of physiologic monitoring modalities performed in a given calendar month.

To report remote therapeutic monitoring treatment management services provided by physician or other qualified health care professional, see 98980, 98981.◄

Do not count any time on a day when the physician or other qualified health care professional reports an E/M service (office or other outpatient services 99202, 99203, 99204, 99205, 99211, 99212, 99213, 99214, 99215, domiciliary, rest home services 99324, 99325, 99326, 99327, 99328, 99334, 99335, 99336, 99337, home services 99341, 99342, 99343, 99344, 99345, 99347, 99348, 99349, 99350, inpatient services 99221, 99222, 99223, 99231, 99232, 99233, 99251, 99252, 99253, 99254, 99255). Do not count any time related to other reported services (eg, 93290, 93793, 99291, 99292).

## Rationale

The remote physiologic monitoring treatment management services guidelines have been revised to clarify the requirement for live, interactive communication with the patient for the time period specified by codes 99457 and 99458.

The revision now states that the interactive communication contributes to the total time, but it does not need to represent the entire cumulative reported time of the treatment management service. The guidelines have also been revised to direct users to codes 98980 and 98981 for remote therapeutic monitoring treatment management services provided by a physician or other qualified health care professional (QHP).

Finally, to accommodate the addition of the new principal care management services codes and other changes made to clarify the reporting of these services, the remote physiologic monitoring treatment management guidelines have been revised with the addition of these codes.

Refer to the codebook and the Rationale for codes 98980, 98981, and 99424-99427 for a full discussion of these changes.

# 99457    Remote physiologic monitoring treatment management services, clinical staff/physician/other qualified health care professional time in a calendar month requiring interactive communication with the patient/caregiver during the month; first 20 minutes

(Report 99457 once each 30 days, regardless of the number of parameters monitored)

(Do not report 99457 for services of less than 20 minutes)

(Do not report 99457 in conjunction with 93264, 99091)

(Do not report 99457 in the same month as 99473, 99474)

#+ 99458    each additional 20 minutes (List separately in addition to code for primary procedure)

(Use 99458 in conjunction with 99457)

▶(For remote therapeutic monitoring treatment management services, see 98980, 98981)◄

(Do not report 99458 for services of less than an additional increment of 20 minutes)

★ = Telemedicine    ✚ = Add-on code    ✔ = FDA approval pending    # = Resequenced code    ⊘ = Modifier 51 exemp

## Rationale

An instructional parenthetical note has been added following code 99458 to direct users to codes 98980 and 98981 to report remote therapeutic monitoring treatment management services.

Refer to the codebook and the Rationale for codes 98980 and 98981 for a full discussion of these changes.

# Inpatient Neonatal Intensive Care Services and Pediatric and Neonatal Critical Care Services

## Pediatric Critical Care Patient Transport

Codes 99466, 99467 are used to report the physical attendance and direct face-to-face care by a physician during the interfacility transport of a critically ill or critically injured pediatric patient 24 months of age or younger. Codes 99485, 99486 are used to report the control physician's non-face-to-face supervision of interfacility transport of a critically ill or critically injured pediatric patient 24 months of age or younger. These codes are not reported together for the same patient by the same physician. For the purpose of reporting 99466 and 99467, face-to-face care begins when the physician assumes primary responsibility of the pediatric patient at the referring facility, and ends when the receiving facility accepts responsibility for the pediatric patient's care. Only the time the physician spends in direct face-to-face contact with the patient during the transport should be reported. Pediatric patient transport services involving less than 30 minutes of face-to-face physician care should not be reported using 99466, 99467. Procedure(s) or service(s) performed by other members of the transporting team may not be reported by the supervising physician.

Codes 99485, 99486 may be used to report control physician's non-face-to-face supervision of interfacility pediatric critical care transport, which includes all two-way communication between the control physician and the specialized transport team prior to transport, at the referring facility and during transport of the patient back to the receiving facility. The "control" physician is the physician directing transport services. These codes do not include pretransport communication between the control physician and the referring facility before or following patient transport. These codes may only be reported for patients 24 months of age or younger who are critically ill or critically injured. The control physician provides treatment advice to a specialized transport team who are present and delivering the hands-on patient care. The control physician does not report any services provided by the specialized transport team. The control physician's non-face-to-face time begins with the first contact by the control physician with the specialized transport team and ends when the patient's care is handed over to the receiving facility team. Refer to 99466 and 99467 for face-to-face transport care of the critically ill/injured patient. Time spent with the individual patient's transport team and reviewing data submissions should be recorded. Code 99485 is used to report the first 16-45 minutes of direction on a given date and should only be used once even if time spent by the physician is discontinuous. Do not report services of 15 minutes or less or any time when another physician is reporting 99466, 99467. Do not report 99485 or 99486 in conjunction with 99466, 99467 when performed by the same physician.

For the definition of the critically injured pediatric patient, see the **Neonatal and Pediatric Critical Care Services** section.

The non-face-to-face direction of emergency care to a patient's transporting staff by a physician located in a hospital or other facility by two-way communication is not considered direct face-to-face care and should not be reported with 99466, 99467. Physician-directed non-face-to-face emergency care through outside voice communication to transporting staff personnel is reported with 99288 or 99485, 99486 based upon the age and clinical condition of the patient.

Emergency department services (99281-99285), initial hospital care (99221-99223), critical care (99291, 99292), initial date neonatal intensive (99477) or critical care (99468) may only be reported after the patient has been admitted to the emergency department, the inpatient floor, or the critical care unit of the receiving facility. If inpatient critical care services are reported in the referring facility prior to transfer to the receiving hospital, use the critical care codes (99291, 99292).

▶The following services are included when performed during the pediatric patient transport by the physician providing critical care and may not be reported separately: routine monitoring evaluations (eg, heart rate, respiratory rate, blood pressure, and pulse oximetry), the interpretation of cardiac output measurements (93598), chest X rays (71045, 71046), pulse oximetry (94760, 94761, 94762), blood gases and information data stored in computers (eg, ECGs, blood pressures, hematologic data), gastric intubation (43752, 43753), temporary transcutaneous pacing (92953), ventilatory management (94002, 94003, 94660, 94662), and vascular access procedures (36000, 36400, 36405, 36406, 36415, 36591, 36600). Any services performed which are not listed above should be reported separately.◀

Services provided by the specialized transport team during non-face-to-face transport supervision are not reported by the control physician.

## Rationale

In accordance with the deletion of code 93562 and the establishment of code 93598, the pediatric critical care patient transport guidelines have been revised to reflect these changes.

Refer to the codebook and the Rationale for code 93598 for a full discussion of these changes.

# Cognitive Assessment and Care Plan Services

▲ **99483**   Assessment of and care planning for a patient with cognitive impairment, requiring an independent historian, in the office or other outpatient, home or domiciliary or rest home, with all of the following required elements:

- Cognition-focused evaluation including a pertinent history and examination,
- Medical decision making of moderate or high complexity,
- Functional assessment (eg, basic and instrumental activities of daily living), including decision-making capacity,
- Use of standardized instruments for staging of dementia (eg, functional assessment staging test [FAST], clinical dementia rating [CDR]),
- Medication reconciliation and review for high-risk medications,
- Evaluation for neuropsychiatric and behavioral symptoms, including depression, including use of standardized screening instrument(s),
- Evaluation of safety (eg, home), including motor vehicle operation,
- Identification of caregiver(s), caregiver knowledge, caregiver needs, social supports, and the willingness of caregiver to take on caregiving tasks,
- Development, updating or revision, or review of an Advance Care Plan,
- Creation of a written care plan, including initial plans to address any neuropsychiatric symptoms, neuro-cognitive symptoms, functional limitations, and referral to community resources as needed (eg, rehabilitation services, adult day programs, support groups) shared with the patient and/or caregiver with initial education and support.

Typically, 50 minutes are spent face-to-face with the patient and/or family or caregiver.

## Rationale

Code 99483 has been editorially revised to replace all semicolons in the code descriptor with commas to be consistent with CPT coding convention for nonparent or nonchild codes. The intent and use of the code remains the same.

# Care Management Services

▶Care management services are management and support services provided by clinical staff, under the direction of a physician or other qualified health care professional, or may be provided personally by a physician or other qualified health care professional to a patient residing at home or in a domiciliary, rest home, or assisted living facility. Services include establishing, implementing, revising, or monitoring the care plan, coordinating the care of other professionals and agencies, and educating the patient or caregiver about the patient's condition, care plan, and prognosis. Care management services improve care coordination, reduce avoidable hospital services, improve patient engagement, and decrease care fragmentation. The physician or other qualified health care professional provides or oversees the management and/or coordination of care management services, which include establishing, implementing, revising, or monitoring the care plan, coordinating the care of other professionals and agencies, and educating the patient or caregiver about the patient's condition, care plan, and prognosis.

There are three general categories of care management services: chronic care management (99437, 99439, 99490, 99491), complex chronic care management (99487, 99489), and principal care management (99424, 99425, 99426, 99427). Complex chronic care management addresses all of the patient's medical conditions, and principal care management services address a single condition. Each of the three categories is further subdivided into those services that are personally performed by the physician or other qualified health care professional and those services that are performed by the clinical staff and overseen by the physician or other qualified health care professional. Code selection for these services is based on time in a calendar month, and time used in reporting these services may not represent time spent in another reported service. Chronic care management services do not require moderate or high-level medical decision making and may be reported for a shorter time threshold than complex chronic care management services. Both chronic care and complex chronic care management address, as needed, all medical conditions, psychosocial needs, and activities of daily living. Principal care management services are disease-specific management services. A patient may have multiple chronic conditions of sufficient severity to warrant complex chronic care management but may receive principal care management if the reporting physician or other qualified health care professional is providing single disease rather than comprehensive care management.◄

—— *Coding Tip* ——

If the treating physician or other qualified health care professional personally performs any of the care management services and those activities are not used to meet the criteria for a separately reported code (99424, 99491), then his or her time may be counted toward the required clinical staff time to meet the elements of 99426, 99487, 99490, as applicable.

## ►Care Planning◄

►A plan of care for health problems is based on a physical, mental, cognitive, social, functional, and environmental evaluation. It is intended to provide a simple and concise overview of the patient, and his or her medical condition(s) and be a useful resource for patients, caregivers, health care professionals, and others, as necessary.

A typical plan of care is not limited to, but may include:

- Problem list
- Expected outcome and prognosis
- Measurable treatment goals
- Cognitive assessment
- Functional assessment
- Symptom management
- Planned interventions
- Medical management
- Environmental evaluation
- Caregiver assessment
- Interaction and coordination with outside resources and health care professionals and others, as necessary
- Summary of advance directives

The above elements are intended to be a guide for creating a meaningful plan of care rather than a strict set of requirements, so each should be addressed only as appropriate for the individual.

The plan of care should include specific and achievable goals for each condition and be relevant to the patient's well-being and lifestyle. When possible, the treatment goals should also be measurable and time bound. The plan should be updated periodically based on status or goal changes. The entire care plan should be reviewed, or revised as needed, but at least annually.◄

An electronic and/or printed plan of care must be documented and shared with the patient and/or caregiver.

►Codes 99424, 99426, 99487, 99490, 99491 are reported only once per calendar month. Codes 99427, 99439 are reported no more than twice per calendar month. Codes 99437, 99439, 99487, 99489, 99490, 99491 may only be reported by the single physician or other qualified health care professional who assumes the care management role with a particular patient for the calendar month. Codes 99424, 99425, 99426, 99427 may be reported by different physicians or qualified health care professionals in the same calendar month for the same patient, and documentation in the patient's medical record should reflect coordination among relevant managing clinicians.

For 99426, 99427, 99439, 99487, 99489, 99490, the face-to-face and non-face-to-face time spent by the clinical staff in communicating with the patient and/or family, caregivers, other professionals, and agencies; creating, revising, documenting, and implementing the care plan; or teaching self-management is used in determining the care management clinical staff time for the month. Only the time of the clinical staff of the reporting professional is counted, and the reporting professional's time is additionally included only if he or she is not otherwise reporting his or her care management time with another service (see Coding Tip on page 63). Only count the time of one clinical staff member or physician or other qualified health care professional when two or more are meeting about the patient at the same time. For 99424, 99425, 99437, 99491, only count the time personally spent by the physician or other qualified health care professional. Time spent by the physician or other qualified health care professional that does not meet the threshold to report 99424, 99425, 99437, 99491 may be used toward the time necessary to report 99426, 99427, 99439, 99487, 99489, 99490. Do not count clinical staff time spent as part of a separately reported service.

Care management activities performed by clinical staff, or personally by the physician or other qualified health care professional, typically include:

- communication and engagement with patient, family members, guardian or caretaker, surrogate decision makers, and/or other professionals regarding aspects of care;
- communication with home health agencies and other community services utilized by the patient;
- collection of health outcomes data and registry documentation;
- patient and/or family/caregiver education to support self-management, independent living, and activities of daily living;
- assessment and support for treatment regimen adherence and medication management;

- identification of available community and health resources;
- facilitating access to care and services needed by the patient and/or family;
- management of care transitions not reported as part of transitional care management (99495, 99496);
- ongoing review of patient status, including review of laboratory and other studies not reported as part of an E/M service, noted above;
- development, communication, and maintenance of a comprehensive or disease-specific (as applicable) care plan.

The care management office/practice must have the following capabilities:

- provide 24/7 access to physicians or other qualified health care professionals or clinical staff including providing patients/caregivers with a means to make contact with health care professionals in the practice to address urgent needs regardless of the time of day or day of week;
- provide continuity of care with a designated member of the care team with whom the patient is able to schedule successive routine appointments;
- provide timely access and management for follow-up after an emergency department visit or facility discharge;
- utilize an electronic health record system for timely access to clinical information;
- be able to engage and educate patients and caregivers as well as coordinate and integrate care among all service professionals, as appropriate for each patient;
- reporting physician or other qualified health care professional oversees activities of the care team;
- all care team members providing services are clinically integrated.

Each minute of service time is counted toward only one service. Do not count any time and activities used to meet criteria for another reported service. However, time of clinical staff and time of a physician or other qualified health care professional are reported separately when each provides distinct services to the same patient at different times during the same calendar month. A list of services not reported in the same calendar month as 99439, 99487, 99489, 99490 is provided in the parenthetical instructions following the care management codes. If the care management services are performed within the postoperative period of a reported surgery, the same individual may not report 99439, 99487, 99489, 99490, 99491.◄

When behavioral or psychiatric collaborative care management services are also provided, 99484, 99492, 99493, 99494 may be reported in addition.

# Chronic Care Management Services

►Chronic care management services are provided when medical and/or psychosocial needs of the patient require establishing, implementing, revising, or monitoring the care plan. Patients who receive chronic care management services have two or more chronic continuous or episodic health conditions that are expected to last at least 12 months, or until the death of the patient, and that place the patient at significant risk of death, acute exacerbation, decompensation, or functional decline. Code 99490 is reported when, during the calendar month, at least 20 minutes of clinical staff time is spent in care management activities. Code 99439 is reported in conjunction with 99490 for each additional 20 minutes of clinical staff time spent in care management activities during the calendar month up to a maximum of 60 minutes total time (ie, 99439 may only be reported twice per calendar month). Code 99491 is reported for at least 30 minutes of physician or other qualified health care professional time personally spent in care management during the calendar month. Code 99437 is reported in conjunction with 99491 for each additional minimum 30 minutes of physician or other qualified health care professional time. If reporting 99437, 99491 do not include any time devoted to the patient and/or family on the date that the reporting physician or other qualified health care professional also performed a face-to-face E/M encounter.◄

#▲ **99490**  Chronic care management services with the following required elements:

- multiple (two or more) chronic conditions expected to last at least 12 months, or until the death of the patient,
- chronic conditions that place the patient at significant risk of death, acute exacerbation/decompensation, or functional decline,
- comprehensive care plan established, implemented, revised, or monitored;

first 20 minutes of clinical staff time directed by a physician or other qualified health care professional, per calendar month.

#+▲ **99439**  each additional 20 minutes of clinical staff time directed by a physician or other qualified health care professional, per calendar month (List separately in addition to code for primary procedure)

(Use 99439 in conjunction with 99490)

(Chronic care management services of less than 20 minutes duration in a calendar month are not reported separately)

(Chronic care management services of 60 minutes or more and requiring moderate or high complexity medical decision making may be reported using 99487, 99489)

(Do not report 99439 more than twice per calendar month)

▶(Do not report 99439, 99490 in the same calendar month with 90951-90970, 99339, 99340, 99374, 99375, 99377, 99378, 99379, 99380, 99424, 99425, 99426, 99427, 99437, 99487, 99489, 99491, 99605, 99606, 99607)◀

(Do not report 99439, 99490 for service time reported with 93792, 93793, 98960, 98961, 98962, 98966, 98967, 98968, 98970, 98971, 98972, 99071, 99078, 99080, 99091, 99358, 99359, 99366, 99367, 99368, 99421, 99422, 99423, 99441, 99442, 99443, 99605, 99606, 99607)

**#▲ 99491** Chronic care management services with the following required elements:

- multiple (two or more) chronic conditions expected to last at least 12 months, or until the death of the patient,
- chronic conditions that place the patient at significant risk of death, acute exacerbation/decompensation, or functional decline,
- comprehensive care plan established, implemented, revised, or monitored;

first 30 minutes provided personally by a physician or other qualified health care professional, per calendar month.

**+● 99437** each additional 30 minutes by a physician or other qualified health care professional, per calendar month (List separately in addition to code for primary procedure)

▶(Use 99437 in conjunction with 99491)◀

▶(Do not report 99437 for less than 30 minutes)◀

▶(Do not report 99437, 99491 in the same calendar month with 90951-90970, 99339, 99340, 99374, 99375, 99377, 99378, 99379, 99380, 99424, 99425, 99426, 99427, 99439, 99487, 99489, 99490, 99605, 99606, 99607)◀

▶(Do not report 99437, 99491 for service time reported with 93792, 93793, 98960, 98961, 98962, 98966, 98967, 98968, 98970, 98971, 98972, 99071, 99078, 99080, 99091, 99358, 99359, 99366, 99367, 99368, 99421, 99422, 99423, 99441, 99442, 99443, 99495, 99496, 99605, 99606, 99607)◀

▶Table for Reporting Chronic Care Management Services◀

| ▶Total Duration Care Management Services | Staff Type | Chronic Care Management |
|---|---|---|
| Less than 20 minutes | Not reported separately | Not reported separately |
| Less than 30 minutes | Physician or other qualified health care professional | Not reported separately or see 99490 |
| 20-39 minutes | Clinical staff | 99490 X 1 |
| 30-59 minutes | Physician or other qualified health care professional | 99491 X 1 |
| 40-59 minutes | Clinical staff | 99490 X 1 and 99439 X 1 |
| 60-89 minutes | Physician or other qualified health care professional | 99491 X 1 and 99437 X 1 |
| 60 minutes or more | Clinical staff | 99490 X 1 and 99439 X 2 |
| 90 minutes or more | Physician or other qualified health care professional | 99491 X 1 and 99437 X 2 as appropriate (see illustrated reporting examples above)◀ |

## Clinical Example (99437)

**Patient 1:** An 11-year-old female with past medical history of meconium aspiration at birth resulting in anoxic brain injury with cerebral palsy, asthma, allergic rhinitis, and global developmental delay, who has already received 59 minutes of physician or other QHP chronic care management (CCM) services during the calendar month, requires additional care management services during the same calendar month. [**Note:** This is an add-on service. Only consider the additional physician or other QHP work beyond the work separately reported with base code 99491.]

**Patient 2:** An 80-year-old male, who has already received 59 minutes of physician or other QHP CCM services during the calendar month, requires additional care management services during the same calendar month. [**Note:** This is an add-on service. Only consider the additional physician or other QHP work beyond the work separately reported with code 99491.]

## Description of Procedure (99437)

A physician or other QHP personally provides CCM services, which are management and support services, to a patient with two or more chronic conditions residing at home or in a domiciliary, rest home, assisted living facility, or nursing home. These services typically include establishing, implementing, revising, or monitoring the patient's care plan; coordinating the care of other professionals and agencies; and educating the patient or caregiver about the patient's condition, care plan, and prognosis. The physician or other QHP provides and/or oversees the coordination of services as needed for all medical conditions, psychosocial needs, and activities of daily living (ADLs), and documents and shares a plan of care with the patient and/or caregiver.

A care plan is based on a physical, mental, cognitive, social, functional, and environmental assessment. It is a comprehensive plan of care for all health problems. It typically includes, but is not limited to, the following elements: problem list; expected outcome and prognosis; measurable treatment goals; symptom management; planned interventions; medication management; community and social services ordered; how the services of agencies and specialists not associated with the practice will be directed and coordinated; identification of the individuals responsible for each intervention; requirements for periodic review; and when applicable, revision of the care plan.

In addition, the care management office or practice must have the following capabilities: provide 24/7 access to physicians, other QHPs, or clinical staff, including providing patients and caregivers with a means to make contact with health care professionals in the practice to address urgent needs regardless of the time of day or day of week; provide continuity of care with a designated member of the care team with whom the patient is able to schedule successive routine appointments; provide timely access and management for follow up after an emergency department visit or facility discharge; use an electronic health record (EHR) system so that care providers have timely access to clinical information; and engage and educate patients and caregivers, as well as coordinate care among all service professionals, as appropriate, for each patient.

## Complex Chronic Care Management Services

►Complex chronic care management services are services that require at least 60 minutes of clinical staff time, under the direction of a physician or other qualified health care professional. Complex chronic care management services require moderate or high medical decision making as defined in the Evaluation and Management (E/M) guidelines.◄

Patients who require complex chronic care management services may be identified by practice-specific or other published algorithms that recognize multiple illnesses, multiple medication use, inability to perform activities of daily living, requirement for a caregiver, and/or repeat admissions or emergency department visits. Typical adult patients who receive complex chronic care management services are treated with three or more prescription medications and may be receiving other types of therapeutic interventions (eg, physical therapy, occupational therapy). Typical pediatric patients receive three or more therapeutic interventions (eg, medications, nutritional support, respiratory therapy). All patients have two or more chronic continuous or episodic health conditions that are expected to last at least 12 months, or until the death of the patient, and that place the patient at significant risk of death, acute exacerbation/decompensation, or functional decline. Typical patients have complex diseases and morbidities and, as a result, demonstrate one or more of the following:

- need for the coordination of a number of specialties and services;
- inability to perform activities of daily living and/or cognitive impairment resulting in poor adherence to the treatment plan without substantial assistance from a caregiver;
- psychiatric and other medical comorbidities (eg, dementia and chronic obstructive pulmonary disease or substance abuse and diabetes) that complicate their care; and/or
- social support requirements or difficulty with access to care.

| Total Duration of Staff Care Management Services | Complex Chronic Care Management |
|---|---|
| less than 60 minutes | Not reported separately |
| 60 to 89 minutes (1 hour - 1 hr. 29 min.) | 99487 X 1 |
| 90 - 119 minutes (1 hr. 30 min. - 1 hr. 59 min.) | 99487 X 1 and 99489 X 1 |
| 120 minutes or more (2 hours or more) | 99487 X 1 and 99489 X 2 and 99489 for each additional 30 minutes |

★ = Telemedicine    ✚ = Add-on code    ⁄⁄ = FDA approval pending    # = Resequenced code    ⊘ = Modifier 51 exempt

▲ **99487**    Complex chronic care management services with the following required elements:

- multiple (two or more) chronic conditions expected to last at least 12 months, or until the death of the patient,
- chronic conditions that place the patient at significant risk of death, acute exacerbation/decompensation, or functional decline,
- comprehensive care plan established, implemented, revised, or monitored,
- moderate or high complexity medical decision making;

first 60 minutes of clinical staff time directed by a physician or other qualified health care professional, per calendar month.

(Complex chronic care management services of less than 60 minutes duration in a calendar month are not reported separately)

▲ **99489**    each additional 30 minutes of clinical staff time directed by a physician or other qualified health care professional, per calendar month (List separately in addition to code for primary procedure)

(Report 99489 in conjunction with 99487)

►(Do not report 99489 for care management service of less than 30 minutes)◄

►(Do not report 99487, 99489 during the same calendar month with 90951-90970, 99339, 99340, 99374, 99375, 99377, 99378, 99379, 99380, 99424, 99425, 99426, 99427, 99437, 99439, 99490, 99491)◄

(Do not report 99487, 99489 for service time reported with 93792, 93793, 98960, 98961, 98962, 98966, 98967, 98968, 98970, 98971, 98972, 99071, 99078, 99080, 99091, 99358, 99359, 99366, 99367, 99368, 99421, 99422, 99423, 99441, 99442, 99443, 99605, 99606, 99607)

## ►Principal Care Management Services◄

►Principal care management represents services that focus on the medical and/or psychological needs manifested by a single, complex chronic condition expected to last at least 3 months and includes establishing, implementing, revising, or monitoring a care plan specific to that single disease. Code 99424 is reported for at least 30 minutes of physician or other qualified health care professional personal time in care management activities during a calendar month. Code 99425 is reported in conjunction with 99424, when at least an additional 30 minutes of physician or other qualified health care professional personal time is spent in care management activities during the calendar month. Code 99426 is reported for the first 30 minutes of clinical staff time spent in care management activities during the calendar month. Code 99427 is reported in

conjunction with 99426, when at least an additional 30 minutes of clinical staff time is spent in care management activities during the calendar month.◄

#● **99424**    Principal care management services, for a single high-risk disease, with the following required elements:

- one complex chronic condition expected to last at least 3 months, and that places the patient at significant risk of hospitalization, acute exacerbation/ decompensation, functional decline, or death,
- the condition requires development, monitoring, or revision of disease-specific care plan,
- the condition requires frequent adjustments in the medication regimen and/or the management of the condition is unusually complex due to comorbidities,
- ongoing communication and care coordination between relevant practitioners furnishing care;

first 30 minutes provided personally by a physician or other qualified health care professional, per calendar month.

#✚● **99425**    each additional 30 minutes provided personally by a physician or other qualified health care professional, per calendar month (List separately in addition to code for primary procedure)

►(Use 99425 in conjunction with 99424)◄

►(Principal care management services of less than 30 minutes duration in a calendar month are not reported separately)◄

►(Do not report 99424, 99425 in the same calendar month with 90951-90970, 99339, 99340, 99374, 99375, 99377, 99378, 99379, 99380, 99426, 99427, 99437, 99439, 99487, 99489, 99490, 99491, 99605, 99606, 99607)◄

►(Do not report 99424, 99425 for service time reported with 93792, 93793, 98960, 98961, 98962, 98966, 98967, 98968, 98970, 98971, 98972, 99071, 99078, 99080, 99091, 99358, 99359, 99366, 99367, 99368, 99421, 99422, 99423, 99441, 99442, 99443, 99605, 99606, 99607)◄

#● **99426**    Principal care management services, for a single high-risk disease, with the following required elements:

- one complex chronic condition expected to last at least 3 months, and that places the patient at significant risk of hospitalization, acute exacerbation/ decompensation, functional decline, or death,
- the condition requires development, monitoring, or revision of disease-specific care plan,
- the condition requires frequent adjustments in the medication regimen and/or the management of the condition is unusually complex due to comorbidities,
- ongoing communication and care coordination between relevant practitioners furnishing care;

first 30 minutes of clinical staff time directed by physician or other qualified health care professional, per calendar month.

Evaluation / Management 99202-99499

**#+● 99427**     each additional 30 minutes of clinical staff time directed by a physician or other qualified health care professional, per calendar month (List separately in addition to code for primary procedure)

►(Use 99427 in conjunction with 99426)◄

►(Principal care management services of less than 30 minutes duration in a calendar month are not reported separately)◄

►(Do not report 99427 more than twice per calendar month)◄

►(Do not report 99426, 99427 in the same calendar mont with 90951-90970, 99339, 99340, 99374, 99375, 99377, 99378, 99379, 99380, 99424, 99425, 99437, 99439, 99487 99489, 99490, 99491, 99605, 99606, 99607)◄

►(Do not report 99426, 99427 for service time reported with 93792, 93793, 98960, 98961, 98962, 98966, 98967, 98968, 98970, 98971, 98972, 99071, 99078, 99080, 99091 99358, 99359, 99366, 99367, 99368, 99421, 99422, 99423 99441, 99442, 99443, 99605, 99606, 99607)◄

### ►Table for Reporting Principal Care Management Services◄

| ►Total Duration Principal Care Management Services | Staff Type | Principal Care Management |
|---|---|---|
| Less than 30 minutes | Not separately reported | Not separately reported |
| 30-59 minutes | Physician or other qualified health care professional | 99424 X 1 |
|  | Clinical staff | 99426 X 1 |
| 60-89 minutes | Physician or other qualified health care professional | 99424 X 1 and 99425 X 1 |
|  | Clinical staff | 99426 X 1 and 99427 X 1 |
| 90-119 minutes | Physician or other qualified health care professional | 99424 X 1 and 99425 X 2 |
|  | Clinical staff | 99426 X 1 and 99427 X 2 |
| 120 minutes or more | Physician or other qualified health care professional | 99424 X 1 and 99425 X 3, as appropriate (see illustrated reporting examples above) |
|  | Clinical staff | 99426 X 1 and 99427 X 2 |

### Care Management Services

| Code | Service | Staff Type | Unit Duration (Time Span) | Unit Max Per Month |
|---|---|---|---|---|
| 99490 | Chronic care management | Clinical staff | 20 minutes (20-39 minutes) | 1 |
| +99439 | Chronic care management | Clinical staff | 40-59 minutes X 1 (60 or more minutes X 2) | 2 |
| 99491 | Chronic care management | Physician or other qualified health care professional | 30 minutes (30-59 minutes) | 1 |
| +99437 | Chronic care management | Physician or other qualified health care professional | 30 minutes (60 minutes or more) | No limit |
| 99487 | Complex chronic care management | Clinical staff | 60 minutes (60-89 minutes) | 1 |
| +99489 | Complex chronic care management | Clinical staff | 30 minutes (≥90 minutes X 1) (≥120 minutes X 2, etc) | No limit |
| 99424 | Principal care management | Physician or other qualified health care professional | 30 minutes (30-59 minutes) | 1 |
| +99425 | Principal care management | Physician or other qualified health care professional | 30 minutes (60 minutes or more) | No limit |
| 99426 | Principal care management | Clinical staff | 30 minutes (30-59 minutes) | 1 |
| +99427 | Principal care management | Clinical staff | 30 minutes (60 minutes or more) | 2◄ |

★ = Telemedicine   ✚ = Add-on code   ✇ = FDA approval pending   # = Resequenced code   ⊘ = Modifier 51 exem

# Rationale

Several changes have been made to the Care Management Services subsection of the E/M section. A new subheading has been added to the care management services guidelines; a new subsection and codes 99424-99427 have been added for reporting principal care management services; guidelines have been added, moved, and revised; a new code (99437) has been added for reporting additional time for chronic care management services; and codes within the Chronic Care Management Services and the Complex Chronic Care Management Services subsections have been revised. In addition, tables have been added, deleted, and moved, and parenthetical notes throughout the E/M and Medicine sections have been added, deleted, and updated to accommodate the addition of the new codes for principal care management services, updated to match other codes and instructions within the subfamily, and to provide better instructions regarding how the new principal care management services codes and other related services (eg, chronic care management services) may be reported, who may report them, and how often these services may be reported.

In the effort to continue to distinguish the different types of E/M services that may be performed and reported, changes continue to be made to the services listed within the E/M Services section. Because many of the services may appear similar or include common components that may not be duplicated when reporting the services (ie, components or time that may not be identified or counted more than once to describe the same work that has already been included as part of a different service), the revisions and additions to the code set help to distinguish these services from one another and provide input for reporting. The additions include definitions for the type of E/M services, how the services are different from other existing codes, instructions regarding which services to report, when certain similar services may be reported together (including reporting for services that utilize different time to complete each service), when certain efforts are excluded from separate reporting, how often these services may be reported, how long they may be reported, and who may report them. This may include the use of tables to exemplify instructions provided within parenthetical notes or guidelines. It may also involve the relocation of information that may apply to more than one type of service. There is also a consistent use of guidelines and parentheticals that cross-reference, restrict, allow concurrent reporting, and educate users regarding how all of these codes work together to provide a bigger picture of the different types of E/M services that

currently exist and how they are used to appropriately capture the work effort that should be reported.

Congruent with this approach, a new subsection, guidelines, codes, parenthetical notes, and tables have been added to the E/M section that provide instructions regarding reporting for principal care management services. The E/M section also includes revisions to guidelines, parenthetical notes, and other instructions for other care management services (ie, chronic care management services and complex chronic care management services) and other services that share similar components of work (eg, digitally stored data services/remote physiologic monitoring, remote physiologic monitoring treatment management services). The changes reflect the addition or revision of instructions regarding reporting of this family of services. The changes also include the addition of the new codes to existing parenthetical notes and guidelines to accommodate the new codes.

Principal care management services focus on establishing, implementing, revising, or monitoring a care plan that is specific to a disease for medical and/or psychological needs that are displayed for a single, complex chronic condition. Note that the condition is expected to last at least 3 months. The codes are specified according to whether the intent is to report the service provided personally by the physician or other QHP (99424, 99425) or to report time spent by the clinical staff providing principal care management as directed by the physician or other QHP (99426, 99427). The services are reported per calendar month.

To provide specific instruction for use of these codes, parenthetical notes have been added to direct and restrict the use of these codes in conjunction with other codes. For example, these codes are mutually exclusive, ie, either the principal care management service provided by the physician or other QHP is reported or the services provided by the clinical staff are reported. This is noted in conditional exclusionary parenthetical notes that restrict the reporting of these codes in conjunction with each other or in conjunction with other services for this type of planning. The phrase, "in the same calendar month," is used, which implies that the codes that follow should not be reported together in the same month for any circumstance.

A different exclusion scenario is also noted in which these codes may not be reported "for service time reported with" other procedures as listed within the parenthetical note. The intent for these instructions is to restrict reporting the noted services together if the time being used to report both services is the same. If *different time* is being used to report each service, then that time may be used to report a different service according to the specific service being provided. (**Note:** Separate guidelines require that the time for each distinct service be documented in order to separately report the service.)

In addition, parenthetical notes have been included after each grouping of principal care codes that restrict reporting services of less than 30 minutes duration during the calendar month.

To reiterate the intended use for principal care management services and other care management services codes, a new subheading titled "Care Planning" has been added to the care management services guidelines. This subheading is intended to combine important instructions regarding care planning for all care management services. It includes content that has been relocated from the general care management services guidelines. It also includes bulleted listings of items that are "commonly included," "may be included," and "must be included" for creating a plan of care. Instruction regarding the number of times the services may be reported and documentation needs for principal care management services provided by different physicians or other QHPs are noted. Special instruction has also been added to this subsection that reiterates time reporting restrictions and how physician time that does not meet the threshold for separate reporting may be captured (eg, by being added to the clinical staff time reported).

In addition to adding the common subheading for care planning, many of the conventions used for principal care management services have been applied to all of the codes, guidelines, and parenthetical notes within the Care Management Services subsection. These updated instructions allow use of similar wording for reporting conventions that match the instruction provided for principal care management services. The instructions include specifications for time restrictions for reporting, exclude reporting when performed with other similar services that inherently include the care management service, allow use for certain services when the time used is separate time, and provide guidance regarding who can report the service, where appropriate.

Note that these instructions have been listed in multiple ways to ensure that the intention is communicated, such as updating both within the guideline and within the parenthetical note following the family of codes. In addition, others have been further exemplified within tables that are used to illustrate important information, such as time reporting, service providers, and how often

the service may be reported. Coding tips have also been added to reinforce the intent.

In agreement with the add-on convention for services in the Care Management Services subsection, code 99437 has been added as an add-on service to be reported for each additional 30 minutes of chronic care management services. Chronic care management services code 99491 has been revised to match the language convention that is now common to codes listed in the Care Management Services subsection. Finally, codes 99439, 99487, 99489, and 99490 have been editorially revised by adding the term "that" to the second bulleted item in the code descriptors.

## Clinical Example (99424)

A patient presents with a single complex chronic condition that places the patient at significant risk of decompensation.

## Description of Procedure (99424)

Principal care management (PCM) represents services that focus on the medical and/or psychological needs manifested by a single complex chronic condition expected to last at least 3 months and includes establishing, implementing, revising, or monitoring a care plan specific to that single disease. Code 99424 is reported for at least 30 minutes of physician or other QHP time in care management activities during a calendar month. PCM services are disease-specific management services. A patient may have multiple chronic conditions of sufficient severity to warrant complex CCM but may receive PCM if the reporting physician or other QHP is providing single-disease management rather than comprehensive care management. Services include establishing, implementing, revising, or monitoring the care plan, coordinating the care of other professionals and agencies, and educating the patient or caregiver about the patient's condition, care plan, and prognosis. A physician or other QHP personally provides these PCM services, which are management and support services, to a patient with a single high-risk disease residing at home or in a domiciliary, rest home, or assisted living facility.

## Clinical Example (99425)

A patient presents with a single complex chronic condition that places the patient at significant risk of decompensation.

## Description of Procedure (99425)

PCM represents services that focus on the medical and/or psychological needs manifested by a single complex chronic condition expected to last at least 3 months and includes establishing, implementing, revising, or monitoring a care plan specific to that single disease. Code 99425 is reported in conjunction with code 99424 when at least an additional 30 minutes of physician or other QHP time is spent in care management activities during the calendar month. PCM services are disease-specific management services. A patient may have multiple chronic conditions of sufficient severity to warrant complex CCM but may receive PCM if the reporting physician or other QHP is providing single-disease management rather than comprehensive care management. Services include establishing, implementing, revising, or monitoring the care plan, coordinating the care of other professionals and agencies, and educating the patient or caregiver about the patient's condition, care plan, and prognosis. A physician or other QHP personally provides these PCM services, which are management and support services, to a patient with a single high-risk disease residing at home or in a domiciliary, rest home, or assisted living facility.

## Clinical Example (99426)

A patient presents with a single complex chronic condition that places the patient at significant risk of decompensation.

## Description of Procedure (99426)

PCM represents services that focus on the medical and/or psychological needs manifested by a single complex chronic condition expected to last at least 3 months and includes establishing, implementing, revising, or monitoring a care plan specific to that single disease. Code 99426 is reported for the first 30 minutes of clinical staff time spent in care management activities during the calendar month. PCM services are disease-specific management services. A patient may have multiple chronic conditions of sufficient severity to warrant complex CCM but may receive PCM if the reporting physician or other QHP is providing single-disease management rather than comprehensive care management. Management and support services are provided by clinical staff under the direction of a physician or other QHP to a patient with a single high-risk disease residing at home or in a domiciliary, rest home, or assisted living facility. These services typically include clinical staff implementing the care plan, coordinating the care of other professionals and agencies, and educating the patient or caregiver about the patient's condition, care plan, and prognosis directed by the physician or other QHP.

## Clinical Example (99427)

A patient presents with a single complex chronic condition that places the patient at significant risk of decompensation.

## Description of Procedure (99427)

PCM represents services that focus on the medical and/or psychological needs manifested by a single complex chronic condition expected to last at least 3 months and includes establishing, implementing, revising, or monitoring a care plan specific to that single disease. Code 99427 is reported in conjunction with code 99426 when at least an additional 30 minutes of clinical staff time is spent in care management activities during the calendar month. PCM services are disease-specific management services. A patient may have multiple chronic conditions of sufficient severity to warrant complex CCM but may receive PCM if the reporting physician or other QHP is providing single-disease management rather than comprehensive care management. Management and support services are provided by clinical staff under the direction of a physician or other QHP to a patient with a single high-risk disease residing at home or in a domiciliary, rest home, or assisted living facility. These services typically include clinical staff implementing the care plan, coordinating the care of other professionals and agencies, and educating the patient or caregiver about the patient's condition, care plan, and prognosis directed by the physician or other QHP.

# Psychiatric Collaborative Care Management Services

▲ 99492 **Initial psychiatric collaborative care management,** first 70 minutes in the first calendar month of behavioral health care manager activities, in consultation with a psychiatric consultant, and directed by the treating physician or other qualified health care professional, with the following required elements:

- outreach to and engagement in treatment of a patient directed by the treating physician or other qualified health care professional,

- initial assessment of the patient, including administration of validated rating scales, with the development of an individualized treatment plan,

- review by the psychiatric consultant with modifications of the plan if recommended,

- entering patient in a registry and tracking patient follow-up and progress using the registry, with appropriate documentation, and participation in weekly caseload consultation with the psychiatric consultant, and

- provision of brief interventions using evidence-based techniques such as behavioral activation, motivational interviewing, and other focused treatment strategies.

**Evaluation / Management  99202-99499**

▲ **99493**  **Subsequent psychiatric collaborative care management,** first 60 minutes in a subsequent month of behavioral health care manager activities, in consultation with a psychiatric consultant, and directed by the treating physician or other qualified health care professional, with the following required elements:

- tracking patient follow-up and progress using the registry, with appropriate documentation,

- participation in weekly caseload consultation with the psychiatric consultant,

- ongoing collaboration with and coordination of the patient's mental health care with the treating physician or other qualified health care professional and any other treating mental health providers,

- additional review of progress and recommendations for changes in treatment, as indicated, including medications, based on recommendations provided by the psychiatric consultant,

- provision of brief interventions using evidence-based techniques such as behavioral activation, motivational interviewing, and other focused treatment strategies,

- monitoring of patient outcomes using validated rating scales, and

- relapse prevention planning with patients as they achieve remission of symptoms and/or other treatment goals and are prepared for discharge from active treatment.

## Rationale

Codes 99492 and 99493 have been editorially revised to replace all semicolons in the code descriptor with commas to be consistent with CPT coding convention for nonparent or nonchild codes. The intent and use of the codes remain the same.

# General Behavioral Health Integration Care Management

#▲ **99484**  Care management services for behavioral health conditions, at least 20 minutes of clinical staff time, directed by a physician or other qualified health care professional, per calendar month, with the following required elements:

- initial assessment or follow-up monitoring, including the use of applicable validated rating scales,

- behavioral health care planning in relation to behavioral/psychiatric health problems, including revision for patients who are not progressing or whose status changes,

- facilitating and coordinating treatment such as psychotherapy, pharmacotherapy, counseling and/or psychiatric consultation, and

- continuity of care with a designated member of the care team.

(Do not report 99484 in conjunction with 99492, 99493, 99494 in the same calendar month)

## Rationale

Code 99484 has been editorially revised to replace all semicolons in the code descriptor with commas to be consistent with CPT coding convention for nonparent or nonchild codes. The intent and use of the code remain the same.

▶(E/M services, including care management services [99424, 99425, 99426, 99427, 99437, 99439, 99487, 99489, 99490, 99491, 99495, 99496], and psychiatric services [90785-90899] may be reported separately by the same physician or other qualified health care professional on the same day or during the same calendar month, but time and activities used to meet criteria for another reported service do not count toward meeting criteria for 99484)◀

## Rationale

To accommodate the addition of the new principal care management services codes and other changes made to clarify the reporting of these services, a parenthetical note following code 99484 has been revised.

Refer to the codebook and the Rationale for codes 99424-99427 for a full discussion of these changes.

# Anesthesia

## Summary of Additions, Deletions, and Revisions

The summary of changes shows the actual changes that have been made to the code descriptors.

New codes appear with a bullet (●) and are indicated as "Code added." Revised codes are preceded with a triangle (▲). Within revised codes, or if a code symbol has been deleted, the deleted language and code symbol appear with a ~~strikethrough~~, while new text appears <u>underlined</u>.

The ✗ symbol is used to identify codes for vaccines that are pending FDA approval. The # symbol is used to identify codes that have been resequenced. CPT add-on codes are annotated by the ✚ symbol. The ⊘ symbol is used to identify codes that are exempt from the use of modifier 51. The ★ symbol is used to identify codes that may be used for reporting telemedicine services. The ✘ symbol is used to identify a proprietary laboratory analyses (PLA) test that has an identical descriptor as another PLA test. A PLA code that satisfies Category I code criteria and has been accepted by the CPT Editorial Panel is annotated with the ↑↓ symbol.

| Code | Description |
|---|---|
| ~~01935~~ | ~~Anesthesia for percutaneous image guided procedures on the spine and spinal cord; diagnostic~~ |
| ~~01936~~ | ~~therapeutic~~ |
| ●01937 | Code added |
| ●01938 | Code added |
| ●01939 | Code added |
| ●01940 | Code added |
| ●01941 | Code added |
| ●01942 | Code added |

# Spine and Spinal Cord

**00600**    Anesthesia for procedures on cervical spine and cord; not otherwise specified

▶(For percutaneous image-guided spine and spinal cord anesthesia procedures, see 01937, 01938, 01939, 01940, 01941, 01942)◀

**00604**    procedures with patient in the sitting position

## Rationale

In support of the establishment of codes 01937-01942, the cross-reference parenthetical note following code 00600 has been revised to include these new codes.

Refer to the codebook and the Rationale for codes 01937-01942 for a full discussion of these changes

# Radiological Procedures

▶(01935, 01936 have been deleted. To report anesthesia for percutaneous image-guided procedures on the spine or spinal cord, see 01937, 01938, 01939, 01940, 01941, 01942)◀

● **01937**    Anesthesia for percutaneous image-guided injection, drainage or aspiration procedures on the spine or spinal cord; cervical or thoracic

● **01938**        lumbar or sacral

▶(For anesthesia for percutaneous image-guided destruction procedures on the spine or spinal cord, see 01939, 01940)◀

● **01939**    Anesthesia for percutaneous image-guided destruction procedures by neurolytic agent on the spine or spinal cord; cervical or thoracic

● **01940**        lumbar or sacral

▶(For anesthesia for percutaneous image-guided injection, drainage or aspiration procedures on the spine or spinal cord, see 01937, 01938)◀

● **01941**    Anesthesia for percutaneous image-guided neuromodulation or intravertebral procedures (eg, kyphoplasty, vertebroplasty) on the spine or spinal cord; cervical or thoracic

● **01942**        lumbar or sacral

## Rationale

A new family of anesthesia codes for percutaneous image-guided procedures (01937-01942) has been established to help clarify when anesthesia is used for percutaneous procedures for anatomical locations of the spine (cervical or thoracic versus lumbar or sacral regions). This new code family will help to address any potential concerns and clarify the use of anesthesia for such procedures.

As part of this change, codes 01935 and 01936 have been deleted. Codes 01935 and 01936 were added to the CPT code set in 2008. However, from 2009 through 2014, the service described by code 01936 was identified on an AMA/Specialty Society Relative Value Scale (RVS) Update Committee (RUC) Relativity Assessment Workgroup (RAW) high-volume growth screen as one that may have been inappropriately reported with other top surgical services.

It was determined that the creation of a new family of codes with more granularities would help clarify when anesthesia is used for percutaneous procedures on the spine (cervical or thoracic versus lumbar or sacral regions). Anesthesia services are reported on the same day for the same patient for a procedure performed by a different physician or other qualified health care professional (QHP) than the one performing the anesthesia service.

In creating the new family of codes, it was determined that categorization by anatomical location on the spine (cervical or thoracic vs lumbar or sacral) was appropriate and consistent with current nomenclature of other CPT codes related to the spine. It was further determined that the new family did not need to be distinguished by diagnostic vs therapeutic procedures as there was no difference in the anesthesia work. Prior to 2022, these codes were distinguished by type of procedure (diagnostic [01935] vs therapeutic [01936]).

First, two new procedures have been established to allow reporting of anesthesia for percutaneous image-guided anesthesia injections, drainage, or aspiration procedures on the spine or spinal cord in the cervical or thoracic region (01937) and the lumbar or sacral region (01938).

Second, two new procedures have been established to allow reporting of anesthesia for percutaneous image-guided destruction procedures by neurolytic agent on the spine or spinal cord in the cervical or thoracic region (01939) and the lumbar or sacral region (01940).

Third, two new procedures have been established to allow reporting of anesthesia for percutaneous image-guided neuromodulation or intravertebral (eg, kyphoplasty, vertebroplasty) procedures on the spine or spinal cord in the cervical or thoracic region (01941) and the lumbar or sacral region (01942).

Finally, additional cross-reference parenthetical notes have been added throughout the family of codes to provide appropriate guidance on how to report the new codes. In addition, the cross-reference parenthetical note following code 00600 has been revised and updated with the new family of codes for reporting anesthesia for percutaneous image-guided procedures on the spine or spinal cord (cervical, thoracic, lumbar, or sacral).

## Clinical Example (01937)

A 67-year-old female presents with chronic neck pain radiating toward her right shoulder. A magnetic resonance imaging (MRI) scan demonstrated facet arthropathy at C4-C5 and multilevel degenerative disc disease. Diagnostic testing with cervical facet blocks under fluoroscopic guidance on the right at the C4-C5 level is indicated.

## Description of Procedure (01937)

In the procedure room, establish monitoring and perform a presurgical review. Place the patient in the prone position. Provide sufficient sedation and analgesia to allow the patient to remain comfortable and cooperative with the procedure. Titrate medications and monitor the patient to preserve stable vital signs and adequate respiratory efforts throughout. At the end of the procedure, turn the patient supine and transfer the patient to the postanesthetic care unit. Provide a postanesthetic report. Document elements of the anesthesia care, including vital signs (at least every 5 minutes), positioning, anesthesia procedures, medications, and significant events, in the anesthetic record.

## Clinical Example (01938)

A 71-year-old male with a history of previous laminectomy at L4-L5 presents with recurrent right leg pain, the ability to stand for only 10 minutes and walk less than one block, and minimal problems sitting. MRI with contrast material shows a small recurrent herniation between L4-L5 with scar tissue and neurodiagnostic studies compatible with L5 radiculopathy. He undergoes a transforaminal epidural injection of an anesthetic and/ or anti-inflammatory agent at the L5-SI level.

## Description of Procedure (01938)

In the procedure room, establish monitoring and perform a presurgical review. Place the patient in the prone position. Provide sufficient sedation and analgesia to allow the patient to remain comfortable and cooperative with the procedure. Titrate medications and monitor the patient to preserve stable vital signs and adequate respiratory efforts throughout. At the end of the procedure, turn the patient supine and transfer the

patient to the postanesthetic care unit. Provide a postanesthetic report. Document elements of the anesthesia care, including vital signs (at least every 5 minutes), positioning, anesthesia procedures, medications, and significant events, in the anesthetic record.

## Clinical Example (01939)

A 65-year-old female with constant neck pain caused by degenerative disc disease and cervical spondylosis has received insufficient relief with conservative treatments. Previous trials of cervical medial branch nerve blocks proved beneficial (separately reported). Radiofrequency neurotomy is performed on two medial branch nerves innervating the unilateral symptomatic facet joint.

## Description of Procedure (01939)

In the procedure room, establish monitoring and perform a presurgical review. Place the patient in the prone position taking special care to avoid positioning injuries. Provide sufficient sedation and analgesia to allow the patient to remain comfortable and cooperative with the procedure. Titrate medications and monitor the patient to preserve stable vital signs and adequate respiratory efforts throughout. At the end of the procedure, turn the patient supine and transfer the patient to the postanesthetic care unit. Provide a postanesthetic report. Document elements of the anesthesia care, including vital signs (at least every 5 minutes), positioning, anesthesia procedures, medications, and significant events, in the anesthetic record.

## Clinical Example (01940)

A 65-year-old male with constant low-back pain due to degenerative disc disease and facet arthropathy has received insufficient relief with conservative treatments. Previous trials of lumbar medial branch nerve blocks proved beneficial (separately reported). He undergoes radiofrequency neurotomy of the two medial branch nerves innervating the unilateral symptomatic facet joint.

## Description of Procedure (01940)

In the procedure room, establish monitoring and perform a presurgical review. Place the patient in the prone position taking special care to avoid positioning injuries. Provide sufficient sedation and analgesia to allow the patient to remain comfortable and cooperative with the procedure. Titrate medications and monitor the patient to preserve stable vital signs and adequate respiratory efforts throughout. At the end of the procedure, turn the patient supine and transfer the patient to the postanesthetic care unit. Provide a postanesthetic report. Document elements of the anesthesia care, including vital signs (at least every 5 minutes), positioning, anesthesia procedures, medications, and significant events, in the anesthetic record.

## Clinical Example (01941)

A 75-year-old female develops sudden, severe mid-back pain after lifting her grandchild. Plain radiographs reveal an acute compression fracture with severe anterior wedging involving T10 and consequent new kyphosis. Pain persists despite a period of conservative care. After referral, percutaneous thoracic vertebral augmentation (and bone biopsy, if indicated) is performed.

## Description of Procedure (01941)

In the procedure room, establish monitoring and perform a presurgical review. Induce general anesthesia and intubate the trachea. After the airway is secured and the patient's vital signs are stable, place the patient in the prone position taking special care to avoid positioning injuries to the eyes, cervical spine, peripheral nerves, and/or soft tissues. Provide anesthesia care, titrate medications, and monitor and reassess the patient throughout the procedure. At the end of the procedure, turn the patient supine. When the patient emerges from anesthesia, extubate when medically appropriate. Transfer the patient to the postanesthetic care unit. Provide a postanesthetic report. Document elements of the anesthesia care, including vital signs (at least every 5 minutes), positioning, anesthesia procedures, medications, and significant events, in the anesthetic record.

## Clinical Example (01942)

A 75-year-old female presents with severe, persistent low-back pain and progressive spinal deformity secondary to osteoporotic vertebral collapse. Plain radiographs reveal an acute compression fracture of L3. Despite conservative medical management, pain persists. Percutaneous lumbar vertebral augmentation (and bone biopsy, if indicated) is performed.

## Description of Procedure (01942)

In the procedure room, establish monitoring and perform a presurgical review. Induce general anesthesia and intubate the trachea. After the airway is secured and the patient's vital signs are stable, place the patient in the prone position taking special care to avoid positioning injuries to the eyes, cervical spine, peripheral nerves, and/or soft tissues. Provide anesthesia care, titrate medications, and monitor and reassess the patient throughout the procedure. At the end of the procedure, turn the patient supine. When the patient emerges from anesthesia, extubate when medically appropriate. Transfer the patient to the postanesthetic care unit. Provide a postanesthetic report. Document elements of the anesthesia care, including vital signs (at least every 5 minutes), positioning, anesthesia procedures, medications, and significant events, in the anesthetic record.

# Surgery

## Summary of Additions, Deletions, and Revisions

The summary of changes shows the actual changes that have been made to the code descriptors.

New codes appear with a bullet (●) and are indicated as "Code added." Revised codes are preceded with a triangle (▲). Within revised codes, or if a code symbol has been deleted, the deleted language and code symbol appear with a ~~strikethrough~~, while new text appears <u>underlined</u>.

The ⩘ symbol is used to identify codes for vaccines that are pending FDA approval. The # symbol is used to identify codes that have been resequenced. CPT add-on codes are annotated by the ✚ symbol. The ⦻ symbol is used to identify codes that are exempt from the use of modifier 51. The ★ symbol is used to identify codes that may be used for reporting telemedicine services. The ✕ symbol is used to identify a proprietary laboratory analyses (PLA) test that has an identical descriptor as another PLA test. A PLA code that satisfies Category I code criteria and has been accepted by the CPT Editorial Panel is annotated with the ⇅ symbol.

| Code | Description |
|---|---|
| ▲11981 | Insertion, ~~non-biodegradable~~ drug-delivery implant <u>(ie, bioresorbable, biodegradable, non-biodegradable)</u> |
| **21310** | ~~Closed treatment of nasal bone fracture without manipulation~~ |
| ▲21315 | Closed treatment of nasal bone fracture <u>with manipulation</u>; without stabilization |
| ▲21320 | with stabilization |
| ▲22600 | Arthrodesis, posterior or posterolateral technique, single ~~level~~<u>interspace</u>; cervical below C2 segment |
| ▲22610 | thoracic (with lateral transverse technique, when performed) |
| ▲22612 | lumbar (with lateral transverse technique, when performed) |
| ✚▲22614 | each additional ~~vertebral segment~~ <u>interspace</u> (List separately in addition to code for primary procedure) |
| ▲22633 | Arthrodesis, combined posterior or posterolateral technique with posterior interbody technique including laminectomy and/or discectomy sufficient to prepare interspace (other than for decompression), single interspace ~~and segment~~; lumbar |
| ✚▲22634 | each additional interspace and segment (List separately in addition to code for primary procedure) |
| #●33267 | Code added |
| #✚●33268 | Code added |
| #●33269 | Code added |
| ✚●33370 | Code added |
| **33470** | ~~Valvotomy, pulmonary valve, closed heart; transventricular~~ |
| ▲33471 | Valvotomy, pulmonary valve, closed heart~~;~~<u>,</u> via pulmonary artery |
| ⦻●33509 | Code added |
| **33722** | ~~Closure of aortico-left ventricular tunnel~~ |

| Code | Description |
|---|---|
| ●33894 | Code added |
| ●33895 | Code added |
| ●33897 | Code added |
| ⊘+▲35600 | Harvest of upper extremity artery, 1 segment, for coronary artery bypass procedure, open (List separately in addition to code for primary procedure) |
| ●42975 | Code added |
| ●43497 | Code added |
| 43850 | Revision of gastroduodenal anastomosis (gastroduodenostomy) with reconstruction; without vagotomy |
| 43855 | with vagotomy |
| ●53451 | Code added |
| ●53452 | Code added |
| ●53453 | Code added |
| ●53454 | Code added |
| ▲54340 | Repair of hypospadias complication(s) (ie, fistula, stricture, diverticula); by closure, incision, or excision, simple |
| ▲54344 | requiring mobilization of skin flaps and urethroplasty with flap or patch graft |
| ▲54348 | requiring extensive dissection, and urethroplasty with flap, patch or tubed graft (includinges urinary diversion, when performed) |
| ▲54352 | Revision of prior hypospadias repair Repair of hypospadias cripple requiring extensive dissection and excision of previously constructed structures including re-release of chordee and reconstruction of urethra and penis by use of local skin as grafts and island flaps and skin brought in as flaps or grafts |
| 59135 | interstitial, uterine pregnancy requiring total hysterectomy |
| ●61736 | Code added |
| ●61737 | Code added |
| +▲63048 | each additional vertebral segment, cervical, thoracic, or lumbar (List separately in addition to code for primary procedure) |
| #+●63052 | Code added |
| #+●63053 | Code added |
| 63194 | Laminectomy with cordotomy, with section of 1 spinothalamic tract, 1 stage; cervical |
| 63195 | thoracic |
| 63196 | Laminectomy with cordotomy, with section of both spinothalamic tracts, 1 stage; cervical |
| ▲63197 | Laminectomy with cordotomy, with section of both spinothalamic tracts, 1 stage;, thoracic |
| 63198 | Laminectomy with cordotomy with section of both spinothalamic tracts, 2 stages within 14 days; cervical |
| 63199 | thoracic |
| ▲64568 | Incision for Open implantation of cranial nerve (eg, vagus nerve) neurostimulator electrode array and pulse generator |
| ▲64575 | Incision for Open implantation of neurostimulator electrode array; peripheral nerve (excludes sacral nerve) |

★ = Telemedicine    + = Add-on code    ⊮ = FDA approval pending    # = Resequenced code    ⊘ = Modifier 51 exempt

| Code | Description |
|------|-------------|
| ▲64580 | neuromuscular |
| ▲64581 | sacral nerve (transforaminal placement) |
| ●64582 | Code added |
| ●64583 | Code added |
| ●64584 | Code added |
| #●64628 | Code added |
| #✚●64629 | Code added |
| #●66989 | Code added |
| #●66991 | Code added |
| ▲67141 | Prophylaxis of retinal detachment (eg, retinal break, lattice degeneration) without drainage, 1 or more sessions; cryotherapy, diathermy |
| ▲67145 | photocoagulation (laser or xenon arc) |
| ●68841 | Code added |
| #▲69714 | Implantation, osseointegrated implant, temporal boneskull, with percutaneous attachment to external speech processor/cochlear stimulator; without mastoidectomywith percutaneous attachment to external speech processor |
| 69715 | Implantation, osseointegrated implant, temporal bone, with percutaneous attachment to external speech processor/cochlear stimulator; with mastoidectomy |
| #●69716 | Code added |
| #▲69717 | Revision or rReplacement (including removal of existing device), osseointegrated implant, temporal boneskull, with percutaneous attachment to external speech processor/cochlear stimulator; with percutaneous attachment to external speech processorwithout mastoidectomy |
| 69718 | Replacement (including removal of existing device), osseointegrated implant, temporal bone, with percutaneous attachment to external speech processor/ cochlear stimulator; with mastoidectomy |
| #●69719 | Code added |
| #●69726 | Code added |
| #●69727 | Code added |

# Surgery Guidelines

## Surgical Destruction

Surgical destruction is a part of a surgical procedure and different methods of destruction are not ordinarily listed separately unless the technique substantially alters the standard management of a problem or condition. Exceptions under special circumstances are provided for by separate code numbers.

## ▶Foreign Body/Implant Definition◀

▶An object intentionally placed by a physician or other qualified health care professional for any purpose (eg, diagnostic or therapeutic) is considered an implant. An object that is unintentionally placed (eg, trauma or ingestion) is considered a foreign body. If an implant (or part thereof) has moved from its original position or is structurally broken and no longer serves its intended purpose or presents a hazard to the patient, it qualifies as a foreign body for coding purposes, unless CPT coding instructions direct otherwise or a specific CPT code exists to describe the removal of that broken/moved implant.◀

### Rationale

The introductory language in the Surgery Guidelines section of the CPT code set has been updated to include a new heading and a definition of "foreign body" and "implant." The definition clarifies the difference between an implant and a foreign body. It also specifies other conditions that qualify an implant as a foreign body for coding purposes. In addition, the definition provides guidance if other instructions or a specific code exists to describe the removal of a broken or moved implant.

# Surgery

## Integumentary System

### Introduction

**11980**   Subcutaneous hormone pellet implantation (implantation of estradiol and/or testosterone pellets beneath the skin)

▲ **11981**   Insertion, drug-delivery implant (ie, bioresorbable, biodegradable, non-biodegradable)

(For manual preparation and insertion of deep [eg, subfascial], intramedullary, or intra-articular drug-delivery device, see 20700, 20702, 20704)

▶(For removal of biodegradable or bioresorbable implant, use 17999)◀

(Do not report 11981 in conjunction with 20700, 20702, 20704)

#### Rationale

Code 11981 has been revised with the relocation of the term "non-biodegradable" into a new itemized list in parentheses, "(ie, bioresorbable, biodegradable, non-biodegradable)," in the code descriptor. The code was revised to allow for reporting of more than non-biodegradable implant insertion. Code 11981 now describes the insertion of a drug-delivery implant such as bioresorbable, biodegradable, or non-biodegradable implants.

In addition, a parenthetical note has been added following code 11981 to instruct users to use unlisted code 17999 for removal of a biodegradable or bioresorbable implant.

### Repair (Closure)

▶Use the codes in this section to designate wound closure utilizing sutures, staples, or tissue adhesives (eg, 2-cyanoacrylate), either singly or in combination with each other, or in combination with adhesive strips. Chemical cauterization, electrocauterization, or wound closure utilizing adhesive strips as the sole repair material are included in the appropriate E/M code.◀

#### Definitions

The repair of wounds may be classified as Simple, Intermediate, or Complex.

▶*Simple repair* is used when the wound is superficial (eg, involving primarily epidermis or dermis, or subcutaneous tissues without significant involvement of deeper structures) and requires simple one-layer closure. Hemostasis and local or topical anesthesia, when performed, are not reported separately.◀

*Intermediate repair* includes the repair of wounds that, in addition to the above, require layered closure of one or more of the deeper layers of subcutaneous tissue and superficial (non-muscle) fascia, in addition to the skin (epidermal and dermal) closure. It includes limited undermining (defined as a distance less than the maximum width of the defect, measured perpendicular to the closure line, along at least one entire edge of the defect). Single-layer closure of heavily contaminated wounds that have required extensive cleaning or removal of particulate matter also constitutes intermediate repair.

*Complex repair* includes the repair of wounds that, in addition to the requirements for intermediate repair, require at least one of the following: exposure of bone, cartilage, tendon, or named neurovascular structure; debridement of wound edges (eg, traumatic lacerations or avulsions); extensive undermining (defined as a distance greater than or equal to the maximum width of the defect, measured perpendicular to the closure line along at least one entire edge of the defect); involvement of free margins of helical rim, vermilion border, or nostril rim; placement of retention sutures. Necessary preparation includes creation of a limited defect for repairs or the debridement of complicated lacerations or avulsions. Complex repair does not include excision of benign (11400-11446) or malignant (11600-11646) lesions, excisional preparation of a wound bed (15002-15005) or debridement of an open fracture or open dislocation.

#### Rationale

The repair (closure) guidelines in the Integumentary System section have been revised to clarify the definition of a simple repair. Prior to 2022, the repair (closure) guidelines stated that simple repair "includes local anesthesia and chemical or electrocauterization of wounds not closed." This statement was often misinterpreted to mean that simple repair codes may be reported when sutures are not used, but rather when electrocauterization is used. This is incorrect. To address this issue, the guidelines have been revised to clarify that chemical cauterization, electrocauterization, or wound closure using adhesive strips as the sole repair material is included in the appropriate evaluation and management (E/M) code. The guidelines have also been revised to clarify that when performed in conjunction with a simple repair, hemostasis and local or topical anesthesia are not reported separately.

# Breast

## Mastectomy Procedures

**19301**　Mastectomy, partial (eg, lumpectomy, tylectomy, quadrantectomy, segmentectomy);

**19302**　　　with axillary lymphadenectomy

(For placement of radiotherapy afterloading balloon/brachytherapy catheters, see 19296-19298)

(Intraoperative placement of clip[s] is not separately reported)

(For the preparation of tumor cavity with placement of an intraoperative radiation therapy applicator concurrent with partial mastectomy, use 19294)

(For radiofrequency spectroscopy, real time, intraoperative margin assessment, at the time of partial mastectomy, with report, use 0546T)

▶(For 3-dimensional volumetric specimen imaging, use 0694T)◀

## Rationale

In accordance with the establishment of Category III code 0694T, a cross-reference parenthetical note has been added following code 19302 directing users to report code 0694T for 3-dimensional volumetric specimen imaging.

Refer to the codebook and the Rationale for code 0694T for a full description of these changes.

# Musculoskeletal System

▶All services that appear in the Musculoskeletal System section include the application and removal of the first cast, splint, or traction device, when performed. Supplies may be reported separately. If a cast is removed by someone other than the physician or other qualified health care professional who applied the cast, report a cast removal code (29700, 29705, 29710).

Subsequent replacement of cast, splint, or strapping (29000-29750) and/or traction device (eg, 20690, 20692) during or after the global period may be reported separately.

A cast, splint, or strapping is not considered part of the preoperative care; therefore, the use of modifier 56 for preoperative management only is not applicable.◀

Codes for obtaining autogenous bone grafts, cartilage, tendon, fascia lata grafts or other tissues through separate incisions are to be used only when the graft is not already listed as part of the basic procedure.

▶**Fracture and/or Dislocation Treatment**

Fracture and dislocation treatment codes appear throughout the Musculoskeletal System section. These codes are categorized by the type of treatment (closed, percutaneous, open) and type of stabilization (fixation, immobilization). There is no coding correlation between the type of fracture/dislocation (eg, open [compound], closed) and the type of treatment (eg, closed, percutaneous, open) provided. For example, a closed fracture may require open treatment.

**Fracture/Dislocation Treatment Definitions**

*Manipulation:* Reduction by the application of manuall applied forces or traction to achieve satisfactory alignment of the fracture or dislocation. If satisfactory alignment (reduction) is not maintained and requires subsequent re-reduction of a fracture or dislocation by th same physician or same qualified health care professional append modifier 76 to the fracture/dislocation treatment code.

*Traction:* The application of a distracting or traction force to the spine or a limb. *Skeletal traction* includes a wire, pin, screw, or clamp that is attached to (penetrates) bone. *Skin traction* is the application of force to a limb using strapping or a device that is applied directly to the skin only.

*Closed treatment:* The treatment site is not surgically opened (ie, not exposed to the external environment nor directly visualized). Closed treatment of a fracture/dislocation may be performed without manipulation (eg, application of cast, splint, or strapping), with manipulation, with skeletal traction, and/or with skin traction.

Casting, splinting, or strapping used solely to temporarily stabilize the fracture for patient comfort is not considered closed treatment.

*Percutaneous skeletal fixation:* Treatment that is neithe open nor closed. In this procedure, the fracture fragment are not visualized, but fixation (eg, pins, screws) is placed across the fracture site, typically with imaging guidance.

*Open treatment:* The site is opened surgically to expose the fracture/dislocation to the external environment for treatment, or the fracture/dislocation is treated through the traumatic wound or an extension thereof or is treated with an intramedullary nail or other internal fixation device placed through a surgical exposure that is remote from the fracture site with or without direct visualization of the fracture site.

*External fixation:* The use of pins and/or wires that penetrate the bone(s) and interconnection devices (eg, clamps, bars, rings) for fracture/dislocation treatment. External fixation may be used for temporary or long-term fracture/dislocation treatment. *Uniplanar external fixation* places all the pins in approximately the same plane but may also include triangular fixation across a joint

*Multiplanar external fixation* uses transosseous wires and threaded pins placed in several planes that are held with interconnected stabilizing and/or tensioning rings and/or half rings. External fixation may be used for all types of fracture/dislocation treatment (ie, closed, percutaneous, open). Codes for external fixation are reported separately only when external fixation is not listed in the code descriptor as inherent to the procedure.

### Reporting Fracture and/or Dislocation Treatment Codes

The physician or other qualified health care professional providing fracture/dislocation treatment should report the appropriate fracture/dislocation treatment codes for the service he or she provided. If the person providing the initial treatment will **not** be providing subsequent treatment, modifier 54 should be appended to the fracture/dislocation treatment codes. If treatment of a fracture as defined above is not performed, report an evaluation and management code.◄

### ►Excision/Resection Soft Tissue Tumors Definitions◄

*Excision of subcutaneous soft connective tissue tumors* (including simple or intermediate repair) involves the simple or marginal resection of tumors confined to subcutaneous tissue below the skin but above the deep fascia. These tumors are usually benign and are resected without removing a significant amount of surrounding normal tissue. Code selection is based on the location and size of the tumor. Code selection is determined by measuring the greatest diameter of the tumor plus that margin required for complete excision of the tumor. The margins refer to the most narrow margin required to adequately excise the tumor, based on the physician's judgment. The measurement of the tumor plus margin is made at the time of the excision. Appreciable vessel exploration and/or neuroplasty should be reported separately. Extensive undermining or other techniques to close a defect created by skin excision may require a complex repair which should be reported separately. Dissection or elevation of tissue planes to permit resection of the tumor is included in the excision. For excision of benign lesions of cutaneous origin (eg, sebaceous cyst), see 11400-11446.

*Excision of fascial or subfascial soft tissue tumors* (including simple or intermediate repair) involves the resection of tumors confined to the tissue within or below the deep fascia, but not involving the bone. These tumors are usually benign, are often intramuscular, and are resected without removing a significant amount of surrounding normal tissue. Code selection is based on size and location of the tumor. Code selection is determined by measuring the greatest diameter of the tumor plus that margin required for complete excision of the tumor. The margins refer to the most narrow margin required to adequately excise the tumor, based on individual judgment. The measurement of the tumor plus

margin is made at the time of the excision. Appreciable vessel exploration and/or neuroplasty should be reported separately. Extensive undermining or other techniques to close a defect created by skin excision may require a complex repair which should be reported separately. Dissection or elevation of tissue planes to permit resection of the tumor is included in the excision.

Digital (ie, fingers and toes) subfascial tumors are defined as those tumors involving the tendons, tendon sheaths, or joints of the digit. Tumors which simply abut but do not breach the tendon, tendon sheath, or joint capsule are considered subcutaneous soft tissue tumors.

*Radical resection of soft connective tissue tumors* (including simple or intermediate repair) involves the resection of the tumor with wide margins of normal tissue. Appreciable vessel exploration and/or neuroplasty repair or reconstruction (eg, adjacent tissue transfer[s], flap[s]) should be reported separately. Extensive undermining or other techniques to close a defect created by skin excision may require a complex repair which should be reported separately. Dissection or elevation of tissue planes to permit resection of the tumor is included in the excision. Although these tumors may be confined to a specific layer (eg, subcutaneous, subfascial), radical resection may involve removal of tissue from one or more layers. Radical resection of soft tissue tumors is most commonly used for malignant connective tissue tumors or very aggressive benign connective tissue tumors. Code selection is based on size and location of the tumor. Code selection is determined by measuring the greatest diameter of the tumor plus that margin required for complete excision of the tumor. The margins refer to the most narrow margin required to adequately excise the tumor, based on individual judgment. The measurement of the tumor plus margin is made at the time of the excision. For radical resection of tumor(s) of cutaneous origin (eg, melanoma), see 11600-11646.

*Radical resection of bone tumors* (including simple or intermediate repair) involves the resection of the tumor with wide margins of normal tissue. Appreciable vessel exploration and/or neuroplasty and complex bone repair or reconstruction (eg, adjacent tissue transfer[s], flap[s]) should be reported separately. Extensive undermining or other techniques to close a defect created by skin excision may require a complex repair which should be reported separately. Dissection or elevation of tissue planes to permit resection of the tumor is included in the excision. It may require removal of the entire bone if tumor growth is extensive (eg, clavicle). Radical resection of bone tumors is usually performed for malignant tumors or very aggressive benign tumors. If surrounding soft tissue is removed during these procedures, the radical resection of soft tissue tumor codes should not be reported separately. Code selection is based solely on the location of the tumor, **not** on the size of the tumor or whether the tumor is benign or malignant, primary or metastatic.

## Rationale

The introductory guidelines in the Musculoskeletal System section have been revised and reorganized to clarify fracture and dislocation treatment services.

The introductory guidelines regarding casts, splints, and traction devices, and obtaining bone grafts have been revised to provide clearer reporting instructions. Specifically, the application and removal of the first cast, splint, or traction device is included in all services in the Musculoskeletal System section. If a cast is removed by someone other than the physician or other qualified health care professional who applied the cast, report a cast removal code (29700, 29705, 29710). Subsequent replacement of a cast, splint or strapping, and/or traction device during or after the global period may be reported separately. Supply of casts, splints, and traction devices is reported separately. Application of casts, splints, and strappings are not considered part of preoperative care, and therefore, modifier 56, *Preoperative Management Only,* is not applicable.

A subheading titled "Fracture and/or Dislocation Treatment" has been added, and the guidelines for fracture and dislocation treatment have been revised to clarify that the treatment codes throughout the Musculoskeletal System section are structured by the type of treatment and the type of stabilization performed, and that there is no correlation between the type of fracture or dislocation injury and the type of treatment performed. For example, a closed fracture may require open treatment.

The definitions for *manipulation, closed treatment,* and *external fixation* have been revised with added clarification of the work that comprises these types of treatment. Specifically, the definition of *manipulation* has been revised to state that if satisfactory alignment (reduction) is not maintained and requires subsequent re-reduction of a fracture or dislocation by the same physician or same qualified health care professional (QHP), then modifier 76, *Repeat Procedure or Service by Same Physician or Other Qualified Health Care Professional,* should be appended to the fracture or dislocation treatment code. The definition of *closed treatment* has been revised to clarify that casting, splinting, or strapping used solely to temporarily stabilize the fracture for patient comfort is not considered closed treatment. The definition of *external fixation* has been revised to clarify what this treatment involves, to clarify the difference between uniplanar and multiplanar external fixation, and to clarify appropriate reporting of external fixation.

A subheading titled "Reporting Fracture and/or Dislocation Treatment Codes" has been added, and the guidelines in this section provide basic instructions on reporting the fraction and/or dislocation treatment codes. Specifically, if the person providing the initial treatment will not be providing subsequent treatment, then modifier 54, *Surgical Care Only,* should be appended to the treatment code. If the fracture treatment provided is not included in the treatment definitions located in the Musculoskeletal System section introductory guidelines, then an E/M code should be reported for the treatment.

# General

## Introduction or Removal

**20615**    Aspiration and injection for treatment of bone cyst

▶(For injection of bone-substitute material for bone marrow lesions, use 0707T)◀

## Rationale

In accordance with the establishment of code 0707T, a cross-reference parenthetical note has been added following code 20615 directing users to report code 0707T for injection of bone-substitute material for bone marrow lesions.

Refer to the codebook and the Rationale for code 0707T for a full description of these changes.

# Head

## Fracture and/or Dislocation

(For operative repair of skull fracture, see 62000-62010)

(To report closed treatment of skull fracture, use the appropriate Evaluation and Management code)

▶(21310 has been deleted. To report closed treatment of nasal bone fracture without manipulation or stabilization, use appropriate E/M code)◀

▲ **21315**    Closed treatment of nasal bone fracture with manipulation; without stabilization

▶(For closed treatment of nasal bone fracture without manipulation or stabilization, use appropriate E/M code)◀

▲ **21320**        with stabilization

## Rationale

Code 21310, *Closed treatment of nasal bone fracture without manipulation,* has been deleted, and codes 21315 and 21320 have been revised to include manipulation. An instructional parenthetical note has been added following code 21315 instructing users to report the appropriate level E/M code for closed treatment of nasal bone fracture without manipulation or stabilization.

Closed treatment of nasal bone fracture can be performed in the following ways: (1) without manipulation; (2) with manipulation and stabilization; and (3) with manipulation, without stabilization. Prior to 2022, the codes 21310, 21315, and 21320 did not specify how to report manipulation when it is performed with closed treatment. In addition, there has been ambiguity regarding the difference in work between the procedure described by code 21310 and E/M services. To address these issues, code 21310 has been deleted, clear instructions have been added in the parenthetical note following code 21315 stating that closed treatment of a nasal bone fracture without manipulation or stabilization should be reported with E/M service codes, and codes 21315 and 21320 have been revised to include manipulation.

## Clinical Example (21315)

A 20-year-old male, who sustained a closed, displaced nasal fracture, undergoes closed reduction of the nasal fracture.

## Description of Procedure (21315)

The physician carefully places the nasal instruments (ie, Goldman elevator) into the nose and realigns the fractured nasal bones into correct anatomic position. Make comparisons between the patient's pre-injury appearance and the reduced nasal fracture, which typically requires multiple manipulations to ensure adequate cosmesis and nasal airflow. Repack the nasal cavity with cottonoids soaked in topical decongestant to ensure hemostasis. Once hemostasis is achieved, remove the cottonoids.

## Clinical Example (21320)

A 20-year-old male, who sustained a closed, displaced nasal fracture, undergoes closed reduction of the nasal fracture.

## Description of Procedure (21320)

The physician carefully places the nasal instruments (ie, Goldman elevator) into the nose and realigns the fractured nasal bones into correct anatomic position. Make comparisons between the patient's pre-injury appearance and the reduced nasal fracture, which typically requires multiple manipulations to ensure adequate cosmesis and nasal airflow. Repack the nasal

cavity with cottonoids soaked in topical decongestant to ensure hemostasis. Once hemostasis is achieved, remove the cottonoids. Pack the nasal cavity with gauze to provide internal support and clean the nasal skin with an alcohol wipe. Apply adhesive to the patient's skin and place adhesive strips to protect the skin. Shape an external splint to conform to the patient's external nose. Place the splint and secure it to the patient's skin with tape.

# Spine (Vertebral Column)

## Percutaneous Vertebroplasty and Vertebral Augmentation

Codes 22510, 22511, 22512, 22513, 22514, 22515 describe procedures for percutaneous vertebral augmentation that include vertebroplasty of the cervical, thoracic, lumbar, and sacral spine and vertebral augmentation of the thoracic and lumbar spine.

For the purposes of reporting 22510, 22511, 22512, 22513, 22514, 22515, "vertebroplasty" is the process of injecting a material (cement) into the vertebral body to reinforce the structure of the body using image guidance. "Vertebral augmentation" is the process of cavity creation followed by the injection of the material (cement) under image guidance. For 0200T and 0201T, "sacral augmentation (sacroplasty)" refers to the creation of a cavity within a sacral vertebral body followed by injection of a material to fill that cavity.

The procedure codes are inclusive of bone biopsy, when performed, and imaging guidance necessary to perform the procedure. Use one primary procedure code and an add-on code for additional levels. When treating the sacrum, sacral procedures are reported only once per encounter.

> ▶(For thermal destruction of intraosseous basivertebral nerve, see 64628, 64629)◀

**22510** Percutaneous vertebroplasty (bone biopsy included when performed), 1 vertebral body, unilateral or bilateral injection, inclusive of all imaging guidance; cervicothoracic

## Rationale

In accordance with the establishment of codes 64628 and 64629, a cross-reference parenthetical note has been added in the Spine (Vertebral Column)/Percutaneous Vertebroplasty and Vertebral Augmentation subsection to direct users to report these codes for thermal destruction of the intraosseous basivertebral nerve.

Refer to the codebook and the Rationale for codes 64628 and 64629 for a full discussion of these changes.

# Arthrodesis

## Anterior or Anterolateral Approach Technique

**22586**  Arthrodesis, pre-sacral interbody technique, including disc space preparation, discectomy, with posterior instrumentation, with image guidance, includes bone graft when performed, L5-S1 interspace

▶(Do not report 22586 in conjunction with 20930-20938, 22840, 22848, 77002, 77003, 77011, 77012)◀

## Rationale

In accordance with the deletion of epidurography code 72275, the exclusionary parenthetical note following code 22586 has been revised to reflect the deletion of code 72275.

Refer to the codebook and the Rationale for code 72275 for a full discussion of these changes.

## Posterior, Posterolateral or Lateral Transverse Process Technique

To report instrumentation procedures, see 22840-22855, 22859. (Report in addition to code[s] for the definitive procedure[s].) Do not append modifier 62 to spinal instrumentation codes 22840-22848, 22850, 22852, 22853, 22854, 22859.

To report bone graft procedures, see 20930-20938. (Report in addition to code[s] for the definitive procedure[s].) Do not append modifier 62 to bone graft codes 20900-20938.

▶**Definitions**

*Corpectomy:* Identifies removal of a vertebral body during spinal surgery.

*Facetectomy:* The excision of the facet joint between two vertebral bodies. There are two facet joints at each vertebral segment (see below).

*Foraminotomy:* The excision of bone to widen the intervertebral foramen. The intervertebral foramen is bordered by the superior notch of the adjacent vertebra, the inferior notch of the vertebra, the facet joint, and the intervertebral disc.

*Hemilaminectomy:* Removal of a portion of a vertebral lamina, usually performed for exploration of, access to, or decompression of the intraspinal contents.

*Lamina:* Pertains to the vertebral arch, the flattened posterior portion of the vertebral arch extending between the pedicles and the midline, forming the dorsal wall of the vertebral forameny, and from the midline junction of which the spinous process extends.

*Laminectomy:* Excision of a vertebral lamina, commonly used to denote removal of the posterior arch.

*Laminotomy:* Excision of a portion of the vertebral lamina, resulting in enlargement of the intervertebral foramen for the purpose of relieving pressure on a spinal nerve root.◀

A vertebral segment describes the basic constituent part into which the spine may be divided. It represents a single complete vertebral bone with its associated articular processes and laminae. A vertebral interspace is the non-bony compartment between two adjacent vertebral bodies which contains the intervertebral disc, and includes the nucleus pulposus, annulus fibrosus, and two cartilaginous endplates.

▶Decompression performed on the same vertebral segment(s) and/or interspace(s) as posterior lumbar interbody fusion that includes laminectomy, facetectomy, and/or foraminotomy may be separately reported using 63052, 63053.

Decompression solely to prepare the interspace for fusion is not separately reported.◀

**22590**  Arthrodesis, posterior technique, craniocervical (occiput-C2)

**22595**  Arthrodesis, posterior technique, atlas-axis (C1-C2)

▲ **22600**  Arthrodesis, posterior or posterolateral technique, single interspace; cervical below C2 segment

▲ **22610**  thoracic (with lateral transverse technique, when performed)

▲ **22612**  lumbar (with lateral transverse technique, when performed)

▶(Do not report 22612 in conjunction with 22630 for the same interspace; use 22633)◀

★ = Telemedicine   ✚ = Add-on code   ✕ = FDA approval pending   # = Resequenced code   ⊘ = Modifier 51 exempt

Surgery / Musculoskeletal System 20100-29999

# Visual Definitions of Spinal Anatomy and Procedures

A. Vertebral interspace (non-bony) and segment (bony)

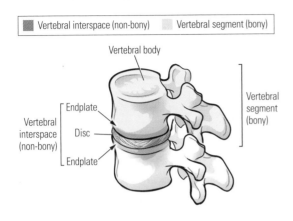

C. Laminotomy, hemilaminectomy, and laminectomy

☐ Area of bone removed during procedure

**Laminotomy** — Vertebral foramen (opening for spinal cord) — Pedicle — Lamina — Spinous process — Lamina

**Hemilaminectomy**

**Laminectomy**

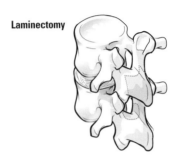

B. Foraminotomy and facetectomy

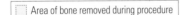

☐ Area of bone removed during procedure

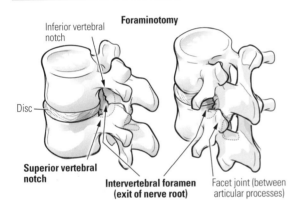

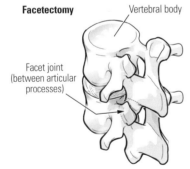

D. Corpectomy

☐ Area of bone removed during procedure

**Corpectomy** *(expanded views)*

Cervical (≥50%)    Thoracic (≥33%)    Lumbar (≥33%)

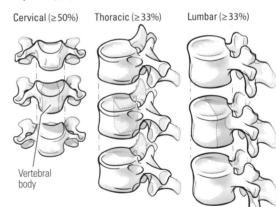

Vertebral body

▲ = Revised code  ● = New code  ▶ ◀ = Contains new or revised text  ✖ = Duplicate PLA test  ⇅ = Category I PLA     American Medical Association  **37**

Surgery / Musculoskeletal System  20100-29999

**+▲ 22614**   each additional interspace (List separately in addition to code for primary procedure)

▶(Use 22614 in conjunction with 22600, 22610, 22612, 22630, or 22633, when performed for arthrodesis at a different interspace. When performing a posterior or posterolateral technique for fusion/arthrodesis at an additional interspace, use 22614. When performing a posterior interbody fusion arthrodesis at an additional interspace, use 22632. When performing a combined posterior or posterolateral technique with posterior interbody arthrodesis at an additional interspace, use 22634)◀

(For facet joint fusion, see 0219T-0222T)

(For placement of a posterior intrafacet implant, see 0219T-0222T)

## Examples of TLIF, PLIF, and Laminectomy Techniques and Procedures
22630, 63052

A. Examples of posterior interbody fusion techniques (22630)

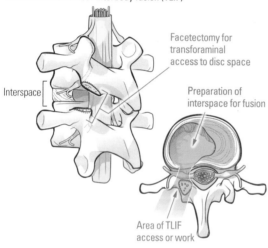

Transforaminal lumbar interbody fusion (TLIF)

Facetectomy for transforaminal access to disc space

Interspace

Preparation of interspace for fusion

Area of TLIF access or work

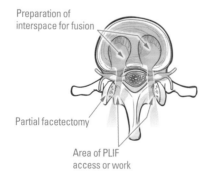

Posterior lumbar interbody fusion (PLIF)

Preparation of interspace for fusion

Partial facetectomy

Area of PLIF access or work

B. Examples of posterior interbody fusion techniques and laminectomy at same interspace (22630, 63052)

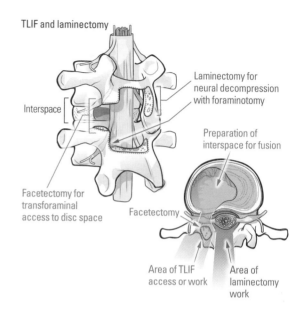

TLIF and laminectomy

Laminectomy for neural decompression with foraminotomy

Interspace

Preparation of interspace for fusion

Facetectomy for transforaminal access to disc space

Facetectomy

Area of TLIF access or work

Area of laminectomy work

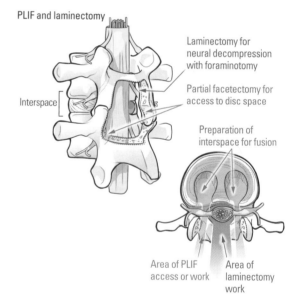

PLIF and laminectomy

Laminectomy for neural decompression with foraminotomy

Partial facetectomy for access to disc space

Interspace

Preparation of interspace for fusion

Area of PLIF access or work

Area of laminectomy work

**22630**   Arthrodesis, posterior interbody technique, including laminectomy and/or discectomy to prepare interspace (other than for decompression), single interspace; lumbar

(Do not report 22630 in conjunction with 22612 for the same interspace and segment, use 22633)

**+ 22632**   each additional interspace (List separately in addition to code for primary procedure)

★ =Telemedicine   ✚ =Add-on code   ✒ =FDA approval pending   # =Resequenced code   ⊘ =Modifier 51 exempt

▶(Use 22632 in conjunction with 22612, 22630, or 22633, when performed at a different interspace. When performing a posterior interbody fusion arthrodesis at an additional interspace, use 22632. When performing a posterior or posterolateral technique for fusion/arthrodesis at an additional interspace, use 22614. When performing a combined posterior or posterolateral technique with posterior interbody arthrodesis at an additional interspace, use 22634)◀

▶(Do not report 22630, 22632 in conjunction with 63030, 63040, 63042, 63047, 63052, 63053, 63056, for laminectomy performed to prepare the interspace on the same spinal interspace[s])◀

▲ **22633**   Arthrodesis, combined posterior or posterolateral technique with posterior interbody technique including laminectomy and/or discectomy sufficient to prepare interspace (other than for decompression), single interspace; lumbar

▶(Do not report with 22612 or 22630 for the same interspace)◀

+▲ **22634**      each additional interspace and segment (List separately in addition to code for primary procedure)

(Use 22634 in conjunction with 22633)

▶(Do not report 22633, 22634 in conjunction with 63030, 63040, 63042, 63047, 63052, 63053, 63056, for laminectomy performed to prepare the interspace on the same spinal interspace[s])◀

▶(For decompression performed on the same interspace[s] as posterior interbody fusion that includes laminectomy, removal of facets, and/or opening/widening of the foramen for decompression of nerves or spinal components, such as spinal cord, cauda equina, or nerve roots, see 63052, 63053)◀

## Rationale

Guidelines and parenthetical notes have been revised and added, and changes have been made to codes for arthrodesis, posterior or posterolateral techniques of the cervical, thoracic, and lumbar bones (22600-22614), for spine fusion procedures that describe posterior interbody fusion techniques (22633, 22634), and for laminectomy code 63048. Codes 63052 and 63053 have been established to provide appropriate reporting for laminectomy when performed in conjunction with fusion of lumbar vertebrae. In addition, definitions for the various terms used to identify anatomy associated with fusion, laminectomy, and other decompression procedures have been added to facilitate better understanding regarding reporting for fusion procedures. New illustrations have also been added to further assist in better understanding of the procedures and reporting.

To provide clarity for reporting, several changes have been made to the instructions and coding for interbody fusion procedures performed with laminectomy to identify: (1) when it is appropriate to separately report laminectomy, facetectomy, and/or foraminotomy procedure(s) performed in conjunction with spine fusion procedures; and (2) the specific fusion or arthrodesis procedures with which laminectomy may be reported. The intent is that new codes 63052 and 63053 may only be reported as add-on services when a decompressive laminectomy (with any other decompressive procedure, such as foraminotomy or facetectomy) is performed in addition to fusion procedures that utilize interbody laminectomy technique (ie, the fusion procedures identified by codes 22630-22634). Codes 63052 and 63053 should not be used in conjunction with other fusion procedures. In addition, these new codes should not be reported if the laminectomy is performed to prepare the interspace for arthrodesis or fusion, such as to allow better access for completing the fusion procedure (ie, if decompression of the neural anatomy is the work being performed, and if the fusion procedure is an interbody technique, codes 63052, 63053 may be reported). This is exemplified within the guideline language that provides instruction regarding the intended use of the codes as follows:

"Decompression performed on the same vertebral segment(s) and/or interspace(s) as posterior lumbar interbody fusion that includes laminectomy, facetectomy, and/or foraminotomy may be separately reported using 63052, 63053.

Decompression solely to prepare the interspace for fusion is not separately reported."

The code descriptors for codes 63052 and 63053 also only note "lumbar" vertebrae as the segments of focus as this interbody technique is only performed on lumbar vertebrae. Codes 63052 and 63053 are included as add-on codes because they are only performed in addition to interbody fusion procedures. The intent is that if decompressive laminectomy is performed by itself (ie, without interbody fusion), the existing laminectomy codes (eg, 63040-63048) may be used to report the service. Parenthetical notes providing instruction on the appropriate use of these codes have been added throughout the Musculoskeletal section, as well as the Nervous System section following codes 63035, 63044, 63048, and 63057.

Other revisions have been made to related sections to address the use of ambiguous terminology. Because the term "level" may be used to reference an individual boney "segment" of the spine or the "interspace" at which work is being performed, to eliminate confusion as to what is specifically being addressed by the code or procedure, the term "level" has been removed from many of the descriptors, parenthetical notes, and guidelines where it was used and replaced with the term "segment," which is used to specify the bone itself as the anatomy of focus. In addition, the term "interspace" may also be used to identify anatomy when multiple segments are involved, such as when identifying the joining of two or more segments to form the fused bones or arthrodesis.

Illustrations have also been added to provide examples of posterior interbody fusion (22630) and examples of posterior interbody fusion and laminectomy at the same interspace (22630, 63052). Other new illustrations provide users with visual representations of the terms within the two sections.

## Spine Deformity (eg, Scoliosis, Kyphosis)

To report instrumentation procedures, see 22840-22855, 22859. (Report in addition to code[s] for the definitive procedure[s].) Do not append modifier 62 to spinal instrumentation codes 22840-22848, 22850, 22852, 22853, 22854, 22859.

To report bone graft procedures, see 20930-20938. (Report in addition to code[s] for the definitive procedure[s].) Do not append modifier 62 to bone graft codes 20900-20938.

A vertebral segment describes the basic constituent part into which the spine may be divided. It represents a single complete vertebral bone with its associated articular processes and laminae.

▶For the following codes, when two surgeons work together as primary surgeons performing distinct part(s) of an arthrodesis for spinal deformity, each surgeon should report his/her distinct operative work by appending modifier 62 to the procedure code. In this situation, modifier 62 may be appended to procedure code(s) 22800-22819 as long as both surgeons continue to work together as primary surgeons. The spinal deformity arthrodesis codes (22800, 22802, 22804, 22808, 22810, 22812) and kyphectomy codes (22818, 22819) should not be reported in conjunction with vertebral body tethering codes (0656T, 0657T).◀

**22800** Arthrodesis, posterior, for spinal deformity, with or without cast; up to 6 vertebral segments

**22802** 7 to 12 vertebral segments

**22804** 13 or more vertebral segments

▶(Do not report 22800, 22802, 22804 in conjunction with 0656T, 0657T)◀

**22808** Arthrodesis, anterior, for spinal deformity, with or without cast; 2 to 3 vertebral segments

**22810** 4 to 7 vertebral segments

**22812** 8 or more vertebral segments

▶(Do not report 22808, 22810, 22812 in conjunction with 0656T, 0657T)◀

**22818** Kyphectomy, circumferential exposure of spine and resection of vertebral segment(s) (including body and posterior elements); single or 2 segments

**22819** 3 or more segments

▶(Do not report 22818, 22819 in conjunction with 0656T, 0657T)◀

(To report arthrodesis, see 22800-22804 and add modifier 51)

## Rationale

In accordance with the establishment of new Category III codes 0656T and 0657T for reporting anterior vertebral body tethering, the spine deformity (eg, scoliosis, kyphosis) guidelines have been revised and updated to provide appropriate guidance for reporting spinal deformity arthrodesis codes 22800, 22802, 22804, 22808, 22810, and 22812, and kyphectomy codes 22818 and 22819 with new codes 0656T and 0657T. Additional exclusionary parenthetical notes have been added following codes 22804, 22812, and 22819 to support accurate reporting of these services in conjunction with codes 0656T and 0657T.

Refer to the codebook and the Rationale for codes 0656T and 0657T for a full discussion of these changes.

## Spinal Instrumentation

**+ 22845** Anterior instrumentation; 2 to 3 vertebral segments (List separately in addition to code for primary procedure)

(Use 22845 in conjunction with 22100-22102, 22110-22114, 22206, 22207, 22210-22214, 22220-22224, 22310-22327, 22532, 22533, 22548-22558, 22590-22612, 22630, 22633, 22634, 22800-22812, 63001-63030, 63040-63042, 63045-63047, 63050-63056, 63064, 63075, 63077, 63081, 63085, 63087, 63090, 63101, 63102, 63170-63290, 63300-63307)

+ **22846**     4 to 7 vertebral segments (List separately in addition
                to code for primary procedure)

                (Use 22846 in conjunction with 22100-22102, 22110-
                22114, 22206, 22207, 22210-22214, 22220-22224, 22310-
                22327, 22532, 22533, 22548-22558, 22590-22612, 22630,
                22633, 22634, 22800-22812, 63001-63030, 63040-63042,
                63045-63047, 63050-63056, 63064, 63075, 63077, 63081,
                63085, 63087, 63090, 63101, 63102, 63170-63290,
                63300-63307)

+ **22847**     8 or more vertebral segments (List separately in
                addition to code for primary procedure)

                (Use 22847 in conjunction with 22100-22102, 22110-
                22114, 22206, 22207, 22210-22214, 22220-22224, 22310-
                22327, 22532, 22533, 22548-22558, 22590-22612, 22630,
                22633, 22634, 22800-22812, 63001-63030, 63040-63042,
                63045-63047, 63050-63056, 63064, 63075, 63077, 63081,
                63085, 63087, 63090, 63101, 63102, 63170-63290,
                63300-63307)

                ▶(For vertebral body tethering of the spine, see 0656T,
                0657T)◀

## Rationale

In accordance with the establishment of codes 0656T and
0657T, a cross-reference parenthetical note has been
added following code 22847 directing users to new
Category III codes 0656T and 0657T for anterior vertebral
body tethering.

Refer to the codebook and the Rationale for codes 0657T
and 0657T for a full discussion of these changes.

# Application of Casts and Strapping

▶All services that appear in the Musculoskeletal System
section include the application and removal of the first
cast, splint, or traction device, when performed. Supplies
are reported separately. If a cast is removed by someone
other than the physician or other qualified health care
professional who applied the cast, report the cast removal
code (29700, 29705, 29710).

Subsequent replacement of cast, splint, or strapping
(29000-29750) and/or traction device (eg, 20690,
20692) during or after the global period may be reported
separately.

A cast, splint, or strapping is not considered part of the
preoperative care; therefore, the use of modifier 56 for
preoperative management only is not applicable.◀

                (For orthotics management and training, see 97760,
                97761, 97763)

## Rationale

In accordance with the revision of the introductory
guidelines in the Musculoskeletal System section, the
application of casts and strapping guidelines have been
revised to reflect these changes.

Refer to the codebook and the Rationale for the
introductory guidelines revisions to the Musculoskeletal
System section for a full discussion of these changes.

# Respiratory System

## Larynx

### Endoscopy

**31575**     Laryngoscopy, flexible; diagnostic

              (Do not report 31575 in conjunction with 31231, unless
              performed for a separate condition using a separate
              endoscope)

              ▶(Do not report 31575 in conjunction with 31572, 31573,
              31574, 31576, 31577, 31578, 42975, 43197, 43198,
              92511, 92612, 92614, 92616)◀

**31576**     with biopsy(ies)

              (Do not report 31576 in conjunction with 31572, 31578)

## Rationale

In accordance with the establishment of new code 42975,
an exclusionary parenthetical note following code 31575
has been revised to preclude users from reporting code
42975 for flexible, diagnostic drug-induced sleep
endoscopy with code 31575.

Refer to the codebook and the Rationale for code 42975
for a full discussion of these changes.

## Lungs and Pleura

### Thoracoscopy (Video-assisted thoracic surgery [VATS])

**32650**     Thoracoscopy, surgical; with pleurodesis (eg, mechanical
              or chemical)

**32651**     with partial pulmonary decortication

**32664**     with thoracic sympathectomy

**32665**     with esophagomyotomy (Heller type)

►(Do not report 32665 in conjunction with 43497)◄

(For exploratory thoracoscopy, and exploratory thoracoscopy with biopsy, see 32601-32609)

## Rationale

In accordance with the establishment of code 43497, an exclusionary parenthetical note has been added following code 32665 to restrict reporting codes 32665 and 43497 together.

Refer to the codebook and the Rationale for code 43497 for a full discussion of these changes.

# Cardiovascular System

## Heart and Pericardium

### Pacemaker or Implantable Defibrillator

A pacemaker system with lead(s) includes a pulse generator containing electronics, a battery, and one or more leads. A lead consists of one or more electrodes, as well as conductor wires, insulation, and a fixation mechanism. Pulse generators are placed in a subcutaneous "pocket" created in either a subclavicular site or just above the abdominal muscles just below the ribcage. Leads may be inserted through a vein (transvenous) or they may be placed on the surface of the heart (epicardial). The epicardial location of leads requires a thoracotomy for insertion.

►A single chamber pacemaker system with lead includes a pulse generator and one electrode inserted in either the atrium or ventricle. A dual chamber pacemaker system with two leads includes a pulse generator and one lead inserted in the right atrium and one lead inserted in the right ventricle. In certain circumstances, an additional lead may be required to achieve pacing of the left ventricle (bi-ventricular pacing). In this event, transvenous (cardiac vein) placement of the lead should be separately reported using code 33224 or 33225. For body surface–activation mapping to optimize electrical synchrony of a biventricular pacing or biventricular pacing-defibrillator system at the time of implant, also report 0695T with the appropriate code (ie, 33224, 33225, 33226). Epicardial placement of the lead should be separately reported using 33202, 33203.◄

A leadless cardiac pacemaker system includes a pulse generator with built-in battery and electrode for implantation in a cardiac chamber via a transcatheter approach. For implantation of a leadless pacemaker system, use 33274. Insertion, replacement, or removal of a leadless pacemaker system includes insertion of a catheter into the right ventricle.

►Right heart catheterization (93451, 93453, 93456, 93457, 93460, 93461) may not be reported in conjunction with leadless pacemaker insertion and removal codes 33274, 33275, unless complete right heart catheterization is performed for an indication distinct from the leadless pacemaker procedure.◄

Like a pacemaker system, an implantable defibrillator system includes a pulse generator and electrodes. Three general categories of implantable defibrillators exist: transvenous implantable pacing cardioverter-defibrillator (ICD), subcutaneous implantable defibrillator (S-ICD), and substernal implantable cardioverter-defibrillator. Implantable pacing cardioverter-defibrillator devices use a combination of antitachycardia pacing, low-energy cardioversion or defibrillating shocks to treat ventricular tachycardia or ventricular fibrillation. The subcutaneous implantable defibrillator uses a single subcutaneous electrode to treat ventricular tachyarrhythmias. The substernal implantable cardioverter-defibrillator uses at least one substernal electrode to perform defibrillation, cardioversion, and antitachycardia pacing. Subcutaneous implantable defibrillators differ from transvenous implantable pacing cardioverter-defibrillators in that subcutaneous defibrillators do not provide antitachycardia pacing or chronic pacing. Substernal implantable defibrillators differ from both subcutaneous and transvenous implantable pacing cardioverter-defibrillators in that they provide antitachycardia pacing, but not chronic pacing.

33224     Insertion of pacing electrode, cardiac venous system, for left ventricular pacing, with attachment to previously placed pacemaker or implantable defibrillator pulse generator (including revision of pocket, removal, insertion, and/or replacement of existing generator)

(When epicardial electrode placement is performed, report 33224 in conjunction with 33202, 33203)

►(Use 33224 in conjunction with 0695T when body surface–activation mapping to optimize electrical synchrony is also performed)◄

+ 33225     Insertion of pacing electrode, cardiac venous system, for left ventricular pacing, at time of insertion of implantable defibrillator or pacemaker pulse generator (eg, for upgrade to dual chamber system) (List separately in addition to code for primary procedure)

(Use 33225 in conjunction with 33206, 33207, 33208, 33212, 33213, 33214, 33216, 33217, 33221, 33223, 33228, 33229, 33230, 33231, 33233, 33234, 33235, 33240, 33249, 33263, 33264)

(Use 33225 in conjunction with 33222 only with pacemaker pulse generator pocket relocation and with 33223 only with implantable defibrillator [ICD] pocket relocation)

▶(Use 33225 in conjunction with 0695T when body surface–activation mapping to optimize electrical synchrony is also performed)◀

**33226** Repositioning of previously implanted cardiac venous system (left ventricular) electrode (including removal, insertion and/or replacement of existing generator)

▶(Use 33226 in conjunction with 0695T when body surface–activation mapping to optimize electrical synchrony is also performed)◀

**# 33275** Transcatheter removal of permanent leadless pacemaker, right ventricular, including imaging guidance (eg, fluoroscopy, venous ultrasound, ventriculography, femoral venography), when performed

(Do not report 33275 in conjunction with 33274)

(Do not report 33274, 33275 in conjunction with femoral venography [75820], fluoroscopy [76000, 77002], ultrasound guidance for vascular access [76937], right ventriculography [93566])

▶(Do not report 33274, 33275 in conjunction with 93451, 93453, 93456, 93457, 93460, 93461, 93593, 93594, 93596, 93597, 93598, unless complete right heart catheterization is performed for indications distinct from the leadless pacemaker procedure)◀

(For subsequent leadless pacemaker device evaluation, see 93279, 93286, 93288, 93294, 93296)

(For insertion, replacement, repositioning, and removal of pacemaker systems with leads, see 33202, 33203, 33206, 33207, 33208, 33212, 33213, 33214, 33215, 33216, 33217, 33218, 33220, 33221, 33227, 33228, 33229, 33233, 33234, 33235, 33236, 33237)

## Rationale

In accordance with the deletion of codes 93530-93533 and the establishment of codes 93593, 93594, and 93596-93598, the pacemaker or implantable defibrillator guidelines and the conditional exclusionary parenthetical note following code 33275 have been revised to reflect these changes.

In addition, in accordance with the establishment of code 0695T, the pacemaker or implantable defibrillator guidelines have been revised to state that when body surface–activation mapping to optimize electrical synchrony of a biventricular pacing or biventricular

pacing-defibrillator system at the time of implant, code 0695T is reported with code 33224, 33225, or 33226, as appropriate. Conditional inclusionary parenthetical notes have been added following codes 33224, 33225, and 33226 instructing users to report code 0695T when body surface–activation mapping to optimize electrical synchrony is also performed.

Refer to the codebook and the Rationale for codes 93593, 93594, 93596-93598, and 0695T for a full description of these changes.

## Electrophysiologic Operative Procedures

This family of codes describes the surgical treatment of supraventricular dysrhythmias. Tissue ablation, disruption, and reconstruction can be accomplished by many methods including surgical incision or through the use of a variety of energy sources (eg, radiofrequency, cryotherapy, microwave, ultrasound, laser). If excision or isolation of the left atrial appendage by any method, including stapling, oversewing, ligation, or plication, is performed in conjunction with any of the atrial tissue ablation and reconstruction (maze) procedures (33254-33259, 33265-33266), it is considered part of the procedure. Codes 33254-33256 are only to be reported when there is no concurrently performed procedure that requires median sternotomy or cardiopulmonary bypass. The appropriate atrial tissue ablation add-on code, 33257, 33258, 33259 should be reported in addition to an open cardiac procedure requiring sternotomy or cardiopulmonary bypass if performed concurrently.

### Definitions

*Limited* operative ablation and reconstruction includes:

Surgical isolation of triggers of supraventricular dysrhythmias by operative ablation that isolates the pulmonary veins or other anatomically defined triggers in the left or right atrium.

*Extensive* operative ablation and reconstruction includes:

1. The services included in *"limited"*
2. Additional ablation of atrial tissue to eliminate sustained supraventricular dysrhythmias. This must include operative ablation that involves either the right atrium, the atrial septum, or left atrium in continuity with the atrioventricular annulus.

▶Codes 33267, 33268, 33269 describe surgical left atrial appendage (LAA) exclusion (eg, excision, isolation via stapling, oversewing, ligation, plication, clip) performed to treat atrial fibrillation and mitigate postoperative thromboembolic complications. Surgical LAA exclusion may be performed as a stand-alone procedure via a sternotomy, thoracotomy, or thoracoscopic approach. It is most commonly performed in conjunction with other procedures requiring a sternotomy or thoracotomy approach. Surgical LAA exclusion is inherent to maze procedures (33254, 33255, 33256, 33257, 33258, 33259, 33265, 33266) and mitral valve repair/replacement procedures (33420, 33422, 33425, 33426, 33427, 33430) and may not be reported separately when performed in the same operative session.

Code 33267 may only be reported when there is no concurrently performed procedure that requires a sternotomy or thoracotomy approach.

Add-on code 33268, if performed concurrently, may be reported in conjunction with a primary procedure performed via a sternotomy or thoracotomy.

Code 33269 may be reported for thoracoscopic LAA exclusion, other than with maze or mitral valve procedures (33254, 33255, 33256, 33257, 33258, 33259, 33265, 33266, 33420, 33422, 33425, 33426, 33427, 33430), when performed during the same operative session.◄

## Rationale

In accordance with the establishment of codes 33267-33269, the electrophysiologic operative procedures guidelines in the Heart and Pericardium subsection of the Cardiovascular System section have been revised to address the new codes. In part, these guidelines indicate that codes 33267-33269 describe surgical left atrial appendage (LAA) exclusion performed to treat atrial fibrillation and mitigate postoperative thromboembolic complications. The guidelines also have been revised to note that surgical LAA exclusion is inherent to maze procedures and mitral valve repair or replacement procedures.

In addition, codes 33267 and 33268 have been added to the Incision subsection, and code 33269 has been added to the Endoscopy subsection of the Heart and Pericardium section of the CPT code set.

Refer to the codebook and the Rationale for codes 33267-33269 for a full discussion of these changes.

### Incision

**+ 33258**   Operative tissue ablation and reconstruction of atria, performed at the time of other cardiac procedure(s), extensive (eg, maze procedure), without cardiopulmonary bypass (List separately in addition to code for primary procedure)

►(Use 33258 in conjunction with 33130, 33250, 33300, 33310, 33320, 33321, 33330, 33365, 33420, 33471, 33501-33503, 33510-33516, 33533-33536, 33690, 33735, 33737, 33750, 33755, 33762, 33764, 33766, 33800-33813, 33820, 33822, 33824, 33840, 33845, 33851, 33852, 33875, 33877, 33915, 33925, 33981, 33982, when the procedure is performed without cardiopulmonary bypass)◄

## Rationale

In accordance with the deletion of code 33470, the inclusionary parenthetical note following code 33258 has been revised with the removal of code 33470.

Refer to the codebook and the Rationale for code 33470 for a full description of these changes.

**33261**   Operative ablation of ventricular arrhythmogenic focus with cardiopulmonary bypass

**#● 33267**   Exclusion of left atrial appendage, open, any method (eg, excision, isolation via stapling, oversewing, ligation, plication, clip)

►(Do not report 33267 in conjunction with 33254, 33255, 33256, 33257, 33258, 33259, 33265, 33266, 33420, 33422, 33425, 33426, 33427, 33430)◄

►(Do not report 33267 in conjunction with other sternotomy or thoracotomy procedures performed during the same session)◄

**#+● 33268**   Exclusion of left atrial appendage, open, performed at the time of other sternotomy or thoracotomy procedure(s), any method (eg, excision, isolation via stapling, oversewing, ligation, plication, clip) (List separately in addition to code for primary procedure)

►(Use 33268 in conjunction with primary procedures performed via sternotomy or thoracotomy approach)◄

►(Do not report 33268 in conjunction with 33254, 33255, 33256, 33257, 33258, 33259, 33265, 33266, 33420, 33422, 33425, 33426, 33427, 33430)◄

### Endoscopy

**#● 33269**   Exclusion of left atrial appendage, thoracoscopic, any method (eg, excision, isolation via stapling, oversewing, ligation, plication, clip)

►(Do not report 33269 in conjunction with 33254, 33255, 33256, 33257, 33258, 33259, 33265, 33266, 33420, 33422, 33425, 33426, 33427, 33430)◄

**33265**   Endoscopy, surgical; operative tissue ablation and reconstruction of atria, limited (eg, modified maze procedure), without cardiopulmonary bypass

★ = Telemedicine   ✦ = Add-on code   ✗ = FDA approval pending   # = Resequenced code   ⊘ = Modifier 51 exempt

**33266**       operative tissue ablation and reconstruction of atria, extensive (eg, maze procedure), without cardiopulmonary bypass

(Do not report 33265-33266 in conjunction with 32551, 33210, 33211)

**33267**       Code is out of numerical sequence. See 33259-33266

**33268**       Code is out of numerical sequence. See 33259-33266

**33269**       Code is out of numerical sequence. See 33259-33266

## Rationale

Codes 33267-33269 have been established to report the exclusion of the LAA. Code 33267 is used to report the exclusion of the LAA by any method via an open approach. Two exclusionary parenthetical notes have been added following code 33267, including one note indicating that code 33267 should not be reported in conjunction with other sternotomy or thoracotomy procedures performed during the same session.

Add-on code 33268 is used to report the exclusion of the LAA by any method via an open approach that is performed at the time of other sternotomy or thoracotomy procedure(s). Two parenthetical notes have also been added following code 33268, including an exclusionary parenthetical note and a parenthetical note indicating that code 33268 should be used in conjunction with primary procedures performed via sternotomy or thoracotomy approaches.

In addition, revisions have been made to the electrophysiologic operative procedures guidelines, and code 33269 has been established in the Endoscopy subsection of the Heart and Pericardium section to report the thorascopic exclusion of the LAA by any method.

## Clinical Example (33267)

A 75-year-old male, who is status post left-lung resection, presents with persistent atrial fibrillation and a $CHADS_2$ (stroke risk) score of 4. Recurrent, significant gastro-intestinal bleeding episodes preclude anticoagulation therapy. He is deemed a poor candidate for a left atrial appendage (LAA) endovascular occlusion device. Because of anticipated dense adhesions within the left chest cavity, a thoracoscopic approach is contraindicated and an open approach to LAA exclusion (eg, ligation, plication, clip) is recommended.

## Description of Procedure (33267)

Under general anesthesia, make a thoracotomy incision and carefully enter the chest over the top of the sixth rib using electrocautery. If necessary, remove a segment of rib to prevent trauma when spreading of the ribs for

exposure. Collapse the left lung and institute single-lung ventilation of the right lung to facilitate exposure. Separate adhesions between the lung and the pericardium to avoid lung parenchymal injury, as well as injury to the phrenic nerve. Open the pericardium posterior to the phrenic nerve. Carefully dissect any adhesions off the LAA and expose and measure the base. Under transesophageal echocardiography (TEE) guidance, staple, clip, or ligate the base of the LAA. Use TEE to confirm there is no flow into the LAA. This can be done either off (most commonly) or on cardiopulmonary bypass (femoral cannulation) (reported separately). Leave the pericardium open. Perform an intercostal nerve block for postoperative analgesia. Place a left chest tube or drain. Expand the left lung. Conduct a careful check for hemostasis and/or lung parenchymal air leaks. Close the thoracotomy incision in layers by approximating the muscles, subcutaneous tissue, and skin. Extubate the patient and transport the patient to the recovery area.

## Clinical Example (33268)

A 50-year-old female, who has severe peripheral vascular disease (PVD) and bicuspid aortic valve with severe stenosis, undergoes surgical aortic valve replacement and surgical LAA exclusion (eg, ligation, plication, clip).

## Description of Procedure (33268)

In addition to performing a procedure via a sternotomy or thoracotomy approach (reported separately), expose the LAA by mobilizing the left ventricle toward the right side. This can be facilitated by dividing the pericardium on the right side to avoid right ventricular compression and decreasing venous return. Use extreme care to avoid injury to the right phrenic nerve. Carefully monitor the hemodynamic stability of the patient. Expose and carefully measure the base of the LAA. Under TEE guidance, staple, clip, or ligate the base of the LAA. Use TEE to confirm there is no flow into the LAA. Once completed, return attention to the final procedural elements of the primary operation.

## Clinical Example (33269)

An 85-year-old female with persistent atrial fibrillation has undergone numerous electrophysiologic procedures in the past and was deemed a poor candidate for an endovascular LAA occlusion device. Thoracoscopic LAA exclusion (eg, ligation, plication, clip) is recommended.

## Description of Procedure (33269)

Under general anesthesia, identify and anesthetize the site for the initial trocar site with local anesthetic. Make an incision, and using a combination of sharp, cautery, and blunt dissection, carefully enter the pleural cavity.

Palpate the parietal pleura, insert a trocar under direct vision, and advance the thoracoscope into the pleural cavity. Perform an initial visual exploration. Identify the sites for all additional trocar incisions (1 or 2) if necessary and anesthetize them with local anesthetic. Make additional trocar incisions in a similar fashion. Place access ports as necessary at each incision site for the passage of instruments. Deflate the left lung. Free adhesions between the lung and chest wall. Take care to avoid decreasing venous return by careful monitoring $CO_2$ flow and pressure (usually kept +/< 6 mmHg) and the patient's blood pressure. Carefully open the pericardium posterior to the phrenic nerve and expose the left atrial appendage. Expose and measure the left atrial appendage base. Clip, staple, or ligate the appendage with TEE guidance to make sure there is no flow into the LAA. Leave the pericardium open. Perform an intercostal nerve block with local anesthetic for postoperative analgesia. Expand the left lung. Insert a chest tube(s) through a separate interspace incision(s) to provide evacuation of air and fluid from the chest. Assess all trocar incisions for hemostasis. Conduct a surgical pause while an instrumentation, needle, and sponge count is completed and confirmed by the surgeon. Close each incision with multiple layers of suture for the muscle, and reapproximate the skin with a subcuticular stitch. Extubate the patient.

## Implantable Hemodynamic Monitors

**33289**    Transcatheter implantation of wireless pulmonary artery pressure sensor for long-term hemodynamic monitoring, including deployment and calibration of the sensor, right heart catheterization, selective pulmonary catheterization, radiological supervision and interpretation, and pulmonary artery angiography, when performed

(For remote monitoring of an implantable wireless pulmonary artery pressure sensor, use 93264)

▶(Do not report 33289 in conjunction with 36013, 36014, 36015, 75741, 75743, 75746, 76000, 93451, 93453, 93456, 93457, 93460, 93461, 93568, 93593, 93594, 93596, 93597, 93598)◀

### Rationale

In accordance with the deletion of heart catheterization codes 93530-93533 and the establishment of heart catheterization codes 93593, 93594, and 93596-93598 for congenital heart defect, the exclusionary parenthetical note following code 33289 has been revised to reflect these changes.

Refer to the codebook and the Rationale for codes 93593, 93594, and 93596-93598 for a full discussion of these changes.

## Heart (Including Valves) and Great Vessels

**33340**    Percutaneous transcatheter closure of the left atrial appendage with endocardial implant, including fluoroscopy, transseptal puncture, catheter placement(s), left atrial angiography, left atrial appendage angiography, when performed, and radiological supervision and interpretation

(Do not report 33340 in conjunction with 93462)

▶(Do not report 33340 in conjunction with 93452, 93453, 93458, 93459, 93460, 93461, 93595, 93596, 93597, 93598, unless catheterization of the left ventricle is performed by a non-transseptal approach for indications distinct from the left atrial appendage closure procedure)◀

▶(Do not report 33340 in conjunction with 93451, 93453, 93456, 93460, 93461, 93593, 93594, 93596, 93597, 93598, unless complete right heart catheterization is performed for indications distinct from the left atrial appendage closure procedure)◀

### Rationale

In accordance with the deletion of codes 93530-93533 and the establishment of codes 93593-93598, the two conditional exclusionary parenthetical notes following code 33340 have been revised to reflect these changes.

Refer to the codebook and the Rationale for codes 93593-93598 for a full discussion of these changes.

## Cardiac Valves

### Aortic Valve

Codes 33361, 33362, 33363, 33364, 33365, 33366 are used to report transcatheter aortic valve replacement (TAVR)/ transcatheter aortic valve implantation (TAVI). TAVR/TAVI requires two physician operators and all components of the procedure are reported using modifier 62.

Codes 33361, 33362, 33363, 33364, 33365, 33366 include the work, when performed, of percutaneous access, placing the access sheath, balloon aortic valvuloplasty, advancing the valve delivery system into position, repositioning the valve as needed, deploying the valve, temporary pacemaker insertion for rapid pacing

★ = Telemedicine    ✚ = Add-on code    ⊮ = FDA approval pending    # = Resequenced code    ⊘ = Modifier 51 exempt

(33210), and closure of the arteriotomy when performed. Codes 33361, 33362, 33363, 33364, 33365, 33366 include open arterial or cardiac approach.

Angiography, radiological supervision, and interpretation performed to guide TAVR/TAVI (eg, guiding valve placement, documenting completion of the intervention, assessing the vascular access site for closure) are included in these codes.

▶Add-on code 33370 may be reported for cerebral embolic protection in conjunction with TAVR/TAVI codes 33361, 33362, 33363, 33364, 33365, 33366. Code 33370 includes percutaneous arterial (eg, right radial or femoral) access, placement of a guiding catheter, and delivery of the embolic protection filter(s) prior to the procedure. Placement of additional/multiple filters is not separately reportable. Code 33370 includes removal of the filter(s) and debris, removal of the arterial sheath, and closure of the arteriotomy by pressure and application of an arterial closure device or standard closure of the puncture by suture. Extensive repair or replacement of an artery may be additionally reported. Code 33370 includes all imaging guidance and radiological supervision and interpretation associated with performing cerebral embolic protection (eg, 75600, 75710, 76937).◀

Diagnostic left heart catheterization codes (93452, 93453, 93458-93461) and the supravalvular aortography code (93567) should **not** be used with TAVR/TAVI services (33361, 33362, 33363, 33364, 33365, 33366) to report:

1. Contrast injections, angiography, roadmapping, and/or fluoroscopic guidance for the TAVR/TAVI,

2. Aorta/left ventricular outflow tract measurement for the TAVR/TAVI, or

3. Post-TAVR/TAVI aortic or left ventricular angiography, as this work is captured in the TAVR/TAVI services codes (33361, 33362, 33363, 33364, 33365, 33366).

Diagnostic coronary angiography performed at the time of TAVR/TAVI may be separately reportable if:

1. No prior catheter-based coronary angiography study is available and a full diagnostic study is performed, or

2. A prior study is available, but as documented in the medical record:

   a. The patient's condition with respect to the clinical indication has changed since the prior study, or

   b. There is inadequate visualization of the anatomy and/or pathology, or

   c. There is a clinical change during the procedure that requires new evaluation.

   d. For same session/same day diagnostic coronary angiography services, report the appropriate diagnostic cardiac catheterization code(s) appended

with modifier 59 indicating separate and distinct procedural service from TAVR/TAVI.

Diagnostic coronary angiography performed at a separate session from an interventional procedure may be separately reportable.

Other cardiac catheterization services may be reported separately when performed for diagnostic purposes not intrinsic to TAVR/TAVI.

Percutaneous coronary interventional procedures are reported separately, when performed.

When transcatheter ventricular support is required in conjunction with TAVR/TAVI, the appropriate code may be reported with the appropriate ventricular assist device (VAD) procedure code (33975, 33976, 33990, 33991, 33992, 33993, 33995, 33997) or balloon pump insertion code (33967, 33970, 33973).

The TAVR/TAVI cardiovascular access and delivery procedures are reported with 33361, 33362, 33363, 33364, 33365, 33366. When cardiopulmonary bypass is performed in conjunction with TAVR/TAVI, codes 33361, 33362, 33363, 33364, 33365, 33366 should be reported with the appropriate add-on code for percutaneous peripheral bypass (33367), open peripheral bypass (33368), or central bypass (33369).

**33361** Transcatheter aortic valve replacement (TAVR/TAVI) with prosthetic valve; percutaneous femoral artery approach

**+ 33367** cardiopulmonary bypass support with percutaneous peripheral arterial and venous cannulation (eg, femoral vessels) (List separately in addition to code for primary procedure)

▶(Use 33367 in conjunction with 33361, 33362, 33363, 33364, 33365, 33366, 33418, 33477, 0483T, 0484T, 0544T, 0545T, 0569T, 0570T, 0643T, 0644T)◀

(Do not report 33367 in conjunction with 33368, 33369)

▶(For cerebral embolic protection, use 33370)◀

**+ 33368** cardiopulmonary bypass support with open peripheral arterial and venous cannulation (eg, femoral, iliac, axillary vessels) (List separately in addition to code for primary procedure)

▶(Use 33368 in conjunction with 33361, 33362, 33363, 33364, 33365, 33366, 33418, 33477, 0483T, 0484T, 0544T, 0545T, 0569T, 0570T, 0643T, 0644T)◀

(Do not report 33368 in conjunction with 33367, 33369)

**+ 33369** cardiopulmonary bypass support with central arterial and venous cannulation (eg, aorta, right atrium, pulmonary artery) (List separately in addition to code for primary procedure)

▶(Use 33369 in conjunction with 33361, 33362, 33363, 33364, 33365, 33366, 33418, 33477, 0483T, 0484T, 0544T, 0545T, 0569T, 0570T, 0643T, 0644T)◀

(Do not report 33369 in conjunction with 33367, 33368)

**+ ● 33370**  Transcatheter placement and subsequent removal of cerebral embolic protection device(s), including arterial access, catheterization, imaging, and radiological supervision and interpretation, percutaneous (List separately in addition to code for primary procedure)

▶(Use 33370 in conjunction with 33361, 33362, 33363, 33364, 33365, 33366)◀

## Rationale

Add-on code 33370 has been established to report percutaneous transcatheter placement and subsequent removal of cerebral embolic protection (CEP) device(s). New guidelines have been added to the Aortic Valve subsection to clarify the work that is included in the procedure and to provide instructions on the appropriate reporting of code 33370.

CEP devices are used in transcatheter aortic valve replacement (TAVR) and transcatheter aortic valve implantation (TAVI) procedures. As such, code 33370 is an add-on code that is reported with TAVR/TAVI codes 33361-33366. During TAVR and TAVI procedures, materials such as valve tissue or calcification fragments may break free and block blood flow, creating a potential for a cerebrovascular accident (CVA). The CEP device captures such embolic material that may be loosened during the TAVR or TAVI procedure to prevent potential CVA. The CEP device(s) is placed through a different access site prior to the TAVR or TAVI procedure and removed at the end of the procedure. Both placement and removal of the device(s) are included in code 33370.

Code 33370 is reported once regardless of the number of devices placed. In addition to placement and removal of the device(s), code 33370 includes arterial access, imaging guidance, and radiological supervision and interpretation for the CEP device protection procedure, placement and removal of the catheter or sheath, removal of the captured debris, and closure of the CEP device access site. A cross-reference parenthetical note has been added following code 33367 directing users to code 33370 for cerebral embolic protection. An inclusionary parenthetical note has been added following code 33370 indicating that code 33370 is reported with codes 33361-33366.

In accordance with the establishment of Category III codes 0643T and 0644T, the inclusionary parenthetical notes following codes 33367-33369 have been revised to include these codes.

Refer to the codebook and the Rationale for codes 0643T and 0644T for a full discussion of these changes.

## Clinical Example (33370)

During a transcatheter aortic valve replacement (TAVR/TAVI) procedure, a 76-year-old male with prior transient ischemic attack (TIA), cerebrovascular accident (CVA), and critical aortic valve stenosis also requires the addition of a cerebral embolic protection device to be placed prior to the TAVR/TAVI and removed after the TAVR/TAVI procedure. [**Note:** This is an add-on service. Only consider the additional work related to the cerebral embolic protection {CEP} device.]

## Description of Procedure (33370)

Assess the stroke risk and baseline neurologic status of the patient. Assess the technical difficulty and risk. Review the computed tomography angiography (CTA) to evaluate patient-specific anatomy of the brachiocephalic artery, the aortic arch, and the origin and course of the left common carotid artery. Evaluate for plaque and calcium burden of the great vessel, another origin. Insert a radial artery sheath.

**CEP Device Insertion:** Navigate the brachial, axillary, and brachiocephalic arteries. Position a guidewire in the ascending aorta. Deploy a proximal filter in the brachiocephalic artery. Flex articulation of the distal segment of the device and direct the guidewire into the left common carotid artery. Advance and deploy a distal filter.

**Device Removal:** Withdraw both filters into the device to capture the embolic debris. Withdraw the device from the vasculature. Remove the radial sheath and place a compression device for hemostasis. Ensure adequacy of hand circulation.

**Device Efficacy Evaluation:** Flush filters and evaluate the captured debris. Perform a neurocognitive assessment. Evaluate the access site.

### Mitral Valve

Codes 33418 and 33419 are used to report transcatheter mitral valve repair (TMVR). Code 33419 should only be reported once per session.

Codes 33418 and 33419 include the work, when performed, of percutaneous access, placing the access sheath, transseptal puncture, advancing the repair device delivery system into position, repositioning the device as needed, and deploying the device(s).

Angiography, radiological supervision, and interpretation performed to guide TMVR (eg, guiding device placement and documenting completion of the intervention) are included in these codes.

★ = Telemedicine    + = Add-on code    � = FDA approval pending    # = Resequenced code    ⊘ = Modifier 51 exempt

►Diagnostic right and left heart catheterization codes (93451, 93452, 93453, 93456, 93457, 93458, 93459, 93460, 93461, 93593, 93594, 93595, 93596, 93597, 93598) should **not** be used with 33418, 33419 to report:

1. Contrast injections, angiography, road-mapping, and/or fluoroscopic guidance for the transcatheter mitral valve repair (TMVR),

2. Left ventricular angiography to assess mitral regurgitation for guidance of TMVR, or

3. Right and left heart catheterization for hemodynamic measurements before, during, and after TMVR for guidance of TMVR.

Diagnostic right and left heart catheterization codes (93451, 93452, 93453, 93456, 93457, 93458, 93459, 93460, 93461, 93593, 93594, 93595, 93596, 93597, 93598) and diagnostic coronary angiography codes (93454, 93455, 93456, 93457, 93458, 93459, 93460, 93461, 93563, 93564) may be reported with 33418, 33419, representing separate and distinct services from TMVR, if:

1. No prior study is available and a full diagnostic study is performed, or

2. A prior study is available, but as documented in the medical record:

    a. There is inadequate visualization of the anatomy and/or pathology, or

    b. The patient's condition with respect to the clinical indication has changed since the prior study, or

    c. There is a clinical change during the procedure that requires new evaluation.◄

Other cardiac catheterization services may be reported separately when performed for diagnostic purposes not intrinsic to TMVR.

For same session/same day diagnostic cardiac catheterization services, report the appropriate diagnostic cardiac catheterization code(s) appended with modifier 59 indicating separate and distinct procedural service from TMVR.

Diagnostic coronary angiography performed at a separate session from an interventional procedure may be separately reportable.

Percutaneous coronary interventional procedures may be reported separately, when performed.

When transcatheter ventricular support is required in conjunction with TMVR, the appropriate code may be reported with the appropriate ventricular assist device (VAD) procedure code (33990, 33991, 33992, 33993, 33995, 33997) or balloon pump insertion code (33967, 33970, 33973).

When cardiopulmonary bypass is performed in conjunction with TMVR, 33418, 33419 may be reported with the appropriate add-on code for percutaneous peripheral bypass (33367), open peripheral bypass (33368), or central bypass (33369).

## Rationale

In accordance with the deletion of codes 93530-93533 and the establishment of codes 93593-93598, the mitral valve guidelines have been revised to reflect these changes.

Refer to the codebook and the Rationale for codes 93593-93598 for a full discussion of these changes.

### Tricuspid Valve

►(For transcatheter tricuspid valve implantation [TTVI]/ replacement, use 0646T)◄

(For transcatheter tricuspid valve repair [TTVr], see 0569T, 0570T)

**33460** Valvectomy, tricuspid valve, with cardiopulmonary bypass

## Rationale

In accordance with the establishment of Category III code 0646T, a cross-reference parenthetical note has been added in the Tricuspid Valve subsection directing users to code 0646T.

Refer to the codebook and the Rationale for code 0646T for a full discussion of these changes

### Pulmonary Valve

Code 33477 is used to report transcatheter pulmonary valve implantation (TPVI). Code 33477 should only be reported once per session.

Code 33477 includes the work, when performed, of percutaneous access, placing the access sheath, advancing the repair device delivery system into position, repositioning the device as needed, and deploying the device(s). Angiography, radiological supervision, and interpretation performed to guide TPVI (eg, guiding device placement and documenting completion of the intervention) are included in the code.

▲ = Revised code  ● = New code  ► ◄ = Contains new or revised text  ✖ = Duplicate PLA test  ↑↓ = Category I PLA       American Medical Association   **49**

Surgery / Cardiovascular System 33016-39599

▶Code 33477 includes all cardiac catheterization(s), intraprocedural contrast injection(s), fluoroscopic radiological supervision and interpretation, and imaging guidance performed to complete the pulmonary valve procedure. Do not report 33477 in conjunction with 76000, 93451, 93453, 93454, 93455, 93456, 93457, 93458, 93459, 93460, 93461,93563, 93566, 93567, 93568, 93593, 93594, 93596, 93597, 93598, for angiography intrinsic to the procedure.◀

Code 33477 includes percutaneous balloon angioplasty of the conduit/treatment zone, valvuloplasty of the pulmonary valve conduit, and stent deployment within the pulmonary conduit or an existing bioprosthetic pulmonary valve, when performed. Do not report 33477 in conjunction with 37236, 37237, 92997, 92998 for pulmonary artery angioplasty/valvuloplasty or stenting within the prosthetic valve delivery site.

Codes 92997, 92998 may be reported separately when pulmonary artery angioplasty is performed at a site separate from the prosthetic valve delivery site. Codes 37236, 37237 may be reported separately when pulmonary artery stenting is performed at a site separate from the prosthetic valve delivery site.

▶Diagnostic right heart catheterization and diagnostic coronary angiography codes (93451, 93453, 93454, 93455, 93456, 93457, 93458, 93459, 93460, 93461, 93563, 93566, 93567, 93568, 93593, 93594, 93596, 93597, 93598) should **not** be used with 33477 to report:

1. Contrast injections, angiography, roadmapping, and/or fluoroscopic guidance for the TPVI,

2. Pulmonary conduit angiography for guidance of TPVI, or

3. Right heart catheterization for hemodynamic measurements before, during, and after TPVI for guidance of TPVI.

Diagnostic right and left heart catheterization codes (93451, 93452, 93453, 93456, 93457, 93458, 93459, 93460, 93461, 93593, 93594, 93595, 93596, 93597, 93598), diagnostic coronary angiography codes (93454, 93455, 93456, 93457, 93458, 93459, 93460, 93461, 93563, 93564), and diagnostic pulmonary angiography code (93568) may be reported with 33477, representing separate and distinct services from TPVI, if:

1. No prior study is available and a full diagnostic study is performed, or

2. A prior study is available, but as documented in the medical record:

   a. There is inadequate visualization of the anatomy and/or pathology, or

   b. The patient's condition with respect to the clinical indication has changed since the prior study, or

   c. There is a clinical change during the procedure that requires new evaluation.◀

Other cardiac catheterization services may be reported separately when performed for diagnostic purposes not intrinsic to TPVI.

For same session/same day diagnostic cardiac catheterization services, report the appropriate diagnostic cardiac catheterization code(s) appended with modifier 59 to indicate separate and distinct procedural services from TPVI.

Diagnostic coronary angiography performed at a separate session from an interventional procedure may be separately reportable, when performed.

Percutaneous coronary interventional procedures may be reported separately, when performed.

Percutaneous pulmonary artery branch interventions may be reported separately, when performed.

When transcatheter ventricular support is required in conjunction with TPVI, the appropriate code may be reported with the appropriate percutaneous ventricular assist device (VAD) procedure codes (33990, 33991, 33992, 33993, 33995, 33997), extracorporeal membrane oxygenation (ECMO) or extracorporeal life support services (ECLS) procedure codes (33946-33989), or balloon pump insertion codes (33967, 33970, 33973).

When cardiopulmonary bypass is performed in conjunction with TPVI, code 33477 may be reported with the appropriate add-on code for percutaneous peripheral bypass (33367), open peripheral bypass (33368), or central bypass (33369).

▶(33470 has been deleted)◀

▲ **33471**   Valvotomy, pulmonary valve, closed heart, via pulmonary artery

(To report percutaneous valvuloplasty of pulmonary valve use 92990)

## Rationale

In accordance with the deletion of codes 93530-93533 and the establishment of codes 93593-93598, the pulmonary valve guidelines have been revised to reflect these changes.

In addition, to ensure the CPT code set reflects current clinical practice, code 33470, *Valvotomy, pulmonary valve, closed heart; transventricular,* has been deleted due to low utilization. The exclusionary parenthetical note restricting use of modifier 63 with code 33470 has also been deleted. Code 33471, which was previously a child code of code 33470, has been revised as a stand-alone code with the deletion of code 33470. A parenthetical note has been added to indicate this deletion.

Refer to the codebook and the Rationale for codes 93593-93598 for a full discussion of these changes.

★ = Telemedicine   ✚ = Add-on code   ✗ = FDA approval pending   # = Resequenced code   ⊘ = Modifier 51 exem

## Endoscopy

▶To report endoscopic harvesting of a vein for coronary artery bypass procedure, use 33508 in addition to the code for the associated bypass procedure. To report endoscopic harvesting of an upper extremity artery for a bypass procedure, use 33509.◀

Surgical vascular endoscopy always includes diagnostic endoscopy.

**+ 33508**    Endoscopy, surgical, including video-assisted harvest of vein(s) for coronary artery bypass procedure (List separately in addition to code for primary procedure)

(Use 33508 in conjunction with 33510-33523)

(For open harvest of upper extremity vein procedure, use 35500)

**⊘● 33509**    Harvest of upper extremity artery, 1 segment, for coronary artery bypass procedure, endoscopic

▶(For open harvest of upper extremity artery, use 35600)◀

▶(For bilateral procedure, report 33509 with modifier 50)◀

### Rationale

Code 33509 has been established to report an endoscopic harvest of the upper extremity (UE) for coronary artery bypass.

In addition to the new code, two new parenthetical notes have been added following code 33509: one to instruct users to use code 35600 to report open harvest of UE artery, and another to instruct users to append modifier 50 for bilateral procedures.

In accordance with the establishment of code 33509, the endoscopy guidelines have been revised to instruct users how to report endoscopic harvesting of a vein for coronary artery bypass procedures and endoscopic harvesting of a UE artery for a bypass procedure.

In addition, with the establishment of code 33509, code 35600 has been revised with the removal of the add-on code symbol and language in the descriptor to reflect that it is not an add-on code.

Finally, codes 35509 and 35600 have been identified as modifier 51 exempt; therefore, the modifier 51 exempt symbol (⊘) has been added to these codes, which means they will be included in in Appendix E (Summary of CPT Codes Exempt from Modifier 51) in the CPT 2022 code set.

### Clinical Example (33509)

A 58-year-old male, who has a history of coronary artery bypass grafting (CABG), presents to the emergency room with unstable angina. Cardiac catheterization reveals multivessel disease requiring several grafts. He is an acceptable candidate for reoperative CABG. The saphenous vein conduit is limited because of the prior CABG, and only a small segment is available. The right internal mammary artery is available, and the left radial artery in this right-handed patient is evaluated and determined to be appropriate for endoscopic harvesting and use for CABG.

### Description of Procedure (33509)

The primary surgeon decides whether to utilize the radial artery as a conduit for CABG, typically during the initial visit with the patient. The primary surgeon performing the CABG obtains a history with attention given to conditions that may mitigate against using the radial, such as renal failure requiring or likely to require dialysis, severe PVD, or history of Reynaud syndrome. Examine the arm and hand and perform an Allen test to assess adequacy of the ulnar circulation and the palmar arch. If available, employ an oxygen-saturation monitor to assess the circulation provided by the ulnar artery. At the time of the CABG procedure (reported separately), the surgeon who will be harvesting the artery checks the radial artery in the operating room (OR). Perform an Allen test utilizing the oxygen-saturation monitor to assess the adequacy of the ulnar circulation and the palmar arch. Discuss any abnormalities or concerns with the primary surgeon, who decides whether to proceed with the harvest. The radial artery is typically harvested simultaneously while other conduits are also being harvested. Position the arm on a surgical arm board and place a tourniquet high on the upper arm in anticipation of later inflation. Set up and test the appropriate endoscopic equipment. Begin a continuous nitroglycerin intravenous infusion to prevent spasm of the radial artery. Make a 3-cm longitudinal incision proximal to the wrist crease over the radial artery. Identify the radial artery by dissection and clamp the artery. Check the pulse oximetry on the index finger to assess integrity of the arterial palmar arch and the adequacy of ulnar artery flow while the radial artery is clamped. Wrap the forearm tightly with a latex-free elastic bandage distal to proximal to evacuate the blood. Inflate the tourniquet to 75 to 100 mmHg over systolic blood pressure, not exceeding 250 mmHg total, and remove the bandage. Dissect the radial artery as a pedicle with the accompanying venae comitantes and the endoscope advanced over the anterior pedicle enough to allow insertion of the port. Inflate the trocar port and insufflate $CO_2$ at a pressure of 10 to 12 mmHg with a flow rate of 3-5 L/min to create a working tunnel. Advance the endoscope to perform the anterior dissection along the pedicle, taking care to secure veins on each side of the radial artery. This is performed while minimizing any contact with the artery itself.

Continue the dissection to the level of the recurrent radial artery or venous plexus in the antecubital fossa, being careful to avoid all nerves and larger vessels. Withdraw the endoscope back to the port, and then advance it posteriorly to the radial artery pedicle. Dissect the posterior arterial branches to the level of the recurrent radial or venous plexus in the antecubital fossa. Withdraw the endoscope again to the port and then advance it laterally for similar dissection. Perform a fasciotomy of the brachioradialis muscle to enhance visualization by opening up the working tunnel using sharp dissection and applying energy from an appropriate power supply (electrocautery) to cut the tissue. Use extreme caution to avoid untoward thermal injury to neural or vascular tissues during brachioradialis fasciotomy. Release the fascia from the distal forearm to the mid or proximal forearm. With the fasciotomy complete, divide the arterial branches using the power source by working proximal to distal. Recheck the pulse oximetry on the thumb. Before dividing the radial artery, place a soft non-occluding clamp across the dissected but still intact radial artery and palpate the ulnar artery to be certain that there is adequate blood supply to the hand. After confirming adequacy of ulnar artery flow, divide and ligate the radial artery pedicle and then withdraw it in a retrograde fashion externally through the port. Withdraw the port and divide and ligate the radial artery at the wrist area using standard technique. Deflate and remove the tourniquet.

Carefully inspect the wound for hemostasis. Close the fascia and subcutaneous tissues at the wrist incision in two layers using absorbable sutures and close the skin by a subcuticular method using monofilament absorbable sutures. Check the hand for warmth and assess circulation with an oxygen-saturation monitor. Wrap the arm and use a methylene blue marking pen to score the artery on its anterior surface so as maintain orientation of the radial artery conduit without inadvertent twisting. Soak and flush the radial artery with papaverine and heparinized patient blood. Check the entire length of the radial artery while flushing it with the heparinized blood and carefully clip or tie the branches per routine. The primary surgeon uses the radial artery to bypass the designated coronary artery. The primary surgeon evaluates the radial artery harvest site at the end of the procedure.

## Combined Arterial-Venous Grafting for Coronary Bypass

The following codes are used to report coronary artery bypass procedures using venous grafts and arterial grafts during the same procedure. These codes may NOT be used alone.

To report combined arterial-venous grafts it is necessary to report two codes: (1) the appropriate combined arterial-venous graft code (33517-33523); and (2) the appropriate arterial graft code (33533-33536).

▶Procurement of the saphenous vein graft is included in the description of the work for 33517-33523 and should not be reported as a separate service or co-surgery. Procurement of the artery for grafting is included in the description of the work for 33533-33536 and should not be reported as a separate service or co-surgery, except when an upper extremity artery (eg, radial artery) is procured. To report harvesting of an upper extremity artery, use 33509 or 35600. To report harvesting of an upper extremity vein, use 35500 in addition to the bypass procedure. To report harvesting of a femoropopliteal vein segment, report 35572 in addition to the bypass procedure. When surgical assistant performs arterial and/or venous graft procurement, add modifier 80 to 33517-33523, 33533-33536, as appropriate. For percutaneous ventricular assist device insertion, removal, repositioning, see 33990, 33991, 33992, 33993, 33995, 33997.◀

+ **33517**    Coronary artery bypass, using venous graft(s) and arterial graft(s); single vein graft (List separately in addition to code for primary procedure)

(Use 33517 in conjunction with 33533-33536)

### Rationale

In accordance with the establishment of code 33509, the combined arterial-venous grafting for coronary bypass guidelines have been revised with the addition of code 33509.

Refer to the codebook and the Rationale for code 33509 for a full discussion of these changes.

## Arterial Grafting for Coronary Artery Bypass

The following codes are used to report coronary artery bypass procedures using either arterial grafts only or a combination of arterial-venous grafts. The codes include the use of the internal mammary artery, gastroepiploic artery, epigastric artery, radial artery, and arterial conduits procured from other sites.

To report combined arterial-venous grafts it is necessary to report two codes: (1) the appropriate arterial graft code (33533-33536); and (2) the appropriate combined arterial-venous graft code (33517-33523).

▶Procurement of the artery for grafting is included in the description of the work for 33533-33536 and should not be reported as a separate service or co-surgery, except when an upper extremity artery (eg, radial artery) is

★ = Telemedicine    ✦ = Add-on code    ✗ = FDA approval pending    # = Resequenced code    ⊘ = Modifier 51 exempt

procured. To report harvesting of an upper extremity artery, use 33509 or 35600. To report harvesting of an upper extremity vein, use 35500 in addition to the bypass procedure. To report harvesting of a femoropopliteal vein segment, report 35572 in addition to the bypass procedure. When surgical assistant performs arterial and/or venous graft procurement, add modifier 80 to 33517-33523, 33533-33536, as appropriate. For percutaneous ventricular assist device insertion, removal, repositioning, see 33990, 33991, 33992, 33993, 33995, 33997.◄

**33548**    Surgical ventricular restoration procedure, includes prosthetic patch, when performed (eg, ventricular remodeling, SVR, SAVER, Dor procedures)

(Do not report 33548 in conjunction with 32551, 33210, 33211, 33310, 33315)

(For Batista procedure or pachopexy, use 33999)

►(For transcatheter left ventricular restoration device implantation, use 0643T)◄

## Rationale

In accordance with the establishment of code 33509, the arterial grafting for coronary bypass guidelines have been revised with the addition of code 33509.

In accordance with the establishment of Category III code 0643T, a cross-reference parenthetical note has been added following code 33548 directing users to code 0643T for transcatheter left ventricular restoration device implantation.

Refer to the codebook and the Rationale for codes 33509 and 0643T for a full discussion of these changes.

## Sinus of Valsalva

►(33722 has been deleted)◄

## Rationale

To ensure the CPT code set reflects current clinical practice, code 33722, *Closure of aortico-left ventricular tunnel,* has been deleted due to low utilization. A parenthetical note has been added to indicate this deletion.

## Shunting Procedures

Codes 33741, 33745 are used to report creation of effective intracardiac blood flow in the setting of congenital heart defects. Code 33741 (transcatheter atrial septostomy) involves the percutaneous creation of improved atrial blood flow (eg, balloon/blade method), typically in infants ≤4 kg with congenital heart disease. Code 33745 is typically used for intracardiac shunt creation by stent placement to establish improved intracardiac blood flow (eg, atrial septum, Fontan fenestration, right ventricular outflow tract, Mustard/Senning/Warden baffles). Code 33746 is used to describe each additional intracardiac shunt creation by stent placement at a separate location during the same session as the primary intervention (33745).

Code 33741 includes percutaneous access, placing the access sheath(s), advancement of the transcatheter delivery system, and creation of effective intracardiac atrial blood flow. Codes 33741, 33745 include, when performed, ultrasound guidance for vascular access and fluoroscopic guidance for the intervention. Code 33745 additionally includes intracardiac stent placement, target zone angioplasty preceding or after stent implantation, and complete diagnostic right and left heart catheterization, when performed.

Diagnostic cardiac catheterization is not typically performed at the same session as transcatheter atrial septostomy (33741) and, when performed, may be separately reported. Diagnostic cardiac catheterization is typically performed at the same session with 33745 and the code descriptor includes this work, when performed.

Cardiovascular injection procedures for diagnostic angiography reported using 93563, 93565, 93566, 93567, 93568 are not typically performed at the same session as 33741. Although diagnostic angiography is typically performed during 33745, target vessels and chambers are highly variable and, when performed, for an evaluation separate and distinct from the shunt creation may be reported separately.

Codes 33745, 33746 are used to describe intracardiac stent placement. Multiple stents placed in a single location may only be reported with a single code. When additional, different intracardiac locations are treated in the same session, 33746 may be reported. Codes 33745, 33746 include any and all balloon angioplasty(ies) performed in the target lesion, including any pre-dilation (whether performed as a primary or secondary dilation), post-dilation following stent placement, or use of larger/smaller balloon to achieve therapeutic result. Angioplasty in a separate and distinct intracardiac lesion may be reported separately. Use 33746 in conjunction with 33745.

Surgery / Cardiovascular System   33016-39599

►Diagnostic right and left heart catheterization codes (93451, 93452, 93453, 93456, 93458, 93460, 93593, 93594, 93595, 93596, 93597) should not be used in conjunction with 33741, 33745 to report:

1. Fluoroscopic guidance for the intervention, or

2. Limited hemodynamic and angiographic data used solely for purposes of accomplishing the intervention (eg, measurement of atrial pressures before and after septostomy, atrial injections to determine appropriate catheter position).

Diagnostic congenital right and left heart catheterization (93593, 93594, 93595, 93596, 93597) performed at the same session as 33741 may be separately reported, if:

1. No prior study is available, and a full diagnostic study is performed, or

2. A prior study is available, but as documented in the medical record:

   a. There is inadequate visualization of the anatomy and/or pathology, or

   b. The patient's condition with respect to the clinical indication has changed since the prior study, or

   c. There is a clinical change during the procedure that requires a more thorough evaluation.

For same-session diagnostic congenital catheterization services, the appropriate diagnostic cardiac catheterization code(s) for congenital anomalies (93593, 93594, 93595, 93596, 93597) may be reported by appending modifier 59, indicating separate and distinct procedural service(s) from 33741. For same-session diagnostic cardiac angiography for an evaluation separate and distinct from the shunt creation, the appropriate contrast injection(s) performed (93563, 93565, 93566, 93567, 93568) may be reported by appending modifier 59, indicating separate and distinct procedural service(s) from 33741, 33745.◄

33745    Transcatheter intracardiac shunt (TIS) creation by stent placement for congenital cardiac anomalies to establish effective intracardiac flow, including all imaging guidance by the proceduralist, when performed, left and right heart diagnostic cardiac catheterization for congenital cardiac anomalies, and target zone angioplasty, when performed (eg, atrial septum, Fontan fenestration, right ventricular outflow tract, Mustard/Senning/Warden baffles); initial intracardiac shunt

+ 33746    each additional intracardiac shunt location (List separately in addition to code for primary procedure)

(Use 33746 in conjunction with 33745)

►(Do not report 33745, 33746 in conjunction with 93593, 93594, 93595, 93596, 93597)◄

## Rationale

In accordance with the deletion of codes 93530-93533 and the establishment of codes 93593-93597, the guidelines for shunting procedures and the exclusionary parenthetical note following code 33746 have been revised to reflect these changes.

Refer to the codebook and the Rationale for codes 93593-93597 for a full discussion of these changes.

## Endovascular Repair of Descending Thoracic Aorta

Codes 33880-33891 represent a family of procedures to report placement of an endovascular graft for repair of the descending thoracic aorta. These codes include all device introduction, manipulation, positioning, and deployment. All balloon angioplasty and/or stent deployment within the target treatment zone for the endoprosthesis, either before or after endograft deployment, are not separately reportable.

Open arterial exposure and associated closure of the arteriotomy sites (eg, 34714, 34715, 34716, 34812, 34820, 34833, 34834), introduction of guidewires and catheters (eg, 36140, 36200-36218), and extensive repair or replacement of an artery (eg, 35226, 35286) may be additionally reported. Transposition of subclavian artery to carotid, and carotid-carotid bypass performed in conjunction with endovascular repair of the descending thoracic aorta (eg, 33889, 33891) may be separately reported. The primary codes, 33880 and 33881, include placement of all distal extensions, if required, in the distal thoracic aorta, while proximal extensions, if needed, may be reported separately.

For fluoroscopic guidance in conjunction with endovascular repair of the thoracic aorta, see codes 75956-75959 as appropriate. Codes 75956 and 75957 include all angiography of the thoracic aorta and its branches for diagnostic imaging prior to deployment of the primary endovascular devices (including all routine components of modular devices), fluoroscopic guidance in the delivery of the endovascular components, and intraprocedural arterial angiography (eg, confirm position, detect endoleak, evaluate runoff). Code 75958 includes the analogous services for placement of each proximal thoracic endovascular extension. Code 75959 includes the analogous services for placement of a distal thoracic endovascular extension(s) placed during a procedure after the primary repair.

Other interventional procedures performed at the time of endovascular repair of the descending thoracic aorta should be additionally reported (eg, innominate, carotid, subclavian, visceral, or iliac artery transluminal angioplasty or stenting, arterial embolization, intravascular ultrasound) when performed before or after deployment of the aortic prostheses.

►For endovascular stenting or balloon angioplasty of congenital coarctation or postsurgical recoarctation of the ascending, transverse, or descending thoracic or abdominal aorta, see 33894, 33895, 33897◄

**33880**    Endovascular repair of descending thoracic aorta (eg, aneurysm, pseudoaneurysm, dissection, penetrating ulcer, intramural hematoma, or traumatic disruption); involving coverage of left subclavian artery origin, initial endoprosthesis plus descending thoracic aortic extension(s), if required, to level of celiac artery origin

(For radiological supervision and interpretation, use 75956 in conjunction with 33880)

## Rationale

In accordance with the establishment of codes 33894-33897, the guidelines for endovascular repair of descending thoracic aorta have been revised with instructions directing users to the new codes for endovascular stenting or balloon angioplasty of congenital coarctation or postsurgical recoarctation of the ascending, transverse, or descending thoracic or abdominal aorta.

Refer to the codebook and the Rationale for codes 33894-33897 for a full discussion of these changes.

## ►Endovascular Repair of Congenital Heart and Vascular Defects◄

►Codes 33894, 33895, 33897 describe transcatheter interventions for revascularization or repair for coarctation of the aorta. Code 33897 describes dilation of the coarctation using balloon angioplasty without stent placement. Codes 33894, 33895 describe stent placement to treat the coarctation. The procedure described in 33894 involves stent placement across one or more major side branches of the aorta. For reporting purposes, the major side branches of the thoracic aorta are the brachiocephalic, carotid, and subclavian arteries, and the major side branches of the abdominal aorta are the celiac, superior mesenteric, inferior mesenteric, and renal arteries.

Codes 33894, 33895, 33897 include all fluoroscopic guidance of the intervention, diagnostic congenital left heart catheterization, all catheter and wire introductions and manipulation, and angiography of the target lesion.

Codes 33894, 33895 include stent introduction, manipulation, positioning, and deployment, temporary pacemaker insertion for rapid pacing (33210) to facilitate stent positioning, when performed, as well as any additional stent delivery in tandem with the initial stent for extension purposes. Balloon angioplasty within the target-treatment zone, either before or after stent deployment, is not separately reportable. For balloon angioplasty of an additional coarctation of the aorta in a segment separate from the treatment zone for the coarctation stent, use 33897.

For balloon angioplasty of the aorta for lesions other than coarctation (eg, atherosclerosis) of the aorta in a segment separate from the coarctation treatment zone, use 37246.

For additional diagnostic right heart catheterization in the same setting as 33894, 33895, see 93593, 93594.

Other interventional procedures performed at the time of endovascular repair of coarctation of the aorta (33894, 33895) may be reported separately (eg, innominate, carotid, subclavian, visceral, iliac, or pulmonary artery balloon angioplasty or stenting, arterial or venous embolization), when performed before or after coarctation stent deployment.◄

● **33894**    Endovascular stent repair of coarctation of the ascending, transverse, or descending thoracic or abdominal aorta, involving stent placement; across major side branches

● **33895**    not crossing major side branches

►(Do not report 33894, 33895 in conjunction with 33210, 34701, 34702, 34703, 34704, 34705, 34706, 36200, 75600, 75605, 75625, 93567, 93595, 93596, 93597)◄

►(Do not report 33894, 33895 in conjunction with 33897, 37236, 37246, for balloon angioplasty of the aorta within the coarctation stent treatment zone)◄

►(For additional atrial, ventricular, pulmonary, coronary, or bypass graft angiography in the same setting, see 93563, 93564, 93565, 93566, 93568)◄

►(For angiography of other vascular structures, use the appropriate code from the Radiology/Diagnostic Radiology section)◄

►(For additional congenital right heart catheterization at same setting as 33894, 33895, see 93593, 93594)◄

● **33897**    Percutaneous transluminal angioplasty of native or recurrent coarctation of the aorta

►(Do not report 33897 in conjunction with 33210, 34701, 34702, 34703, 34704, 34705, 34706, 36200, 37236, 37246, 75600, 75605, 75625, 93567, 93595, 93596, 93597)◄

►(Do not report 33897 in conjunction with 33894, 33895 for balloon angioplasty of the aorta within the coarctation stent treatment zone)◄

▶(For additional congenital right heart diagnostic catheterization performed in same setting as 33897, see 93593, 93594)◀

▶(For angioplasty and other transcatheter revascularization interventions of additional upper or lower extremity vessels in same setting, use the appropriate code from the Surgery/Cardiovascular System section)◀

## Rationale

A new subsection (Endovascular Repair of Congenital Heart and Vascular Defects) with three new codes (33894, 33895, 33897) and guidelines has been added.

Codes 33894 and 33895 describe endovascular stent repair of coarctation of the ascending, transverse, or descending thoracic or abdominal aorta. Both codes include stent placement. Code 33894 is reported when the procedure is performed across major side branches, and code 33895 is reported when the procedure is not performed across major side branches. Code 33897 describes endovascular angioplasty of native or recurrent aortic coarctation without the use of a stent.

Codes 33840, 33845, and 33851 describe open procedures for excision of coarctation of the aorta. Prior to 2022, there were no CPT codes that described endovascular procedures to repair coarctation of the aorta.

Coarctation can occur in the ascending, transverse, or descending thoracic or abdominal aorta. In certain cases, it is necessary to place the stent across one or more of the major side branches of the thoracic or abdominal aorta. For reporting purposes, the major side branches of the thoracic aorta are the brachiocephalic, carotid, and subclavian arteries, and the major side branches of the abdominal aorta are the celiac, superior mesenteric, inferior mesenteric, and renal arteries.

Code 33894 is reported when the stent is placed across major side branches. Code 33895 is reported when stent placement does not cross any of the major side branches. Code 33897 is reported when the coarctation is dilated using balloon angioplasty and the procedure does not involve stent placement. It is important to review the new guidelines carefully as they indicate the work that is included in each of the procedures (eg, fluoroscopic guidance, catheter introduction, etc), which should not be reported separately.

The guidelines also clarify that balloon angioplasty of the aorta for lesions other than coarctation in a separate treatment zone, additional right heart catheterization, and other interventional procedures performed at the time of endovascular coarctation repair, when performed before or after coarctation stent deployment, may be reported

separately. Several parenthetical notes have been added following codes 33895 and 33897 that further clarify the appropriate reporting of these codes and codes for other procedures that may be performed at the time of the coarctation repair procedure.

## Clinical Example (33894)

A 4-year-old male with hypoplastic left heart syndrome and prior history of Norwood arch reconstruction is suspected of having complex transverse arch coarctation of the surgical site. He is brought to the cardiac catheterization laboratory for further diagnostic evaluation and to identify if it meets criteria for intervention and possible treatment with percutaneous stent placement.

## Description of Procedure (33894)

Conduct the procedure under general anesthesia and under fluoroscopic guidance. Apply lidocaine for local analgesia. Obtain access percutaneously, typically into the femoral vein and artery. As necessary, obtain additional arterial access in the radial, brachial, or axillary artery for simultaneous pre- and postcoarctation pressure evaluation during the procedure. Place a sheath in the femoral vein and artery to establish secure access. Administer intravenous heparin to achieve therapeutic anticoagulation. Monitor the activated clotting time thereafter and administer additional heparin as needed. Pass a pacing catheter through the venous sheath and position it in the right ventricle for transvenous pacing during stent delivery. Introduce a pigtail catheter through the arterial sheath and manipulate it into the descending aorta, ascending aorta, and across the aortic valve into the left ventricle. Record baseline pressures and conduct blood sampling in each of these locations to be used for hemodynamic calculations. If the coarctation is severe, exchange the pigtail catheter for another end-hole catheter and specialty wire to cross the severe stenosis. Once the wire is across the stenosis, perform multiple catheter and wire exchanges between the end-hole catheter and angiographic catheter to obtain hemodynamic data and perform all necessary angiograms. As needed, obtain multiple angiograms to clearly delineate the lesion, paying particular attention to the origins of the subclavian and carotid arteries. The procedure may involve stenting across either only select head and neck vessels, or the entire transverse aorta, and careful evaluation of all branches is crucial. Use the angiograms to obtain measurements of the lesion as well as the healthy vessel, which are used for appropriate stent selection. Use the diagnostic catheter to secure wire position with a more rigid interventional guidewire as needed to support the balloon and stent delivery.

Prepare and de-air the appropriately sized balloon. Prepare and mount the stent on the balloon catheter. Replace the short access sheath in the artery over the wire with a larger and longer sheath, and advance the longer sheath across the lesion. Remove the dilator and allow the sheath to bleed back. Flush the sheath. Advance the balloon with the mounted stent over the wire into position across the coarctation. Periodically perform additional angiograms through the side-port to evaluate proper positioning and make adjustments. Once in the appropriate position, pull back the sheath to fully expose the stent and balloon. Initiate transvenous cardiac pacing to decrease the cardiac output and pulsatility in the aorta. The anesthesiologist holds mechanical ventilation temporarily to minimize respiratory variation in the position of the stent on fluoroscopy. Deploy the stent by inflating the delivery balloon(s). Resume mechanical ventilation and discontinue cardiac pacing. Remove the delivery balloon and insert another appropriately sized balloon to fully expand and seat the stent (not additionally reportable). Perform postprocedure angiography to assess postprocedural success. If necessary, deploy a second stent to extend the initial stent length (not additionally reportable). Remove all catheters and sheaths and achieve hemostasis either by manual compression or via a closure device prior to transferring the patient to recovery. Ensure adequate circulation distal to the arterial access site prior to transferring the patient to the recovery area.

## Clinical Example (33895)

A 16-year-old male with hypertension is found to have severe native coarctation of the aorta by echocardiography and/or CT angiogram. He is brought to the cardiac catheterization laboratory for further diagnostic evaluation and to identify if it meets criteria for intervention and possible repair with percutaneous stent placement.

## Description of Procedure (33895)

Conduct the procedure under general anesthesia and perform all steps under fluoroscopic guidance. Administer lidocaine for local analgesia. Obtain access percutaneously, typically into the femoral vein and artery. Obtain additional arterial access in the radial, brachial, or axillary artery for simultaneous pre- and postcoarctation pressure evaluation during the procedure. Place a sheath in the femoral vein and artery to establish secure access. Administer intravenous heparin to achieve therapeutic anticoagulation. Monitor the activated clotting time thereafter and administer additional heparin as needed. Pass a pacing catheter through the venous sheath and position it in the right ventricle for temporary transvenous pacing during stent delivery. Introduce a pigtail catheter through the arterial sheath and manipulate it into the descending aorta, ascending aorta, and across the aortic valve into the left ventricle. Record baseline pressures and conduct blood sampling in each of these locations to be used for hemodynamic calculations. If the coarctation is severe,

exchange the pigtail catheter for another end-hole catheter and specialty wire to cross the severe stenosis. Once the wire is across the stenosis, perform multiple catheter and wire exchanges between the end-hole catheter and angiographic catheter to obtain hemo-dynamic data and perform all necessary angiograms. As needed, obtain multiple angiograms above and below the lesion to identify the complete anatomy. Use the angiograms to obtain measurements of the lesion as well as the healthy vessel, which are used for appropriate stent selection. Use a diagnostic guide catheter to secure wire position with a more rigid interventional guidewire as needed to support the balloon and stent delivery.

Prepare and de-air the appropriately sized balloon. Prepare and mount the stent on the balloon catheter. Place the short access sheath in the artery over the wire with a larger and longer sheath; advance the longer sheath across the lesion. Remove the dilator and allow the sheath to bleed back. Flush the sheath. Advance the balloon with the mounted stent over the wire into position across the coarctation. Perform additional angiograms through the long sheath side-port or from an additional arterial access site to evaluate proper positioning and make adjustments, and to ensure the stent will not encroach on the origins of any vital side branches. Once in the appropriate position, pull back the sheath to fully expose the stent and balloon. The anesthesiologist holds mechanical ventilation to minimize stent position movement on fluoroscopy. Initiate rapid transvenous cardiac pacing to reduce aortic pulsatility and cardiac output. Deploy the stent by inflating the delivery balloon(s). Resume mechanical ventilation and discontinue cardiac pacing. Deflate and reposition the balloon slightly and perform a second inflation. Remove the delivery balloon and insert another appropriately sized balloon to fully expand and seat the stent (not additionally reportable). Perform postprocedure angiography to assess postprocedural success. If necessary, deploy a second stent to extend the initial stent length (not additionally reportable). Remove all catheters and sheaths and achieve hemostasis either by manual compression or via a closure device prior to transferring the patient to recovery. Ensure adequate circulation distal to the arterial access site prior to transferring the patient to the recovery area.

## Clinical Example (33897)

A 2-year-old female with prior surgical repair of coarctation of the aorta in infancy is suspected to have recurrent coarctation of the aorta by echocardiography and physical examination. She is brought to the cardiac catheterization laboratory for further diagnostic evaluation to identify if she meets criteria for intervention and possible percutaneous angioplasty of the aorta.

## Description of Procedure (33897)

Conduct the procedure under general anesthesia and perform all steps under fluoroscopic guidance. Apply local anesthetic to the access site and obtain access percutaneously, typically into the femoral artery and vein. As necessary, perform additional arterial monitoring from the radial artery for simultaneous pre- and postcoarctation pressure evaluation. For neonates, this additional access is typically obtained in the common carotid artery. Place a sheath in the vein and artery to establish secure access. Administer intravenous heparin to achieve therapeutic anticoagulation. Monitor the activated clotting time thereafter and administer additional heparin as needed. Obtain venous access for either resuscitation purposes for emergent situations or for transvenous ventricular pacing, when performed. Introduce a pigtail catheter through the arterial sheath and manipulate it into the descending aorta, ascending aorta, and across the aortic valve into the left ventricle. Record baseline pressures and conduct blood sampling in each of these locations to be used for hemodynamic calculations. If the coarctation is severe, exchange the pigtail catheter for another end-hole catheter and specialty wire to cross the severe stenosis. Multiple exchanges are often required between the pigtail catheter and end-hole catheter to obtain hemodynamic data and perform all necessary angiograms. As needed, obtain multiple angiograms of the aorta above and below the lesion to identify the complete anatomy. Use the angiograms to obtain measurements of the lesion as well as the healthy vessel, which are used for appropriate balloon selection. Use a diagnostic guide catheter to secure wire position with a more rigid guidewire as needed to support the balloons.

Prepare and de-air the appropriately sized balloon. Exchange the sheath in the artery for a larger sheath to accommodate the angioplasty balloon. Advance the balloon over the wire into position across the coarctation. Once in the appropriate position, inflate the balloon to the appropriate pressure. Adjust the balloon catheter position slightly and inflate the balloon again. Remove the balloon and obtain post angioplasty angiograms from multiple angles to closely examine for the presence of any vascular injury. Repeat hemodynamic evaluation to assess postprocedural success. It is often necessary to repeat this process with a larger balloon to achieve optimal success (not additionally reported). Remove all catheters and sheaths and apply manual compression to achieve hemostasis prior to transferring the patient to recovery. Ensure adequate circulation distal to the arterial access site prior to transferring the patient to the recovery area.

## Pulmonary Artery

**+ 33924**  Ligation and takedown of a systemic-to-pulmonary artery shunt, performed in conjunction with a congenital heart procedure (List separately in addition to code for primary procedure)

▶(Use 33924 in conjunction with 33471, 33474, 33475, 33476, 33477, 33478, 33600-33617, 33622, 33684-33688, 33692-33697, 33735-33767, 33770-33783, 33786, 33917, 33920, 33922, 33925, 33926, 33935, 33945)◀

## Rationale

In accordance with the deletion of code 33470, the inclusionary parenthetical note following code 33924 has been revised with the removal of code 33470.

Refer to the codebook and the Rationale for code 33470 for a full description of these changes.

# Arteries and Veins

## Endovascular Repair of Abdominal Aorta and/or Iliac Arteries

**+ 34714**  Open femoral artery exposure with creation of conduit for delivery of endovascular prosthesis or for establishment of cardiopulmonary bypass, by groin incision, unilateral (List separately in addition to code for primary procedure)

▶(Use 34714 in conjunction with 32852, 32854, 33031, 33120, 33251, 33256, 33259, 33261, 33305, 33315, 33322, 33335, 33390, 33391, 33404, 33405, 33406, 33410, 33411, 33412, 33413, 33414, 33415, 33416, 33417, 33422, 33425, 33426, 33427, 33430, 33440, 33460, 33463, 33464, 33465, 33468, 33474, 33475, 33476, 33478, 33496, 33500, 33502, 33504, 33505, 33506, 33507, 33510, 33511, 33512, 33513, 33514, 33516, 33533, 33534, 33535, 33536, 33542, 33545, 33548, 33600-33688, 33692, 33694, 33697, 33702, 33710, 33720, 33724, 33726, 33730, 33732, 33736, 33750, 33755, 33762, 33764, 33766, 33767, 33770-33783, 33786, 33788, 33802, 33803, 33814, 33820, 33822, 33824, 33840, 33845, 33851, 33853, 33858, 33859, 33863, 33864, 33871, 33875, 33877, 33880, 33881, 33883, 33884, 33886, 33910, 33916, 33917, 33920, 33922, 33926, 33935, 33945, 33975, 33976, 33977, 33978, 33979, 33980, 33983, 33990, 33991, 34701, 34702, 34703, 34704, 34705, 34706, 34707, 34708, 34710, 34712, 34718, 34841, 34842, 34843, 34844, 34845, 34846, 34847, 34848)◀

(34714 may only be reported once per side. For bilateral procedure, report 34714 twice. Do not report modifier 50 in conjunction with 34714)

Surgery / Cardiovascular System   33016-39599

(Do not report 34714 in conjunction with 33362, 33953, 33954, 33959, 33962, 33969, 33984, 34812 when performed on the same side)

**#+ 34833** Open iliac artery exposure with creation of conduit for delivery of endovascular prosthesis or for establishment of cardiopulmonary bypass, by abdominal or retroperitoneal incision, unilateral (List separately in addition to code for primary procedure)

▶(Use 34833 in conjunction with 32852, 32854, 33031, 33120, 33251, 33256, 33259, 33261, 33305, 33315, 33322, 33335, 33390, 33391, 33404, 33405, 33406, 33410, 33411, 33412, 33413, 33414, 33415, 33416, 33417, 33422, 33425, 33426, 33427, 33430, 33440, 33460, 33463, 33464, 33465, 33468, 33474, 33475, 33476, 33478, 33496, 33500, 33502, 33504, 33505, 33506, 33507, 33510, 33511, 33512, 33513, 33514, 33516, 33533, 33534, 33535, 33536, 33542, 33545, 33548, 33600-33688, 33692, 33694, 33697, 33702, 33710, 33720, 33724, 33726, 33730, 33732, 33736, 33750, 33755, 33762, 33764, 33766, 33767, 33770-33783, 33786, 33788, 33802, 33803, 33814, 33820, 33822, 33824, 33840, 33845, 33851, 33853, 33858, 33859, 33863, 33864, 33871, 33875, 33877, 33880, 33881, 33883, 33884, 33886, 33910, 33916, 33917, 33920, 33922, 33926, 33935, 33945, 33975, 33976, 33977, 33978, 33979, 33980, 33983, 33990, 33991, 34701, 34702, 34703, 34704, 34705, 34706, 34707, 34708, 34710, 34712, 34718, 34841, 34842, 34843, 34844, 34845, 34846, 34847, 34848)◀

(34833 may only be reported once per side. For bilateral procedure, report 34833 twice. Do not report modifier 50 in conjunction with 34833)

(Do not report 34833 in conjunction with 33364, 33953, 33954, 33959, 33962, 33969, 33984, 34820 when performed on the same side)

## Rationale

In accordance with the deletion of code 33722, the inclusionary parenthetical notes following codes 34714 and 34833 have been revised with the removal of code 33722.

Refer to the codebook and the Rationale for code 33722 for a full description of these changes.

**+ 34715** Open axillary/subclavian artery exposure for delivery of endovascular prosthesis by infraclavicular or supraclavicular incision, unilateral (List separately in addition to code for primary procedure)

(Use 34715 in conjunction with 33880, 33881, 33883, 33884, 33886, 33990, 33991, 34701, 34702, 34703, 34704, 34705, 34706, 34707, 34708, 34710, 34712, 34718, 34841, 34842, 34843, 34844, 34845, 34846, 34847, 34848)

(34715 may only be reported once per side. For bilateral procedure, report 34715 twice. Do not report modifier 50 in conjunction with 34715)

▶(Do not report 34715 in conjunction with 33363, 33953, 33954, 33959, 33962, 33969, 33984)◀

## Rationale

In accordance with the deletion of Category III codes 0451T, 0452T, 0455T, and 0456T, the exclusionary parenthetical note following code 34715 has been revised with the removal of these codes.

Refer to the codebook and the Rationale for codes 0451T-0463T for a full discussion of these changes

**+ 34716** Open axillary/subclavian artery exposure with creation of conduit for delivery of endovascular prosthesis or for establishment of cardiopulmonary bypass, by infraclavicular or supraclavicular incision, unilateral (List separately in addition to code for primary procedure)

▶(Use 34716 in conjunction with 32852, 32854, 33031, 33120, 33251, 33256, 33259-33261, 33305, 33315, 33322, 33335, 33390, 33391, 33404, 33405, 33406, 33410, 33411, 33412, 33413, 33414, 33415, 33416, 33417, 33422, 33425, 33426, 33427, 33430, 33440, 33460, 33463, 33464, 33465, 33468, 33474, 33475, 33476, 33478, 33496, 33500, 33502, 33504, 33505, 33506, 33507, 33510, 33511, 33512, 33513, 33514, 33516, 33533, 33534, 33535, 33536, 33542, 33545, 33548, 33600-33688, 33692, 33694, 33697, 33702, 33710, 33720, 33724, 33726, 33730, 33732, 33736, 33750, 33755, 33762, 33764, 33766, 33767, 33770-33783, 33786, 33788, 33802, 33803, 33814, 33820, 33822, 33824, 33840, 33845, 33851, 33853, 33858, 33859, 33863, 33864, 33871, 33875, 33877, 33880, 33881, 33883, 33884, 33886, 33910, 33916, 33917, 33920, 33922, 33926, 33935, 33945, 33975, 33976, 33977, 33978, 33979, 33980, 33983, 33990, 33991, 34701, 34702, 34703, 34704, 34705, 34706, 34707, 34708, 34710, 34712, 34718, 34841, 34842, 34843, 34844, 34845, 34846, 34847, 34848)◀

(34716 may only be reported once per side. For bilateral procedure, report 34716 twice. Do not report modifier 50 in conjunction with 34716)

## Rationale

In accordance with the deletion of code 33722, the inclusionary parenthetical note following code 34716 has been revised with the removal of code 33722.

Refer to the codebook and the Rationale for code 33722 for a full description of these changes.

## Bypass Graft

### Other Than Vein

⊘▲ **35600**   Harvest of upper extremity artery, 1 segment, for coronary artery bypass procedure, open

▶(For endoscopic approach, see 33508, 33509, 37500)◀

▶(For bilateral procedure, report 35600 with modifier 50)◀

## Rationale

In accordance with the establishment of code 33509, code 35600 has been revised with the removal of the add-on code symbol and language in the descriptor to reflect that it is not an add-on code.

In addition, the parenthetical note instructing users to use code 35600 in conjunction with codes 33533 and 33536 has been deleted and replaced with two new parenthetical notes: one to instruct users that code 35600 should be reported with modifier 50 for bilateral procedures, and another to instruct users to see codes 33508, 33509, and 37500 for endoscopic approach.

Finally, codes 33509 and 35600 have been identified as modifier 51 exempt; therefore, the modifier 51 exempt symbol (⊘) has been added to these codes, which means they will be included in Appendix E (Summary of CPT Codes Exempt from Modifier 51) in the CPT 2022 code set.

Refer to the codebook and the Rationale for code 33509 for a full discussion of these changes.

## Clinical Example (35600)

A 58-year-old male, who has a history of coronary artery bypass grafting (CABG), presents to the emergency room (ER) with unstable angina. Cardiac catheterization reveals multivessel disease requiring several grafts. He is an acceptable candidate for reoperative CABG. The saphenous vein conduit is limited because of the prior CABG, and only a small segment is available. The right internal mammary artery is available, and the left radial artery in this right-handed individual is evaluated and determined to be appropriate for open harvesting and used for the CABG.

## Description of Procedure (35600)

The primary surgeon decides whether to utilize the radial artery as a conduit for CABG, typically during the initial visit with the patient. The primary surgeon performing the CABG obtains a history with attention given to conditions that may mitigate against using the radial, such as renal failure requiring or likely to require dialysis, severe PVD, or history of Reynaud syndrome. Examine the arm and hand and preform an Allen test to assess adequacy of the ulnar circulation and the palmar arch. If available, employ an oxygen-saturation monitor to assess the circulation provided by the ulnar artery. At the time of the CABG procedure (reported separately), the provider who will be harvesting the artery checks the radial artery in the operating room. Perform an Allen test using the oxygen-saturation monitor to assess the adequacy of the ulnar circulation and the palmar arch. Discuss any abnormalities or concerns with the primary surgeon and decide whether to proceed with the harvest. Begin a continuous intravenous nitroglycerin infusion to prevent spasm of the radial artery. Harvest the radial artery simultaneously with the other conduits by making a curvilinear incision at the edge of the hairline of the left forearm, following the brachioradialis muscle lateral to the biceps tendon and down to a midway point between the tendon of the flexor carpi radialis muscle and the radial styloid at the wrist crease. Obtain hemostasis using a microdissection needle coagulator or a harmonic scalpel and continue dissection, taking care to avoid nerves and larger vessels. Divide the fascia between the bellies of the brachioradialis and flexor carpi radialis muscle. Visualize the radial artery and dissect by beginning at the middle of the forearm proximally, keeping the venous vascular pedicle intact. Divide the vasa vasorum of the radial artery posteriorly using the harmonic scalpel or silk sutures proximally and metallic clips distally. As the dissection approaches the wrist, numerous small vessels usually require meticulous identification and separation. Recheck pulse oximetry on the thumb. Before dividing the radial artery, place a soft non-occluding clamp across the dissected, but still intact, radial artery and palpate the ulnar artery to be certain blood supply to the hand is adequate. Only after adequacy of ulnar artery flow is confirmed, ligate and divide the radial artery pedicle. Inspect the wound for hemostasis and ligate and divide the artery. Close the fascia and subcutaneous tissues throughout the length of the forearm incision in two layers using absorbable sutures. Close the entire forearm skin incision using a subcuticular method and monofilament absorbable sutures. Check the hand for warmth and assess circulation with an oxygen-saturation monitor. Wrap the arm and score the artery on its anterior surface with a methylene blue marking pen to maintain orientation of the radial artery conduit without inadvertent twisting. Soak and flush the radial artery with papaverine and heparinized patient blood. Check

★ =Telemedicine   ✚ =Add-on code   𝒩 =FDA approval pending   # =Resequenced code   ⊘ =Modifier 51 exempt

the entire length of the radial artery while flushing it with the heparinized blood, and carefully clip or tie the branches per routine. The primary surgeon uses the radial artery to bypass the designated coronary artery. The primary surgeon evaluates the radial artery–harvest site at the end of the procedure.

## Vascular Injection Procedures

### Intra-Arterial—Intra-Aortic

**36215** Selective catheter placement, arterial system; each first order thoracic or brachiocephalic branch, within a vascular family

(For catheter placement for coronary angiography, see 93454-93461)

**+ 36218** additional second order, third order, and beyond, thoracic or brachiocephalic branch, within a vascular family (List in addition to code for initial second or third order vessel as appropriate)

(Use 36218 in conjunction with 36216, 36217, 36225, 36226)

(For angiography, see 36222-36228, 75600-75774)

(For transluminal balloon angioplasty [except lower extremity artery[ies] for occlusive disease, intracranial, coronary, pulmonary, or dialysis circuit], see 37246, 37247)

(For transcatheter therapies, see 37200, 37211, 37213, 37214, 37236, 37237, 37238, 37239, 37241, 37242, 37243, 37244, 61624, 61626)

▶(When arterial [eg, internal mammary, inferior epigastric or free radial artery] or venous bypass graft angiography is performed in conjunction with cardiac catheterization, see the appropriate cardiac catheterization, injection procedure, and imaging supervision code[s] [93454, 93455, 93456, 93457, 93458, 93459, 93460, 93461, 93564, 93593, 93594, 93595, 93596, 93597] in the **Medicine** section. When internal mammary artery angiography only is performed without a concomitant cardiac catheterization, use 36216 or 36217 as appropriate)◀

### Rationale

In accordance with the deletion of codes 93530-93533 and the establishment of codes 93593-93597, the cross-reference parenthetical note following code 36218 has been revised to reflect these changes, and to include coronary artery catheter placement codes 93454, 93456, 93458, and 93460.

Refer to the codebook and the Rationale for codes 93593-93597 for a full discussion of these changes.

### Venous

**36522** Photopheresis, extracorporeal

(For dialysis services, see 90935-90999)

▶(For therapeutic ultrafiltration, use 0692T)◀

(For therapeutic apheresis for white blood cells, red blood cells, platelets and plasma pheresis, see 36511, 36512, 36513, 36514)

(For therapeutic apheresis extracorporeal adsorption procedures, use 36516)

### Rationale

In accordance with the establishment of code 0692T for reporting therapeutic ultrafiltration, a cross-reference parenthetical note has been revised following code 36522 with instructions to use the new code instead of an unlisted code.

Refer to the codebook and the Rationale for code 0692T for a full discussion of these changes.

# Mediastinum and Diaphragm

## Diaphragm

### Other Procedures

**39599** Unlisted procedure, diaphragm

▶(For laparoscopic insertion or replacement of a permanent synchronized diaphragmatic stimulation system, see 0674T, 0675T, 0680T)◀

### Rationale

In accordance with the addition of a new subsection, guidelines, parenthetical notes, and codes for reporting laparoscopic services for use of a permanent implantable synchronized diaphragmatic stimulation system for augmentation of cardiac function (0674T-0685T) and associated services, a cross-reference parenthetical note has been added following code 39599 to direct users to codes 0674T- 0680T for laparoscopic insertion or replacement procedures.

Refer to the codebook and the Rationale for codes 0674T-0685T for a full discussion of these changes.

# Digestive System

## Pharynx, Adenoids, and Tonsils

### Other Procedures

**42970** Control of nasopharyngeal hemorrhage, primary or secondary (eg, postadenoidectomy); simple, with posterior nasal packs, with or without anterior packs and/or cautery

**42971** complicated, requiring hospitalization

**42972** with secondary surgical intervention

● **42975** Drug-induced sleep endoscopy, with dynamic evaluation of velum, pharynx, tongue base, and larynx for evaluation of sleep-disordered breathing, flexible, diagnostic

▶(Do not report 42975 in conjunction with 31231, unless performed for a separate condition [ie, other than sleep-disordered breathing] and using a separate endoscope)◀

▶(Do not report 42975 in conjunction with 31575, 92511)◀

**42999** Unlisted procedure, pharynx, adenoids, or tonsils

### Rationale

A new code (42975) has been established to report flexible, diagnostic drug-induced sleep endoscopy. Two parenthetical notes have been added to provide appropriate reporting guidance for the use of this code in conjunction with codes 31231, 31575, and 92511.

Currently, drug-induced sleep endoscopy is reported with code 31575, *Laryngoscopy, flexible; diagnostic*, 31622, *Bronchoscopy, rigid or flexible, including fluoroscopic guidance, when performed; diagnostic, with cell washing, when performed (separate procedure),* or 92502, *Otolaryngologic examination under general anesthesia.* These codes alone or in combination do not accurately capture the work involved in examining the dynamic nature and site(s) of airway obstruction within the nasal cavity, nasopharynx, oropharynx, hypopharynx, and larynx while under anesthesia in an operative setting, nor are they inclusive of the examination of the effects of positional and head and neck manipulation on the obstruction.

Code 42975 describes drug-induced sleep endoscopy designed to evaluate sleep-disordered breathing. Two parenthetical notes following code 42975 have been added to provide instruction on how to report this code in conjunction with codes 31231, 31575, and 92511: one to restrict reporting code 42975 in conjunction with code 31231, unless performed for a separate condition for other than sleep-disordered breathing and using a separate

endoscope, and another to restrict reporting codes 31575 and 92511 with code 42975.

In accordance with the establishment of code 42975, two exclusionary parenthetical notes following codes 31575 and 92511 have been revised to include new code 42975.

## Clinical Example (42975)

A 45-year-old male with moderate to severe obstructive sleep apnea has been unable to tolerate positive airway pressure (PAP) therapy. Sleep endoscopy is performed to identify anatomic and physiologic factors contributing to his obstructive sleep apnea and the selection of noncontinuous PAP treatment options.

## Description of Procedure (42975)

Prepare the nasal passages with application of a decongestant and/or topical anesthesia. Provide light intravenous sedation, which is typically provided by a separate health care professional, to a point in which the patient is nonresponsive to verbal stimuli, has snoring or partial upper airway–flow limitation, and observed oxygen desaturations. The performing physician places a flexible endoscope through the nose and advances it to the pharynx. Perform endoscopic evaluation of the nasopharynx, oropharynx, hypopharynx, and larynx during sleep or sedation over multiple cycles of airway narrowing and/or obstruction. The velopharynx is the term for the distal (nonmuscular) component of the soft palate and uvula, which is the predominant site of upper pharyngeal collapse. The physician notes the anatomic site of obstruction (velopharynx, oropharynx, tongue, epiglottis), the severity of the obstruction (non, partial, complete), and the pattern of obstruction (anteroposterior, circular, lateral). The physician then repositions the patient and/or performs manipulation of the head and neck and repeats endoscopy to determine effect of body position (supine versus lateral), jaw lift, tongue protrusion, or hyoid lift on airway obstruction. Place and titrate a patient's existing oral appliance (mandibular advancement device) to optimal effect. In certain cases, a CPAP mask may be applied to determine sites on ongoing obstruction in regular CPAP users who fail to improve with CPAP therapy.

★ = Telemedicine ✚ = Add-on code ✗ = FDA approval pending # = Resequenced code ⊘ = Modifier 51 exempt

# Esophagus

## Endoscopy

### Esophagoscopy

**43191**   Esophagoscopy, rigid, transoral; diagnostic, including collection of specimen(s) by brushing or washing when performed (separate procedure)

▶(Do not report 43191 in conjunction with 43192, 43193, 43194, 43195, 43196, 43197, 43198, 43210, 43497)◀

(For diagnostic transnasal esophagoscopy, see 43197, 43198)

(For diagnostic flexible transoral esophagoscopy, use 43200)

**43197**   Esophagoscopy, flexible, transnasal; diagnostic, including collection of specimen(s) by brushing or washing, when performed (separate procedure)

▶(Do not report 43197 in conjunction with 31575, 43191, 43192, 43193, 43194, 43195, 43196, 43198, 43200-43232, 43235-43259, 43266, 43270, 43497, 92511, 0652T, 0653T, 0654T)◀

(Do not report 43197 in conjunction with 31231 unless separate type of endoscope [eg, rigid endoscope] is used)

(For transoral esophagoscopy, see 43191, 43200)

**43198**      with biopsy, single or multiple

▶(Do not report 43198 in conjunction with 31575, 43191, 43192, 43193, 43194, 43195, 43196, 43197, 43200-43232, 43235-43259, 43266, 43270, 92511, 0652T, 0653T, 0654T)◀

(Do not report 43198 in conjunction with 31231 unless separate type of endoscope [eg, rigid endoscope] is used)

(For transoral esophagoscopy with biopsy, see 43193, 43202)

**43200**   Esophagoscopy, flexible, transoral; diagnostic, including collection of specimen(s) by brushing or washing, when performed (separate procedure)

▶(Do not report 43200 in conjunction with 43197, 43198, 43201-43232, 43497)◀

(For diagnostic rigid transoral esophagoscopy, use 43191)

(For diagnostic flexible transnasal esophagoscopy, use 43197)

(For diagnostic flexible esophagogastroduodenoscopy, use 43235)

## Rationale

In accordance with the establishment of Category III codes 0652T, 0653T, and 0654T, the exclusionary parenthetical notes following codes 43197 and 43198 have been revised with the addition of the new codes.

In accordance with the establishment of code 43497, the exclusionary parenthetical notes following codes 43191, 43197, and 43200 have been revised with the addition of code 43497 to restrict reporting these codes with code 43497.

Refer to the codebook and the Rationale for codes 0652T, 0653T, 0654T, and 43497 for a full discussion of these changes.

### Esophagogastroduodenoscopy

**43235**   Esophagogastroduodenoscopy, flexible, transoral; diagnostic, including collection of specimen(s) by brushing or washing, when performed (separate procedure)

▶(Do not report 43235 in conjunction with 43197, 43198, 43210, 43236-43259, 43266, 43270, 43497, 44360, 44361, 44363, 44364, 44365, 44366, 44369, 44370, 44372, 44373, 44376, 44377, 44378, 44379)◀

## Rationale

In accordance with the establishment of code 43497, the exclusionary parenthetical note following code 43235 has been revised with the addition of code 43497 to restrict reporting code 43235 with code 43497.

Refer to the codebook and the Rationale for code 43497 for a full discussion of these changes.

## Other Procedures

**43496**   Free jejunum transfer with microvascular anastomosis

(Do not report code 69990 in addition to code 43496)

● **43497**   Lower esophageal myotomy, transoral (ie, peroral endoscopic myotomy [POEM])

▶(Do not report 43497 in conjunction with 32665, 43191, 43197, 43200, 43235)◀

Surgery / Digestive System  40490-49999

## Rationale

Code 43497 has been established to report transoral lower esophageal myotomy, which is also known as peroral endoscopic myotomy (POEM). Prior to 2022, there was no CPT code to report the POEM procedure. The POEM procedure is performed for disorders such as achalasia, which is the inability to pass food from the esophagus to the stomach.

Three existing CPT codes (32665, 43279, 43330) describe esophagomyotomy via different approaches. Code 32665 describes esophagomyotomy via thoracoscopy; code 43279 describes laparoscopic esophagomyotomy; and code 43330 describes esophagomyotomy via an open abdominal approach. The esophagomyotomy performed in the POEM procedure is similar to the procedures described in codes 32665, 43279, and 43330; however, it is performed via endoscope using a peroral approach.

An exclusionary parenthetical note has been added following code 43497 restricting reporting code 43497 with codes 32665, 43191, 43197, 43200, and 43235.

## Clinical Example (43497)

A 48-year-old male presents with progressive dysphagia for solids and liquids. Testing has confirmed achalasia. The patient is referred for peroral endoscopic myotomy (POEM).

## Description of Procedure (43497)

Place a bite-block in the patient's mouth. Confirm with anesthesiology that an adequate level of anesthesia is in place to begin intubation of the esophagus. Insert a flexible upper endoscope through the mouth into the oropharynx and into the esophagus to assess for esophageal anatomy, retained food, infections (candidiasis), and degree of esophageal dilation/tortuosity, removing and reinserting the scope. Pay meticulous attention to suctioning and removing solid and liquid debris and secretions from the esophagus to allow complete visualization of the esophageal mucosa and anatomy. Advance the endoscope through the lower esophageal sphincter into the proximal stomach. Insufflate the stomach with $CO_2$. Perform an examination of the entire stomach in the forward and retroflexed position. Advance the endoscope through the pylorus into the duodenal bulb. Perform circumferential inspection of the duodenum after insufflation. Once initial examination confirms that there are no contraindications to proceeding, it is optional to lavage the esophagus with antibiotics and/or place an esophageal overtube. During this detailed endoscopic examination, record careful measurements of critical landmarks (teeth and overtube, squamocolumnar junction, proximal gastric folds). Observe esophageal motility and mucosa and make final adjustments to planned endpoints and length of myotomy as

appropriate. Instill water into the esophageal lumen to determine anterior vs posterior wall, because approach may differ in each case. Once initial examination and landmarks are noted, and anterior vs posterior approach determined, remove the endoscope, and fit and securely fix the endoscope with a clear cap. Reinsert the cap-fitted endoscope into the esophagus and position the endoscope in the esophageal lumen at the anticipated proximal end of the myotomy and perform a submucosal injection with appropriate lifting solution using an injection needle. After an adequate fluid cushion is achieved, create a mucosal incision using the electrocautery dissection knife selected at the appropriate energy settings to create a submucosal entry tunnel for the endoscope. Incision should be several centimeters proximal to planned proximal myotomy. Once the esophageal submucosal space has been entered, carefully dissect the layers of submucosal tissue to further expand the submucosal tunnel and expose the inner circular esophageal muscle below it. It is essential to ensure meticulous hemostasis of submucosal vessels as encountered during creation of the tunnel, and, as needed, use alternative instruments, settings, and interventions. Extend the tunnel distally until the tunnel has reached 1.5 to 3 cm onto the gastric cardia below the gastroesophageal (GE) junction. Perform continuous monitoring of the patient's vital signs and physical examination of the chest and abdomen to assess the presence and impact of extraluminal $CO_2$ extravasation. Once the submucosal tunnel creation is complete and its adequacy documented, incise and divide the circular muscle fibers, extending the full length of the myotomy. Once the myotomy is complete, repeat the endoscopy to evaluate the adequacy of the myotomy and patency of the GE junction. Carefully examine the esophageal mucosa to rule out any mucosal injury. Close the mucosal defect at the entry point of the submucosal tunnel using endoclips. Perform careful inspection of the incision site to assure adequate closure and hemostasis. After suctioning to deflate the stomach and esophagus, withdraw the endoscope.

## Stomach

## Other Procedures

▶(43850, 43855 have been deleted)◀

## Rationale

Codes 43850, *Revision of gastroduodenal anastomosis (gastroduodenostomy) with reconstruction; without vagotomy*, and 43855, *Revision of gastroduodenal anastomosis (gastroduodenostomy) with reconstruction; with vagotomy*, have been deleted due to low utilization. A parenthetical note has been added to indicate these deletions.

★ = Telemedicine   ✚ = Add-on code   ✗ = FDA approval pending   # = Resequenced code   ⊘ = Modifier 51 exempt

# Urinary System

## Urethra

### Repair

**53450** Urethromeatoplasty, with mucosal advancement

    (For meatotomy, see 53020, 53025)

● **53451** Periurethral transperineal adjustable balloon continence device; bilateral insertion, including cystourethroscopy and imaging guidance

    ▶(Do not report 53451 in conjunction with 52000, 53452, 53453, 53454, 76000)◀

● **53452**     unilateral insertion, including cystourethroscopy and imaging guidance

    ▶(Do not report 53452 in conjunction with 52000, 53451, 53453, 53454, 76000)◀

● **53453**     removal, each balloon

    ▶(Do not report 53453 in conjunction with 53451, 53452, 53454)◀

● **53454**     percutaneous adjustment of balloon(s) fluid volume

    ▶(Do not report 53454 in conjunction with 53451, 53452, 53453)◀

    ▶(Report 53454 only once per patient encounter)◀

**53460** Urethromeatoplasty, with partial excision of distal urethral segment (Richardson type procedure)

### Rationale

In accordance with the conversion of Category III codes 0548T-0551T to Category I codes 53451-53454, codes 0548T-0551T have been deleted, and codes 53451-53454 have been established to report periurethral transperineal balloon–continence device procedures.

To assist in appropriate reporting of this new family of codes, (1) several exclusionary parenthetical notes have been added throughout the code family; (2) deletion parenthetical notes have been added in the Category III section; (3) instructional parenthetical notes have been added in the Category III section to direct users to report codes 53451-53454 for bilateral insertion, unilateral insertion, removal, or fluid adjustment of a periurethral adjustable balloon–continence device; and (4) a parenthetical note has been added to indicate that code 53454 should only be reported once per patient encounter.

Codes 53451 and 53452 describe periurethral transperineal bilateral and unilateral insertion of a single adjustable balloon device. These codes also include the performance of a cystourethroscopy and imaging guidance. Code 53453 is reported for the removal of each balloon. Code 53454 is reported for percutaneous adjustment of the fluid volume of the balloon(s).

## Clinical Example (53451)

A 70-year-old male underwent radical prostatectomy 4 years ago. His prostate-specific antigen is undetectable; however, he has intractable stress incontinence secondary to intrinsic sphincter deficiency and has failed all conservative measures. After appropriate counseling, it was decided to perform implantation of two permanent, adjustable balloon-continence devices.

## Description of Procedure (53451)

N/A

## Clinical Example (53452)

A 70-year-old male with post-prostatectomy urinary stress incontinence underwent implantation of two permanent, adjustable balloon devices 1 year ago, followed by removal of the left balloon 10 months later due to balloon migration and recurrence of his incontinence. After sufficient healing, he has elected to undergo reimplantation of a single permanent, adjustable balloon-continence device on the left side.

## Description of Procedure (53452)

N/A

## Clinical Example (53453)

A 65-year-old male with post-prostatectomy urinary stress incontinence underwent implantation of two permanent, adjustable balloon-continence devices 2 years ago with excellent initial results. The patient noticed a recurrence of his incontinence. Upon examination, the left balloon has migrated from its original location, and he is to undergo removal of the left balloon.

## Description of Procedure (53453)

N/A

## Clinical Example (53454)

A 66-year-old male with post-prostatectomy urinary stress incontinence underwent implantation of two permanent, adjustable balloon-continence devices 6 weeks ago. Postoperatively his continence is improved; however, he still has bothersome leakage. In the office, he will undergo the addition of fluid to both balloons to increase urethral resistance and decrease urinary leakage.

## Description of Procedure (53454)

N/A

# Male Genital System

## Penis

### Repair

▲ **54340**   Repair of hypospadias complication(s) (ie, fistula, stricture, diverticula); by closure, incision, or excision, simple

▲ **54344**   requiring mobilization of skin flaps and urethroplasty with flap or patch graft

▲ **54348**   requiring extensive dissection, and urethroplasty with flap, patch or tubed graft (including urinary diversion, when performed)

▲ **54352**   Revision of prior hypospadias repair requiring extensive dissection and excision of previously constructed structures including re-release of chordee and reconstruction of urethra and penis by use of local skin as grafts and island flaps and skin brought in as flaps or grafts

▶(Do not report 54352 in conjunction with 15275, 15574, 15740, 53235, 53410, 54300, 54336, 54340, 54344, 54348, 54360)◀

### Rationale

Existing codes 54340, 54344, 54348 have been editorially revised with the addition of "(s)" to the word "complication" in the parent code descriptor to indicate that there may be more than one complication when reporting these codes. Child code 54348 has been further revised with the addition of the term "when performed" to the descriptor, as it relates to urinary diversion.

Code 54352 has been editorially revised with the replacement of the phrase "Repair of hypospadias cripple" with "Revision of prior hypospadias repair" in the descriptor to more accurately describe the procedure performed.

In addition, an exclusionary parenthetical note has been added following code 54352 to list the services that code 54352 may not be reported in conjunction with, which includes three integumentary system codes (15275, 15574, 15740), two urinary system codes (53235, 53410), and several male genital system codes (54300, 54336, 54340, 54344, 54348, 54360).

# Maternity Care and Delivery

## Excision

▶(59135 has been deleted)◀

### Rationale

To ensure the CPT code set reflects current clinical practice, code 59135, *Surgical treatment of ectopic pregnancy; interstitial, uterine pregnancy requiring total hysterectomy,* has been deleted due to low utilization. A parenthetical note has been added to indicate this deletion.

# Nervous System

## Skull, Meninges, and Brain

### Stereotaxis

**61720**   Creation of lesion by stereotactic method, including burr hole(s) and localizing and recording techniques, single or multiple stages; globus pallidus or thalamus

**61735**   subcortical structure(s) other than globus pallidus or thalamus

● **61736**   Laser interstitial thermal therapy (LITT) of lesion, intracranial, including burr hole(s), with magnetic resonance imaging guidance, when performed; single trajectory for 1 simple lesion

▶(Do not report 61736 in conjunction with 20660, 61737, 61781, 70551, 70552, 70553, 70557, 70558, 70559, 77021, 77022)◀

● **61737**   multiple trajectories for multiple or complex lesion(s)

▶(Do not report 61737 in conjunction with 20660, 61736, 61781, 70551, 70552, 70553, 70557, 70558, 70559, 77021, 77022)◀

### Rationale

Two new codes (61736, 61737) have been established to report laser interstitial thermal therapy (LITT) for treatment of intracranial lesions. In addition, new parenthetical notes have been added to guide users in the appropriate reporting of these services.

LITT involves the stereotactic placement of a laser fiber into an intracranial target lesion. It is followed with thermal treatment of the target lesion under real-time magnetic resonance imaging (MRI) thermographic

★=Telemedicine   ✚=Add-on code   ✒=FDA approval pending   #=Resequenced code   ⊘=Modifier 51 exempt

monitoring. Adjustment of the laser position with multiple laser firings is often vital for the completion of a patient's treatment. Some larger or more complex lesions may require multiple laser trajectories at the same sitting.

Code 61736 is reported when LITT is performed for a single trajectory for one simple lesion, intracranial, including burr hole(s), using MRI guidance. Code 61737 is reported when LITT is performed for multiple trajectories for multiple or complex lesion(s).

Two exclusionary parenthetical notes have been added to guide users in the appropriate reporting of these services with other services within the CPT code set. It is important to note that codes 61736 and 61737 should not be reported together.

## Clinical Example (61736)

A 45-year-old male with a 10-year history of seizures due to an intracranial tumor that was identified on magnetic resonance imaging (MRI) has failed to respond to medication adjustments to control his weekly seizures. An image-guided stereotactic interstitial laser ablation procedure is performed.

## Description of Procedure (61736)

Set a sterile stereotactic frame arc to appropriate frame coordinates as needed and mount it over the sterile-draped base ring. Alternately, attach a sterile frameless navigation arm or robotic instrument holder to the head holder or the previously draped stereotactic robot, respectively, as appropriate. Inject the scalp over the entry site with local anesthetic. Make a 2-cm incision and clear the soft tissue from the skull using monopolar cautery. Lower a drill guide tube into the incision and brace it against the bone. Measure the thickness of the skull along the planned trajectory on the navigation plan and set the twist drill depth to the corresponding length. Create a twist drill hole using a twist drill of appropriate diameter for the size of the laser bolt. Replace the guide with a reducing cannula, and carefully open the dura and pia using a long monopolar cautery that has been measured to the appropriate depth. Obtain the distance to the target from the robot, navigation system, or frame, measure a thin stylet to this distance, and then insert the stylet to verify that the pia and dura have been opened to create a path for the laser. Screw the threaded laser bolt into the skull through the chosen targeting device using the correct number of rotations to ensure that it is securely seated. Measure the stereotactic alignment rod to the target distance and insert it through the anchor bolt and into the brain. Use fluoroscopic imaging as appropriate to verify the accuracy of the trajectory. Calculate the distance to the target from the top of the bolt. After removing the alignment rod from the anchor bolt, mark the laser apparatus components at the distance-to-target.

These may be slowly and carefully inserted through the anchor bolt either at this point or after transporting the patient to the MRI suite, as appropriate. Remove the drapes and carefully detach the patient from the table, making sure to protect the anchor bolt and laser (if inserted) from both movement and for sterility.

Carefully transport the patient to the MRI suite and place the patient supine within the magnet, turning the patient's head treatment-side up to protect the laser assembly and anchor bolt. If necessary, remove any sterile covering of the anchor bolt and then measure the laser probe apparatus to the appropriate length and deliver it to the intended target in the brain. Acquire a volumetric image to confirm the placement of the laser tip at the intended target. Co-register the image with the preoperative imaging in the laser ablation–software workstation in the MRI control room. Use the software to identify the intended ablation target boundary(s) and verify the location of the probe on imaging. Mark temperature reference points and safety limits on the laser-ablation software. Initiate and stream continuous MRI thermometry to the workstation, where thermal maps are superimposed over static images of the target area. Deliver laser energy to the target, while continuously monitoring subsequent thermal-dose damage contour lines created by the program software, as tissue is heated to the required temperatures. Alter the laser position as necessary and deliver laser energy to the target, while continuously monitoring subsequent thermal-dose damage contour lines created by the program software, as tissue is heated to the required temperatures. Repeat this process as many times as is necessary to create the entire lesion. Once the intended lesion is created, conduct a final MRI scan. Transfer these images to the laser workstation and merge them with the previous imaging sets. Compare the lesion to the plan and the lesion as estimated by the laser software. Once the lesion is declared complete, withdraw the patient from the MRI scanner, completely remove the laser applicators and anchor bolts, and close the incisions.

## Clinical Example (61737)

A 25-year-old male with a 15-year history of seizures due to a large complex hypothalamic hamartoma identified on MRI has failed to respond to medication adjustments to control his weekly seizures. An image-guided stereotactic interstitial laser ablation procedure, including multiple laser trajectories, is performed.

## Description of Procedure (61737)

Set a sterile stereotactic frame arc to appropriate frame coordinates as needed and mount it over the sterile-draped base ring. Alternately, attach a sterile frameless navigation arm or robotic instrument holder to the head holder or the previously draped stereotactic robot, respectively, as appropriate. Inject the scalp over the entry site with local anesthetic. Make a 2-cm incision and clear the soft tissue from the skull using monopolar cautery. Lower a drill guide tube into the incision and brace it against the bone. Measure the thickness of the skull along the planned trajectory on the navigation plan and set the twist drill depth to the corresponding length. Create a twist drill hole with a twist drill of appropriate diameter for the size of the laser bolt. Replace the guide with a reducing cannula, and carefully open the dura and pia using a long monopolar cautery that has been measured to the appropriate depth. Obtain the distance to the target from the robot, navigation system, or frame, measure a thin stylet to this distance, and then insert the stylet to verify that the pia and dura have been opened to create a path for the laser. Screw the threaded laser bolt into the skull through the chosen targeting device using the correct number of rotations to ensure that it is securely seated. Measure the stereotactic alignment rod to the target distance and insert it through the anchor bolt and into the brain. Use fluoroscopic imaging as appropriate to verify the accuracy of the trajectory. Calculate the distance to the target from the top of the bolt. After removing the alignment rod from the anchor bolt, mark the laser apparatus components at the distance-to-target. These may be slowly and carefully inserted through the anchor bolt either at this point or after transporting the patient to the MRI suite, as appropriate. Align the navigation system to the next trajectory and mark the next entry point. Infiltrate local anesthetic in this region, make another incision, and insert the next anchor bolt and laser in similar fashion to the first. Repeat this process for each subsequent required laser trajectory. Remove the drapes and carefully detach the patient from the table, making sure to protect the anchor bolt and laser (if inserted) from both movement and for sterility.

After all anchor bolts have been placed, carefully transport the patient to the MRI suite and place the patient supine within the magnet, turning the patient's head treatment-side up to protect the laser assemblies and anchor bolts. If necessary, remove any sterile coverings of the anchor bolts, and then measure each laser probe apparatus to the appropriate length and deliver it to the intended target in the brain through the corresponding anchor bolt. Acquire a volumetric image to confirm the placement of each of the laser tips at the intended target. Co-register the image with the preoperative imaging in the laser ablation–software workstation in the MRI control room. Use the software to identify the intended ablation target boundary(ies) and verify the location of each probe on imaging. Select the first laser trajectory and align the imaging to this trajectory. Mark temperature reference points and safety limits on the laser-ablation software. Initiate and stream continuous MRI thermometry to the workstation, where thermal maps are superimposed over static images of the target area. Deliver laser energy to the target, while continuously monitoring subsequent thermal-dose damage contour lines created by the program software, as tissue is heated to the required temperatures. Alter the laser position as necessary and deliver laser energy to the target, while continuously monitoring subsequent thermal-dose damage contour lines created by the program software, as tissue is heated to the required temperatures. Repeat this process as many times as is necessary to create the entire lesion. Repeat this process for each subsequent laser trajectory. Once all the intended lesions are created with the multiple laser trajectories, conduct a final MRI scan. Transfer and merge these images to the laser workstation with the previous imaging sets. Compare the set of lesions to the plan and the estimate from the laser software. Once the set of lesions is declared complete, withdraw the patient from the MRI scanner, completely remove the laser applicators and anchor bolts, and close the incisions.

# Spine and Spinal Cord

## Injection, Drainage, or Aspiration

▶Injection of contrast during fluoroscopic guidance and localization is an inclusive component of 62263, 62264, 62267, 62273, 62280, 62281, 62282, 62302, 62303, 62304, 62305, 62321, 62323, 62325, 62327, 62328, 62329. Fluoroscopic guidance and localization is reported with 77003, unless a formal contrast study (myelography or arthrography) is performed, in which case the use of fluoroscopy is included in the supervision and interpretation codes or the myelography via lumbar injection code. Image guidance and the injection of contrast are inclusive components and are required for the performance of myelography, as described by codes 62302, 62303, 62304, 62305.◀

Code 62263 describes a catheter-based treatment involving targeted injection of various substances (eg, hypertonic saline, steroid, anesthetic) via an indwelling epidural catheter. Code 62263 includes percutaneous insertion and removal of an epidural catheter (remaining in place over a several-day period), for the administration of multiple injections of a neurolytic agent(s) performed during serial treatment sessions (ie, spanning two or more treatment days). If required, adhesions or scarring may also be lysed by mechanical means. Code 62263 is **not** reported for each adhesiolysis treatment, but should be reported **once** to describe the entire series of injections/infusions spanning two or more treatment days.

▶Codes 62263 and 62264 include fluoroscopic guidance and localization (77003) during initial or subsequent sessions.

Fluoroscopy or CT and any injection of contrast are inclusive components of 62321, 62323, 62325, 62327.◀

The placement and use of a catheter to administer one or more epidural or subarachnoid injections on a single calendar day should be reported in the same manner as if a needle had been used, ie, as a single injection using either 62320, 62321, 62322, or 62323. Such injections should not be reported with 62324, 62325, 62326, or 62327.

Threading a catheter into the epidural space, injecting substances at one or more levels and then removing the catheter should be treated as a single injection (62320, 62321, 62322, 62323). If the catheter is left in place to deliver substance(s) over a prolonged period (ie, more than a single calendar day) either continuously or via intermittent bolus, use 62324, 62325, 62326, 62327 as appropriate.

**62263** Percutaneous lysis of epidural adhesions using solution injection (eg, hypertonic saline, enzyme) or mechanical means (eg, catheter) including radiologic localization (includes contrast when administered), multiple adhesiolysis sessions; 2 or more days

▶(62263 includes code 77003)◀

**62264** 1 day

(Do not report 62264 with 62263)

▶(62264 includes code 77003)◀

## Rationale

In accordance with the deletion of epidurography code 72275, the injection, drainage, or aspiration guidelines have been revised, and several parenthetical notes have been revised and/or deleted as they are no longer applicable to epidurography code 72275.

Refer to the codebook and the Rationale for code 72275 for a full discussion of these changes.

## Posterior Extradural Laminotomy or Laminectomy for Exploration/ Decompression of Neural Elements or Excision of Herniated Intervertebral Discs

**63020** Laminotomy (hemilaminectomy), with decompression of nerve root(s), including partial facetectomy, foraminotomy and/or excision of herniated intervertebral disc; 1 interspace, cervical

(For bilateral procedure, report 63020 with modifier 50)

**63030** 1 interspace, lumbar

**+ 63035** each additional interspace, cervical or lumbar (List separately in addition to code for primary procedure)

(Use 63035 in conjunction with 63020-63030)

▶(Do not report 63030, 63035 in conjunction with 22630, 22632, 22633, 22634, for laminotomy performed to prepare the interspace for fusion on the same spinal interspace[s])◀

▶(For decompression performed on the same interspace and vertebral segment[s] as posterior interbody fusion that includes laminectomy, removal of facets, and/or opening/widening of the foramen for decompression of nerves or spinal components, such as spinal cord, cauda equina, or nerve roots, see 63052, 63053)◀

(For bilateral procedure, report 63035 twice. Do not report modifier 50 in conjunction with 63035)

(For percutaneous endoscopic approach, see 0274T, 0275T)

**63040** Laminotomy (hemilaminectomy), with decompression of nerve root(s), including partial facetectomy, foraminotomy and/or excision of herniated intervertebral disc, reexploration, single interspace; cervical

(For bilateral procedure, report 63040 with modifier 50)

**63042** lumbar

(For bilateral procedure, report 63042 with modifier 50)

**+ 63043** each additional cervical interspace (List separately in addition to code for primary procedure)

(Use 63043 in conjunction with 63040)

(For bilateral procedure, report 63043 twice. Do not report modifier 50 in conjunction with 63043)

**+ 63044** each additional lumbar interspace (List separately in addition to code for primary procedure)

(Use 63044 in conjunction with 63042)

▶(Do not report 63040, 63042, 63043, 63044 in conjunction with 22630, 22632, 22633, 22634, for laminotomy to prepare the interspace for fusion on the same interspace[s] and vertebral segment[s])◀

▶(For decompression performed on the same vertebral segment[s] and/or interspace[s] as posterior interbody fusion that includes laminectomy, removal of facets, and/or opening/widening of the foramen for decompression of nerves or spinal components, such as spinal cord, cauda equina, or nerve roots, see 63052, 63053)◀

(For bilateral procedure, report 63044 twice. Do not report modifier 50 in conjunction with 63044)

▶Decompression performed on the same vertebral segment(s) and/or interspace(s) as posterior interbody fusion that includes laminectomy, facetectomy, or foraminotomy may be separately reported using 63052.

Codes 63052, 63053 may only be reported for decompression at the same anatomic site(s) when posterior interbody fusion (eg, 22630) requires decompression beyond preparation of the interspace(s) for fusion.◀

**63045** Laminectomy, facetectomy and foraminotomy (unilateral or bilateral with decompression of spinal cord, cauda equina and/or nerve root[s], [eg, spinal or lateral recess stenosis]), single vertebral segment; cervical

**63046** thoracic

**63047** lumbar

+▲ **63048** each additional vertebral segment, cervical, thoracic, or lumbar (List separately in addition to code for primary procedure)

(Use 63048 in conjunction with 63045-63047)

▶(Do not report 63047, 63048 in conjunction with 22630, 22632, 22633, 22634, for laminectomy performed to prepare the interspace for fusion on the same vertebral segment[s] and/or interspace[s])◀

▶(For decompression performed on the same vertebral segment[s] and/or interspace[s] as posterior interbody fusion that includes laminectomy, removal of facets, and/or opening/widening of the foramen for decompression of nerves or spinal components, such as spinal cord, cauda equina, or nerve roots, see 63052, 63053)◀

---

### Example of Laminectomy at Single Interspace
63047

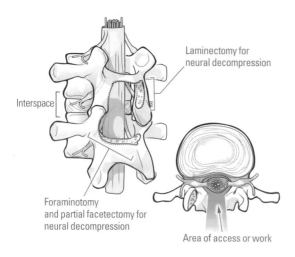

Laminectomy for neural decompression

Interspace

Foraminotomy and partial facetectomy for neural decompression

Area of access or work

---

#+● **63052** Laminectomy, facetectomy, or foraminotomy (unilateral or bilateral with decompression of spinal cord, cauda equina and/or nerve root[s] [eg, spinal or lateral recess stenosis]), during posterior interbody arthrodesis, lumbar; single vertebral segment (List separately in addition to code for primary procedure)

#+● **63053** each additional segment (List separately in addition to code for primary procedure)

▶(Use 63053 in conjunction with 63052)◀

▶(Use 63052, 63053 in conjunction with 22630, 22632, 22633, 22634)◀

**63050** Laminoplasty, cervical, with decompression of the spinal cord, 2 or more vertebral segments;

**63051** with reconstruction of the posterior bony elements (including the application of bridging bone graft and non-segmental fixation devices [eg, wire, suture, mini-plates], when performed)

(Do not report 63050 or 63051 in conjunction with 22600, 22614, 22840-22842, 63001, 63015, 63045, 63048, 63295 for the same vertebral segment(s))

**63052** Code is out of numerical sequence. See 63047-63051

**63053** Code is out of numerical sequence. See 63047-63051

---

## Transpedicular or Costovertebral Approach for Posterolateral Extradural Exploration/Decompression

**63055** Transpedicular approach with decompression of spinal cord, equina and/or nerve root(s) (eg, herniated intervertebral disc), single segment; thoracic

**63056** lumbar (including transfacet, or lateral extraforamina approach) (eg, far lateral herniated intervertebral disc)

+ **63057** each additional segment, thoracic or lumbar (List separately in addition to code for primary procedure)

(Use 63057 in conjunction with 63055, 63056)

▶(Do not report 63056, 63057 for a herniated disc in conjunction with 22630, 22632, 22633, 22634 for decompression to prepare the interspace on the same interspace[s])◀

▶(For decompression performed on the same interspace[s] as posterior interbody fusion that includes laminectomy, removal of facets, and/or opening/widening of the foramen for decompression of nerves or spinal components, such as spinal cord, cauda equina, or nerve roots, see 63052, 63053)◀

---

### Rationale

Guidelines and parenthetical notes have been added, code 63048 has been editorially revised with the addition of the term "vertebral" to the descriptor, and codes 63052 and 63053 have been established to provide better instruction regarding the appropriate reporting of these and related procedures. In addition, new illustrations have been added to enable users to visually identify the anatomy defined in the new definitions.

Refer to the codebook and the Rationale for codes 22600-22614 and 22630-22634 for a full discussion of these changes.

★ = Telemedicine  ✚ = Add-on code  ✎ = FDA approval pending  # = Resequenced code  ⊘ = Modifier 51 exempt

## Clinical Example (63052)

A 63-year-old female, through advanced imaging demonstrated central canal and bilateral lateral recess and foraminal stenosis at the L4-L5 level that requires bilateral laminectomy with extensive decompression of the cauda equina and/or nerve root(s), during posterior lumbar interbody arthrodesis (separately reported) for L4-L5 spondylolisthesis with axial mechanical back pain and worsening neurogenic claudication and/or radiculopathy (extremity symptoms) refractory to nonoperative treatment. This more extensive decompression is beyond the typical dissection needed to complete the interbody arthrodesis approach and intervention. [**Note:** This is an add-on service. Only consider the additional work related to bilateral laminectomy with decompression of the cauda equina and/or nerve root(s)].

## Description of Procedure (63052)

Following bony and soft tissue resection and exposure of the L4-L5 disc space for the interbody access and preparation for interbody arthrodesis, turn attention to the additional bone and nervous system work required for decompression, beyond what is required to access the disc space for the interbody arthrodesis. Remove additional portions of the laminae at the L4 and L5 vertebral segments with a drill or bone-biting instruments and resect the inferior and superior facets. Expand the neural foramina with bone-biting instruments. Dissect and completely remove the ligamentum flavum off the dura and completely removed to allow for decompression and mobilization of the neural elements. Confirm the neural elements are mobilized and decompressed. Document the additional work in the patient's medical record.

## Clinical Example (63053)

A 68-year-old male, through advanced imaging demonstrated central canal and bilateral lateral recess and foraminal stenosis at the L4-L5 and L5-S1 levels that require bilateral laminectomy with extensive decompression of the cauda equina and/or nerve root(s), during posterior lumbar interbody arthrodesis (separately reported) for L4-L5 and L5-S1 spondylolisthesis with axial mechanical back pain and worsening neurogenic claudication and/or radiculopathy (extremity symptoms) refractory to nonoperative treatment. This more extensive decompression is beyond the typical dissection needed to complete the interbody arthrodesis approach and intervention at each level. [**Note:** This is an add-on service. Only consider the additional work related to bilateral laminectomy with decompression of the cauda equina and/or nerve root(s)].

## Description of Procedure (63053)

After bony and soft tissue resection and exposure of the L4-L5 and L5-S1 disc spaces for the interbody access and preparation for arthrodesis is completed (separately reported), along with the decompression of neural elements at the L4-L5 interspace (separately reported), turn attention to the additional bone and nervous system work required for decompression of the L5-S1 interspace, beyond what is required to access the disc space for the interbody arthrodesis. Remove additional portions of the laminae at the L5 and S1 vertebral segments with the drill or bone-biting instruments and resect the inferior and superior facets. Expand the neural foramina with bone-biting instruments. Dissect and completely remove the ligamentum flavum off the dura to allow for decompression and mobilization of the neural elements. Confirm the neural elements are mobilized and decompressed. Document the additional work in the patient's medical record.

## Incision

▶(63194, 63195 have been deleted)◀

▶(63196 has been deleted)◀

▲ **63197**  Laminectomy with cordotomy, with section of both spinothalamic tracts, 1 stage, thoracic

▶(63198, 63199 have been deleted)◀

### Rationale

To ensure the CPT code set reflects current clinical practice, codes 63194, *Laminectomy with cordotomy, with section of 1 spinothalamic tract, 1 stage; cervical;* 63195, *Laminectomy with cordotomy, with section of 1 spinothalamic tract, 1 stage; thoracic;* 63196, *Laminectomy with cordotomy, with section of both spinothalamic tracts, 1 stage; cervical;* 63198, *Laminectomy with cordotomy with section of both spinothalamic tracts, 2 stages within 14 days; cervical;* and 63199, *Laminectomy with cordotomy with section of both spinothalamic tracts, 2 stages within 14 days; thoracic,* have been deleted due to low utilization.

Code 63197 was previously a child code of code 63196. With the deletion of code 63196, code 63197 has been revised as a stand-alone code. Parenthetical notes have been added to indicate that codes 63194-63196, 63198, and 63199 have been deleted.

# Extracranial Nerves, Peripheral Nerves, and Autonomic Nervous System

## Introduction/Injection of Anesthetic Agent (Nerve Block), Diagnostic or Therapeutic

### Somatic Nerves

**64400**    Injection(s), anesthetic agent(s) and/or steroid; trigeminal nerve, each branch (ie, ophthalmic, maxillary, mandibular)

**64455**        plantar common digital nerve(s) (eg, Morton's neuroma)

(Do not report 64455 in conjunction with 64632)

(64470-64476 have been deleted. To report, see 64490-64495)

**+ 64484**        transforaminal epidural, with imaging guidance (fluoroscopy or CT), lumbar or sacral, each additional level (List separately in addition to code for primary procedure)

(Use 64484 in conjunction with 64483)

(64479-64484 are unilateral procedures. For bilateral procedures, report 64479, 64483 with modifier 50. Report add-on codes 64480, 64484 twice, when performed bilaterally. Do not report modifier 50 in conjunction with 64480, 64484)

▶(Imaging guidance [fluoroscopy or CT] and any injection of contrast are inclusive components of 64479-64484. Imaging guidance and localization are required for the performance of 64479-64484)◀

### Rationale

Prior to 2022, the parenthetical note following code 64455 was misplaced as it did not reference code 64455. Therefore, it has been relocated to more appropriately follow code 64484.

## Neurostimulators (Peripheral Nerve)

▲ **64568**    Open implantation of cranial nerve (eg, vagus nerve) neurostimulator electrode array and pulse generator

(Do not report 64568 in conjunction with 61885, 61886, 64570)

**64569**    Revision or replacement of cranial nerve (eg, vagus nerve) neurostimulator electrode array, including connection to existing pulse generator

(Do not report 64569 in conjunction with 64570 or 61888)

(For replacement of pulse generator, use 61885)

**64570**    Removal of cranial nerve (eg, vagus nerve) neurostimulator electrode array and pulse generator

(Do not report 64570 in conjunction with 61888)

(For laparoscopic implantation, revision, replacement, or removal of vagus nerve blocking neurostimulator electrode array and/or pulse generator at the esophagogastric junction, see 0312T-0317T)

▲ **64575**    Open implantation of neurostimulator electrode array; peripheral nerve (excludes sacral nerve)

▲ **64580**        neuromuscular

▲ **64581**        sacral nerve (transforaminal placement)

● **64582**    Open implantation of hypoglossal nerve neurostimulator array, pulse generator, and distal respiratory sensor electrode or electrode array

● **64583**    Revision or replacement of hypoglossal nerve neurostimulator array and distal respiratory sensor electrode or electrode array, including connection to existing pulse generator

▶(Do not report 64583 in conjunction with 64582, 64584)◀

▶(For replacement of pulse generator, use 61886)◀

▶(For revision or replacement of either the hypoglossal nerve stimulator electrode array or distal respiratory sensor, use modifier 52)◀

● **64584**    Removal of hypoglossal nerve neurostimulator array, pulse generator, and distal respiratory sensor electrode or electrode array

▶(Do not report 64584 in conjunction with 61888, 64582, 64583)◀

▶(For removal of one or two components of the hypoglossal nerve stimulator electrode array, pulse generator, or distal respiratory sensor, use modifier 52)◀

### Rationale

Category III codes 0466T-0468T have been deleted, and Category I codes 64582-64584 have been established to report hypoglossal nerve stimulation services. Parenthetical notes have also been deleted, added, and revised throughout the Surgery, Medicine, and Category III sections. In addition, codes 64568, 64575, 64580, and 64581 have been revised for consistency in language with the new codes.

Codes 64582-64584 have been established to identify open implantation, revision or replacement, and removal services for hypoglossal nerve stimulator systems. These procedures differ from the procedures described by the Category III codes (0466T-0468T) that were previously used to report chest wall respiratory sensor electrode or electrode array services.

Codes 0466T-0468T were originally added because they represented the effort of inserting, revising, or removing neurostimulator sensor electrodes or electrode arrays for chest wall nerve stimulation. However, the new Category I codes (64582-64584) do identify the effort to implant a neurostimulator system for the hypoglossal nerve that includes both sensor components and stimulation components.

Although the hypoglossal nerve is considered a cranial nerve for which codes exist (61885, 61886, 61888), the work necessary for placing a hypoglossal nerve stimulator system is more extensive. This is because work for hypoglossal nerve placements requires more dissection of the nerve to identify the branches that protrude the tongue. The new Category I codes (64582-64584) capture the extra service performed when placing the inspiratory sensor, as well as its replacement or removal. As a result, these codes appropriately represent the total effort necessary to report the services for these neurostimulation services.

Code 64582 is used to report the open insertion of a hypoglossal nerve neurostimulator system. This includes the work of implanting neurostimulator array, the pulse generator, and sensor electrode or electrode array.

Code 64583 is used to report the revision or replacement services performed for both the hypoglossal nerve stimulator array and the distal respiratory sensor electrode or electrode array. It includes any efforts necessary to attach the arrays to an existing pulse generator.

Code 64584 is used to report the efforts necessary to remove the entirety of the hypoglossal nerve neurostimulator system.

Parenthetical notes have been added to direct users on the appropriate reporting of these services, such as when only one hypoglossal nerve stimulator electrode array or respiratory sensor electrode or electrode array is revised or replaced, or when individual components of the neurostimulator system are removed, modifier 52 should be used either in conjunction with the revision or replacement (64583) or with the removal (64584) code.

Parenthetical notes have also been added to direct users on the appropriate reporting of replacement or revision services performed for the chest components of the system (ie, pulse generator). Exclusionary parenthetical notes have been added to restrict reporting any of these complete services together with each other. In addition, an exclusionary parenthetical note has been added to restrict reporting the removal of the complete

neurostimulator system (64584) in conjunction with removal of just the pulse generator (61888).

Other changes have also been made to clarify the reporting of these services and related services. To accommodate the removal of the previous Category III codes and eliminate confusion regarding reporting chest wall sensor electrodes or electrode arrays, all references to the insertion, revision or replacement, and removal of the chest wall sensors have been deleted.

In addition, codes 64568, 64575, 64580, and 64581 have been editorially revised with the replacement of the term "Incision for" with the term "Open" to match the language used for similar services.

This update has also been incorporated in illustrations included within the code set for visual instruction. The illustration titled, "Implantation Neurostimulator Electrodes, Cranial Nerve (Vagus Nerve Stimulation) 64568-64570," has been revised with the addition of the term "Open" to the title. The illustration titled, "Implantation of Sacral Nerve Neurostimulator," has been revised with the replacement of the term "Incisional" with the term "Open" in the title.

## Clinical Example (64582)

A 46-year-old male with moderate to severe obstructive sleep apnea presents after failing positive airway pressure (PAP) therapy. Examination shows base of tongue airway collapse without complete concentric collapse at the palate.

## Description of Procedure (64582)

Make an incision in the neck and bring it through the platysma and deep fascia. Raise the subplatysmal flaps and identify and retract the submandibular gland. Identify and preserve the lingual nerve and marginal mandibular nerve. Take care to achieve meticulous hemostasis to avoid injuries to these, as well as the contents of the carotid sheath. Identify the posterior belly of the digastric muscle and identify the carotid artery through palpation. Identify the hypoglossal nerve by dissecting through the deep cervical fascia and following it distally until the branch(s) that extrudes the tongue is identified through electrical stimulation. A microscope is typically used to identify these distal branches. Attach the stimulatory array to these distal branch(s) and secure the stimulatory array to the digastric muscle. Make an upper chest incision and create a pocket. Bury the pulse generator in the created pocket and sew it to the pectoralis muscle. Make a tunnel between the hypoglossal lead and the upper chest incision. Make a horizontal incision in the lateral chest wall. Take the incision through the skin and subcutaneous tissue until the serratus anterior and pectoralis major muscles are identified. Proceed with dissection between these structures to the sixth intercostal space, identifying external and internal intercostal muscles. Extend blunt dissection between the intercostal muscles, avoiding the neurovascular bundle. Place a sensor lead between the intercostal muscles and secure it with multiple permanent sutures to the fascia overlying the chest wall. Create a subcutaneous tunnel to connect the sensor-lead incision to the generator pocket. Attach the sensor lead to the generator and verify the respiratory sensing. Reposition the sensor lead if the sensor waveform is not adequate. Irrigate all sites. Close the surgical incisions in a layered fashion and apply dressings.

## Clinical Example (64583)

A 48-year-old male, who underwent placement of a hypoglossal nerve stimulator, develops a malfunctioning device. He undergoes replacement of the hypoglossal nerve neurostimulator electrode array, pulse generator, and distal respiratory sensor electrode or electrode array.

## Description of Procedure (64583)

Make incisions to access the stimulator array, chest wall sensor, and generator sites. Proceed with dissection to the sensor lead placed between the intercostal muscles. Once identified, remove the sensor and dissect its lead from its subcutaneous tunnel to the generator pocket. Detach and remove the old sensor lead from the generator. Remove the old generator after it is disconnected from the stimulator array. Carefully dissect the stimulator array free of the hypoglossal nerve and replace it with a new stimulator array that is attached to the distal hypoglossal branches that only protrude into the tongue as identified through direct stimulation. A microscope is typically utilized to visualize these distal branches. Place a new respiratory sensor into the intercostal muscles and place a new generator into the previously created generator pocket. Attach both the new respiratory sensor and new stimulator array to the pulse generator and test the system to ensure functional integrity. Irrigate the wounds. Close the surgical incisions in a layered fashion and apply dressings.

## Clinical Example (64584)

A 48-year-old male, who underwent placement of a hypoglossal nerve stimulator, develops an intolerance to the system. He undergoes removal of the hypoglossal nerve neurostimulator electrode array, pulse generator, and distal respiratory sensor electrode or electrode array.

## Description of Procedure (64584)

Make incisions to access the stimulator array, chest wall sensor, and generator sites. Proceed with dissection to the

sensor lead placed between the intercostal muscles. Once identified, remove the sensor and dissect its lead from its subcutaneous tunnel to the generator pocket. Detach and remove the old sensor lead from the generator. Remove the old generator after it is disconnected from the stimulator array. Carefully dissect the stimulator array free of the hypoglossal nerve. Irrigate the wounds. Close the surgical incisions in a layered fashion and apply dressings.

# Destruction by Neurolytic Agent (eg, Chemical, Thermal, Electrical or Radiofrequency), Chemodenervation

### Somatic Nerves

**# 64625** Radiofrequency ablation, nerves innervating the sacroiliac joint, with image guidance (ie, fluoroscopy or computed tomography)

(Do not report 64625 in conjunction with 64635, 77002, 77003, 77012, 95873, 95874)

(For radiofrequency ablation, nerves innervating the sacroiliac joint, with ultrasound, use 76999)

(For bilateral procedure, report 64625 with modifier 50)

**#● 64628** Thermal destruction of intraosseous basivertebral nerve, including all imaging guidance; first 2 vertebral bodies, lumbar or sacral

**#+● 64629** each additional vertebral body, lumbar or sacral (List separately in addition to code for primary procedure)

▶(Use 64629 in conjunction with 64628)◀

▶(Do not report 64628, 64629 in conjunction with 77003, 77012)◀

**64611** Chemodenervation of parotid and submandibular salivary glands, bilateral

(Report 64611 with modifier 52 if fewer than four salivary glands are injected)

**64628** Code is out of numerical sequence. See 64610-64612

**64629** Code is out of numerical sequence. See 64610-64612

**# 64633** Destruction by neurolytic agent, paravertebral facet joint nerve(s), with imaging guidance (fluoroscopy or CT); cervical or thoracic, single facet joint

## Rationale

Two codes (64628, 64629) have been added to the Somatic Nerve subsection to describe a new surgical procedure: thermal destruction of the intraosseous basivertebral nerve. Parenthetical instructional notes have

★ = Telemedicine   ✚ = Add-on code   ✗ = FDA approval pending   # = Resequenced code   ⊘ = Modifier 51 exempt

also been added to provide guidance on the appropriate reporting of these codes when these procedures are performed.

Codes 64628 and 64629 have been added to describe procedures that may provide effective relief for patients suffering from certain types of chronic low-back pain.

Code 64628 describes the primary procedure and is intended to describe the thermal destruction of intraosseous basivertebral nerve for the first two vertebral bodies at the lumbar or sacral level.

Code 64629 describes the add-on procedure, when performed. Thus, code 64629 describes the thermal destruction of the intraosseous basivertebral nerve for each additional vertebral body, when performed.

Codes 64628 and 64629 include all imaging guidance and should not be reported in conjunction with Radiology codes 77003 and 77012. An exclusionary parenthetical note has been added following code 64629 to reflect this instruction. Add-on code 64629 should be reported in conjunction with primary code 64628, and a parenthetical note has been added to reflect this reporting instruction.

In accordance with the establishment of these new procedures (64628, 64629) and to aid users in locating the new codes, an additional cross-reference parenthetical note has been added in the Musculoskeletal section to direct users to the new codes to report thermal destruction of the intraosseous basivertebral nerve.

## Clinical Example (64628)

A 50-year-old female, who failed a minimum of 6 months of traditional conservative therapies including active physical therapy or chiropractic care, spinal injections, and/or medications, presents with more than 6 months of chronic axial low-back pain. MRI demonstrates degenerative disc disease at L5-S1 with associated endplate changes consistent with Modic Type I in the L5 and S1 vertebral bodies.

## Description of Procedure (64628)

Make an incision and insert an introducer trocar with a mallet to access the vertebral body via a transpedicular approach. After breaching the posterior vertebral body with the trocar at the junction of the pedicle and vertebral body, use a curved cannula assembly within the vertebral body to navigate toward the basivertebral nerve, which is located in the posterior one-third of the vertebral body. Use a straight channeling stylet if needed to extend the channel to the midline location of the basivertebral nerve. Remove the straight channeling stylet. Once accurate placement is confirmed, insert a bipolar probe that is connected to the radiofrequency

generator into the posterior half of the vertebral body. Apply radiofrequency energy for 15 minutes to destroy the basivertebral nerve. Access the next vertebral body sequentially using the same technique with additional instrumentation required. Apply energy for 15 minutes to destroy the basivertebral nerve in this adjacent vertebral body. At the completion of the procedure, remove all instruments and close the incisions. (Report code 64628 for the destruction of the intraosseous basivertebral nerve within two consecutive vertebral bodies [1 motion segment] and code 64629 for each additional destruction of intraosseous basivertebral nerve within each additional vertebral body.)

## Clinical Example (64629)

A 50-year-old female, who failed a minimum of 6 months of traditional conservative therapies including active physical therapy or chiropractic care, spinal injections, and/or medications, presents with more than 6 months of chronic axial low-back pain. MRI demonstrates degenerative disc disease at L5-S1 with associated endplate changes consistent with Modic Type I in the L5 and S1 vertebral bodies. [**Note:** This is an add-on service. Only consider the additional work related to the primary procedure.]

## Description of Procedure (64629)

Make an incision and insert an introducer trocar with a mallet to access the vertebral body via a transpedicular approach. After breaching the posterior vertebral body with the trocar at the junction of the pedicle and vertebral body, use a curved cannula assembly within the vertebral body and navigate toward the basivertebral nerve, which is located in the posterior one-third of the vertebral body. Use a straight channeling stylet if needed to extend the channel to the midline location of the basivertebral nerve. Remove the straight channeling stylet. Once accurate placement is confirmed, insert a bipolar probe that is connected to the radiofrequency generator into the posterior half of the vertebral body. Apply radiofrequency energy for 15 minutes to destroy the basivertebral nerve. Access the next vertebral body sequentially using the same technique with additional instrumentation required. Apply energy for 15 minutes to destroy the basivertebral nerve in this adjacent vertebral body. At the completion of the procedure, remove all instruments and close the incisions. (Report code 64628 for the destruction of the intraosseous basivertebral nerve within two consecutive vertebral bodies [1 motion segment] and code 64629 for each additional destruction of intraosseous basivertebral nerve within each additional vertebral body.)

# Eye and Ocular Adnexa

## Anterior Segment

### Anterior Sclera

#### Excision

**66174** Transluminal dilation of aqueous outflow canal; without retention of device or stent

▶(Do not report 66174 in conjunction with 65820)◀

---

### Rationale

To provide clarity in reporting, a new parenthetical instructional note has been added following code 66174. After a review by the AMA/Specialty Society Relative Value Scale (RVS) Update Committee (RUC) Relativity Assessment Workgroup (RAW) of the utilization of codes 66174 and 65820, *Goniotomy,* it was determined that these procedures should not be reported together because code 65820 is considered an inherent component of code 66174. This guidance has been added in a new exclusionary parenthetical note following code 66174 to clarify that these services should not be reported together.

---

### Intraocular Lens Procedures

**66982** Extracapsular cataract removal with insertion of intraocular lens prosthesis (1-stage procedure), manual or mechanical technique (eg, irrigation and aspiration or phacoemulsification), complex, requiring devices or techniques not generally used in routine cataract surgery (eg, iris expansion device, suture support for intraocular lens, or primary posterior capsulorrhexis) or performed on patients in the amblyogenic developmental stage; without endoscopic cyclophotocoagulation

(For complex extracapsular cataract removal with concomitant endoscopic cyclophotocoagulation, use 66987)

▶(For complex extracapsular cataract removal with intraocular lens implant and concomitant intraocular aqueous drainage device by internal approach, use 66989)◀

(For insertion of ocular telescope prosthesis including removal of crystalline lens, use 0308T)

#● **66989** with insertion of intraocular (eg, trabecular meshwork, supraciliary, suprachoroidal) anterior segment aqueous drainage device, without extraocular reservoir, internal approach, one or more

▶(For complex extracapsular cataract removal with intraocular lens implant without concomitant aqueous drainage device, use 66982)◀

▶(For insertion of intraocular anterior segment drainage device into the trabecular meshwork without concomitant cataract removal with intraocular lens implant, use 0671T)◀

# **66987** with endoscopic cyclophotocoagulation

(For complex extracapsular cataract removal without endoscopic cyclophotocoagulation, use 66982)

(For insertion of ocular telescope prosthesis including removal of crystalline lens, use 0308T)

**66983** Intracapsular cataract extraction with insertion of intraocular lens prosthesis (1 stage procedure)

(Do not report 66983 in conjunction with 0308T)

**66984** Extracapsular cataract removal with insertion of intraocular lens prosthesis (1 stage procedure), manual or mechanical technique (eg, irrigation and aspiration or phacoemulsification); without endoscopic cyclophotocoagulation

(For complex extracapsular cataract removal, use 66982)

(For extracapsular cataract removal with concomitant endoscopic cyclophotocoagulation, use 66988)

▶(For extracapsular cataract removal with concomitant intraocular aqueous drainage device by internal approach, use 66989)◀

(For insertion of ocular telescope prosthesis including removal of crystalline lens, use 0308T)

▶(For insertion of intraocular anterior segment drainage device into the trabecular meshwork without concomitant cataract removal with intraocular lens implant, use 0671T)◀

#● **66991** with insertion of intraocular (eg, trabecular meshwork, supraciliary, suprachoroidal) anterior segment aqueous drainage device, without extraocular reservoir, internal approach, one or more

▶(For extracapsular cataract removal with intraocular lens implant without concomitant aqueous drainage device, use 66984)◀

▶(For insertion of intraocular anterior segment drainage device into the trabecular meshwork without concomitant cataract removal with intraocular lens implant, use 0671T)◀

# **66988** with endoscopic cyclophotocoagulation

(For extracapsular cataract removal without endoscopic cyclophotocoagulation, use 66984)

(For complex extracapsular cataract removal with endoscopic cyclophotocoagulation, use 66987)

(For insertion of ocular telescope prosthesis, including removal of crystalline lens, use 0308T)

★ = Telemedicine   ✚ = Add-on code   ✗ = FDA approval pending   # = Resequenced code   ⊘ = Modifier 51 exempt

**66989**     Code is out of numerical sequence. See 66940-66984

**66991**     Code is out of numerical sequence. See 66983-66986

## Rationale

Category III codes 0191T and 0376T have been deleted, and new Category III code 0671T and Category I codes 66989 and 66991 have been added to report various insertion procedures for the placement of an anterior segment aqueous drainage device into the trabecular meshwork without an external reservoir. New guidelines and parenthetical notes have also been added to provide instruction regarding the intent and use of the new codes.

The AMA RAW recommended a review of codes 0191T and 0376T due to increased utilization. As a result of this review and the Food and Drug Administration (FDA) approval of the procedure described by codes 0191T and 0376T when performed with the removal of cataracts, these Category III codes have been deleted to accommodate (1) the addition of code 66989 to identify complex insertion of the drainage device with cataract removal, (2) the addition of code 66991 to identify extracapsular cataract removal with intraocular lens implant and concomitant intraocular aqueous drainage device by internal approach, and (3) the addition of code 0671T to identify the insertion of the drainage device only without removal of cataracts.

New Category III code 0671T is intended to be used in place of the deleted Category III codes and is only reported once regardless of the number of devices implanted.

Code 66989 describes a complex version of the procedure described by code 66991 because code 66989 also includes extracapsular cataract removal with insertion of intraocular lens prosthesis, which requires the use of devices or techniques that are not generally used in routine cataract surgery, such as use of an iris-expansion device, suture support for the intraocular lens, or primary posterior capsulorrhexis. The complex procedure could also involve the performance of the procedure on patients in the amblyogenic developmental stage. This language is noted in the parent portion of the descriptor for code 66989.

To provide further instruction regarding the intent and use of all three codes, new parenthetical notes have been added that provide input regarding the appropriate code to use for each specific procedure. An exclusionary parenthetical note has also been added following code 0671T to restrict the reporting of multiple services together (ie, restricts the use of code 0671T in conjunction with codes 66989 and 66991).

An illustration in the Category III section that references the deleted codes has been revised to accommodate the noted deletions and addition of new code 0671T.

## Clinical Example (66989)

A 74-year-old male, who requires cataract removal and replacement with an intraocular lens (IOL), presents with a cortical cataract severe enough to no longer allow vision for reading. He has a history of use of systemic medications, which cause floppy iris syndrome, and the intraoperative use of an iris retraction device is planned. In addition, his increased intraocular pressure (IOP) is not well controlled on two topical medications so placement of an aqueous drainage device through an internal approach is planned at the same time.

## Description of Procedure (66989)

Insert a lid speculum. Position the microscope. Make a side-port incision 45° to 90° away from the intended site of the surgical incision. Fill the anterior chamber with a viscoelastic. Create a temporal multiplanar limbal corneal incision into the anterior chamber. Make four additional 1-mm incisions at the limbus to place iris hooks in a diamond pattern around the eye. One by one, insert the iris hooks into the incisions and manipulate to retract the iris. Reposition the iris hooks in the areas of loose zonules to better support the iris and the capsule during subsequent steps of cataract removal. Enter the eye through the main incision with a sharp bent needle to open the anterior capsule, followed by forceps to fashion a circular opening in the anterior capsule of the cataract. Insert a cannula into the eye to perform hydrodissection by injecting balanced salt solution between the lens cortex and capsule, loosening the nuclear and cortical layers of the lens in the process, while maintaining the integrity of the capsule. Hydrodelineate as needed by injecting balanced salt solution between the lens cortex and nucleus. Inject additional viscoelastic into the anterior chamber of the eye prior to phacoemulsification. Check the function of the phacoemulsification handpiece and the machine settings. Remove bubbles by tapping the handpiece with irrigation on. Insert the phacoemulsification tip into the eye and a second instrument through the side-port incision. Using both hands and foot-actuated phacoemulsification pedal, carefully perform phacoemulsification with simultaneous aspiration of the lens nuclear material. Rotate and disassemble the lens to avoid inadvertent trauma to the cornea, lens capsule, or iris. Add viscoelastic as needed to maintain a safe working space. Remove the phacoemulsification tip and the second instrument from the eye once all the nuclear material has been removed. Introduce an irrigation and aspiration tip into the eye to aspirate the remainder of the cortical lens material. Then carefully vacuum and polish the interior surface of the thin lens capsule to avoid future secondary membrane formation.

Assess the integrity of the capsule and zonules and determine how much additional support the capsular bag and IOL will require. Enlarge incisions and create scleral flaps as needed for the IOL and support system chosen. Insert and suture a capsular tension ring or segment as needed. While maintaining traction on the eye via the side-port incision, insert the tip of the IOL-injection device into the main incision and place the IOL in the eye. Once in the eye, allow the IOL to unfold without damage to the cornea. Properly position and center the IOL using a lens hook. Suture the IOL and/or capsular bag and zonular complex as needed. Remove the iris hooks one by one. Perform a peripheral iridectomy as necessary. Deepen the anterior chamber with additional viscoelastic. Apply viscoelastic to the corneal surface, apply a goniolens, and locate collector channels to identify sites for drainage device insertion. Lift the patient's head off the head rest and rotate 30° away from the surgeon. Rotate the operating microscope 30° toward the surgeon. Re-apply the goniolens and adjust the microscope to visualize the chamber angle and nasal trabecular meshwork. Insert the drainage device inserter through the main incision and across the anterior chamber toward the nasal chamber angle. Retract the protective sleeve. Position the drainage device at the trabecular meshwork and insert into Schlemm's canal. Release the device from the injector. Tap the tip of the device to seat it firmly. Observe for blood reflux. Remove the injector and deepen the chamber with additional viscoelastic as needed. Re-insert the injector, retract the protective sleeve, and position and insert the second drainage device approximately 2 clock-hours from the first. Tap to seat firmly, observe for blood reflux, and remove the injector. Reposition the head and microscope vertically. Irrigate excess viscoelastic from the surface of the cornea. Reposition the IOL. Aspirate viscoelastic from the anterior chamber with the irrigation and aspiration handpiece. Inject a miotic drug into the anterior chamber to produce pupillary miosis as needed. Reform the eye with balanced salt solution and adjust the intraocular pressure to a physiologic range. Test the incisions for leaks and hydrate or suture any that leak. Remove the lid speculum. Place an antibiotic ointment on the eye as necessary. Place a soft patch and a rigid shield on the operative eye.

## Clinical Example (66991)

A 69-year-old female with a posterior subcapsular cataract, who is no longer able to drive, requires cataract removal and replacement with an IOL. In addition, her increased IOP is not well controlled so placement of an aqueous drainage device through an internal approach is planned for the same time.

## Description of Procedure (66991)

Insert a lid speculum. Position the microscope. Make a side-port incision 45° to 90° away from the intended site of the surgical incision. Fill the anterior chamber with a viscoelastic. Create a temporal multiplanar limbal corneal incision into the anterior chamber. Enter the eye through the main incision with a sharp bent needle to open the anterior capsule, followed by forceps to fashion a circular opening in the anterior capsule of the cataract. Insert a cannula into the eye to perform hydrodissection by injecting balanced salt solution between the lens cortex and capsule, loosening the nuclear and cortical layers of the lens in the process, while maintaining the integrity of the capsule. Hydrodelineate as needed by injecting fluid between the lens cortex and nucleus. Inject additional viscoelastic into the anterior chamber prior to phacoemulsification. Check the function of the phacoemulsification handpiece and the machine settings. Remove bubbles by tapping the handpiece with irrigation on. Insert the phacoemulsification tip into the eye and a second instrument through the side-port incision. Using both hands and the foot-actuated phacoemulsification pedal, carefully perform phacoemulsification with simultaneous aspiration of the lens nuclear material. Rotate and disassemble the lens to avoid inadvertent trauma to the cornea, lens capsule, or iris. Add viscoelastic as needed to maintain a safe working space. Remove the phacoemulsification tip and second instrument from the eye. Introduce an irrigation and aspiration tip into the eye to aspirate the remainder of the cortical lens material. Then carefully vacuum and polish the interior surface of the thin lens capsule to avoid future secondary membrane formation.

Adjust the size of the incision as needed to accommodate the IOL. While maintaining traction on the eye via the side-port incision, insert the tip of the IOL injection device into the main incision and place the IOL in the eye. Once in the eye, allow the IOL to unfold without damage to the cornea. Properly position and center the IOL into the capsular bag using a lens hook. Deepen the anterior chamber with additional viscoelastic. Apply viscoelastic to the corneal surface, apply a goniolens, and locate collector channels to identify sites for drainage device insertion. Lift the patient's head off the head rest and rotate 30° away from the surgeon. Rotate the operating microscope 30° toward the surgeon. Re-apply the goniolens and adjust the microscope to visualize the chamber angle and nasal trabecular meshwork. Insert the drainage device inserter through the main incision and across the anterior chamber towards the nasal chamber angle. Retract the protective sleeve. Position the drainage device at the trabecular meshwork and insert into Schlemm's canal. Release the device from the injector. Tap the tip of the device to seat it firmly. Observe for blood reflux. Remove the injector and deepen the chamber with additional viscoelastic as needed. Re-insert the injector, retract the protective sleeve, and position and insert the second drainage device approximately 2 clock-hours from the first. Tap to seat firmly, observe for blood reflux, and remove the injector and goniolens. Reposition the head and microscope vertically. Irrigate excess viscoelastic from the surface of the cornea. Reposition the IOL. Aspirate viscoelastic from the anterior chamber with the irrigation and aspiration handpiece. Inject a miotic drug into the anterior chamber to produce pupillary miosis as needed. Reform the eye with balanced salt solution and adjust the intraocular pressure to a physiologic range. Test the incisions for leaks and hydrate or suture any that leak. Remove the lid speculum. Place an antibiotic ointment on the eye as necessary. Place a soft patch and a rigid shield on the operative eye.

## Posterior Segment

## Retina or Choroid

### Prophylaxis

▲ **67141** Prophylaxis of retinal detachment (eg, retinal break, lattice degeneration) without drainage; cryotherapy, diathermy

▲ **67145** photocoagulation

### Rationale

Codes 67141 and 67145 have been revised to align with other retinal laser photocoagulation codes.

The AMA/RAW identified codes 67141 and 67145 for Medicare utilization screen of a code greater than 30,000 and never surveyed. In an effort to ensure codes 67141 and 67145 are being used properly, the descriptors have been revised by removing the number of sessions and removing "laser or xenon arc."

Along with these revisions, the prefatory guidelines for this section have also been deleted because the number of sessions has been removed from the code descriptors.

## Clinical Example (67141)

A 66-year-old male, who has a retinal tear with a vitreous hemorrhage without retinal detachment, has cryotherapy to the retina around the tear.

## Description of Procedure (67141)

Place a lid speculum in the eye. Re-examine the retina to localize the retinal tear and lattice degeneration. Place lubrication on the ocular surface and apply the cryopexy probe directly to the sclera overlying the retinal tear. Place multiple transscleral freezes with the cryopexy probe to surround the retinal tear and associated lattice degeneration while monitoring the freezes with the indirect ophthalmoscope. Reposition the patient's head

as needed throughout the treatment. Remove the lid speculum. Apply a topical ointment and place a patch over the eye.

## Clinical Example (67145)

A 72-year-old female, who has a retinal tear without a retinal detachment, has photocoagulation of the retina around the tear.

## Description of Procedure (67145)

Re-examine the retina to localize the tear and determine the extent of the treatment. Multiple rows of laser photocoagulation surrounding the retinal tear are applied with the indirect ophthalmoscope laser delivery system using scleral depression. Reposition the patient's head and eye during the treatment to visualize the entire extent of the pathology and ensure that it is completely surrounded.

## Conjunctiva

## Lacrimal System

### Repair

**68760** Closure of the lacrimal punctum; by thermocauterization, ligation, or laser surgery

**68761** by plug, each

▶(For insertion and removal of drug-eluting implant into lacrimal canaliculus for intraocular pressure, use 68841)◀

(For placement of drug-eluting insert under the eyelid[s], see 0444T, 0445T)

### Rationale

In accordance with the deletion of Category III code 0356T and the establishment of code 68841, the cross-reference parenthetical note following code 68761 has been revised to reflect these changes.

Refer to the codebook and the Rationale for code 68841 for a full discussion of these changes.

### Probing and/or Related Procedures

**68810** Probing of nasolacrimal duct, with or without irrigation;

(For bilateral procedure, report 68810 with modifier 50)

**68811** requiring general anesthesia

(For bilateral procedure, report 68811 with modifier 50)

**68815**      with insertion of tube or stent

(See also 92018)

(For bilateral procedure, report 68815 with modifier 50)

►(For insertion and removal of drug-eluting implant into lacrimal canaliculus for intraocular pressure, use 68841)◄

(For placement of drug-eluting insert under the eyelid[s], see 0444T, 0445T)

**68816**      with transluminal balloon catheter dilation

(Do not report 68816 in conjunction with 68810, 68811, 68815)

(For bilateral procedure, report 68816 with modifier 50)

**68840**      Probing of lacrimal canaliculi, with or without irrigation

● **68841**      Insertion of drug-eluting implant, including punctal dilation when performed, into lacrimal canaliculus, each

►(For placement of drug-eluting ocular insert under the eyelid[s], see 0444T, 0445T)◄

►(Report drug-eluting implant separately with 99070 or appropriate supply code)◄

## Rationale

Category III code 0356T has been converted to Category I code 68841. Code 68841 describes the insertion of a drug-eluting implant into the lacrimal canaliculus. The lacrimal canaliculus is a canal through which lacrimal fluid (tears) is drained from the lacrimal punctum to the lacrimal sac.

Drug-eluting implants are used to administer medication, such as for the treatment of pain and inflammation following cataract surgery, and are designed to dissolve on their own over time. The drug-eluting implant is inserted through the lacrimal punctum and into the canaliculus. It may be necessary to dilate the punctum to accommodate the insertion of the implant. Dilation of the punctum is included in code 68841, when performed.

Code 68841 is reported for each lacrimal canaliculus (ie, each eye) in which an implant is inserted. Therefore, if a drug-eluting implant is inserted into the lacrimal canaliculus of both eyes, code 68841 would be reported twice.

Supply of the implant is reported separately with code 99070 or the appropriate supply code. A cross-reference parenthetical note has been added following code 68841 directing users to Category III codes 0444T and 0445T for the placement of a drug-eluting ocular insert under the eyelid(s). An instructional parenthetical note has also been added instructing users to report the supply of the implant separately.

The cross-reference parenthetical note following code 68815 has also been revised to reflect these changes.

## Clinical Example (68841)

A 67-year-old female presents for cataract removal. A drug-eluting implant is placed in conjunction with the cataract removal.

## Description of Procedure (68841)

Insert a punctal dilator and advance into the canaliculus, dilating the punctum, then remove. Dry the punctum and surrounding tissue with a cotton-tipped applicator. Grasp the drug-eluting implant with forceps and insert it through the punctum into the canaliculus. Bury the tip of the implant below the surface of the punctum opening.

# Auditory System

## Middle Ear

### ►Osseointegrated Implants◄

►The following codes are for implantation of an osseointegrated implant into the skull. These devices treat hearing loss through surgical placement of an abutment or device into the skull that facilitates transduction of acoustic energy to be received by the better-hearing inner ear or both inner ears when the implant is coupled to a speech processor and vibratory element. This coupling may occur in a percutaneous or a transcutaneous fashion. Other reparative middle ear and mastoid procedures (69501-69676) may be performed for different indications and may be reported separately, when performed.◄

\#▲ **69714**      Implantation, osseointegrated implant, skull; with percutaneous attachment to external speech processor

►(69715 has been deleted. To report mastoidectomy performed at the same operative session as osseointegrated implant placement, revision, replacement, or removal, see 69501-69676)◄

\#● **69716**      with magnetic transcutaneous attachment to external speech processor

\#▲ **69717**      Revision or replacement (including removal of existing device), osseointegrated implant, skull; with percutaneous attachment to external speech processor

►(69718 has been deleted. To report mastoidectomy performed at the same operative session as osseointegrated implant placement, revision, replacement, or removal, see 69501-69676)◄

\#● **69719**      with magnetic transcutaneous attachment to external speech processor

#● **69726**   Removal, osseointegrated implant, skull; with percutaneous attachment to external speech processor

#● **69727**   with magnetic transcutaneous attachment to external speech processor

## Rationale

Two codes (69714, 69717) have been revised and four codes (69716, 69719, 69726, 69727) have been established to report the implantation of an osseointegrated implant into the skull.

Codes 69716 and 69719 have been added as child codes to codes 69714 and 69717 to report the magnetic transcutaneous attachment to an external speech processor for implantation or revision or replacement of an osseointegrated implant.

Code 69726 has been established to report the removal of an osseointegrated implant, and child code 69727 has been established to report the magnetic transcutaneous attachment to an external speech processor.

Codes 69714 and 69717 have been revised with the removal of the term "temporal bones" and the phrase "cochlear stimulator without mastoidectomy."

In addition, a new heading with new introductory guidelines have been added and codes 69714 and 69717 have been resequenced under this new subsection for osseointegrated implants. Codes 69715 and 69718 (and all related references) have been deleted, and two parenthetical notes have been added to guide users in the appropriate reporting of these services.

## Clinical Example (69714)

A 56-year-old male suffers from chronic otitis media resulting in otorrhea and mixed-hearing loss. He is unable to wear traditional hearing aids. Implantation of an osseointegrated bone-anchored device with a percutaneous attachment to an external speech processor is performed.

## Description of Procedure (69714)

Create an incision and meticulously dissect to the pericranium. Incise and dissect the pericranium away from the cranial bone to expose an area for implant placement. Drill a pilot guide hole through the cranium, and "instrument" the deep portion of the guide hole to ascertain the possible presence of dural contact and lack of sigmoid sinus exposure. Deepen the pilot hole, if necessary. Widen the final guide hole with spiral drilling to achieve a larger opening to receive the implant. Install the implanted fixture in the cranial bone to very specific torque settings. Secure the implanted fixture to the transcutaneous abutment. Thin the overlying flap and surrounding soft tissues to a maximal thickness to allow for transcutaneous attachment to the processor. Make a separate incision in the overlying skin of the flap to allow the percutaneous abutment to extend through the soft tissue flap. Irrigate the wound and obtain hemostasis. Close the wound in a layered fashion. Create a small bolster immediately surrounding the abutment and fix a locking cap to the abutment to keep the bolster in place and with appropriate pressure.

## Clinical Example (69716)

A 48-year-old male with left mixed-hearing loss seeks intervention for improved quality of life at work and socially. Placement of a magnetic transcutaneous bone-anchored hearing device is performed.

## Description of Procedure (69716)

Make an incision and meticulously dissect through the pericranium. Dissect subpericranially and create a subpericranial pocket for the implant coil and magnet. Identify and mark the area for the transducer using the template on the outer table of the skull in the region of the sinodural angle. Drill surgical guide and fixation holes, taking care not to penetrate the sigmoid sinus or the dura overlying the temporal lobe of the brain. Measure this area for appropriate depth to accommodate the fixation screw. Drill the skull overlying the sinodural angle to create a well in the bone to accommodate the transducer device, again staying just superficial to the dura and sigmoid sinus. Place the entire device, including the coil, magnet, and transducer portions, and then fix the device to the skull using the fixation screw to a specific torque setting. Carefully measure the thickness of the flap overlying the magnet and coil portion of the device and trim it to a specific thickness to allow for transcutaneous transmission. Irrigate the wound and obtain hemostasis. Close the wound in a layered fashion.

## Clinical Example (69717)

A 16-year-old female, who has chronic otitis media and conductive hearing loss with previous percutaneous bone-anchored implant, has chronic inflammation at the abutment site that has been unresponsive to medical therapy. The device is removed and a new device is placed at a different site.

## Description of Procedure (69717)

Create an incision and meticulously dissect to the pericranium. Perform a subpericranial dissection and remove the previous implant abutment. Drill the cranial bone surrounding the osseointegrated titanium fixture in the patient's skull around the implant. Remove the fixture. Thoroughly inspect the wound for the cause of the patient's original complication related to the implant.

Identify, template, and mark on the outer table of the skull the area for the new placement of the implant. Incise and dissect the pericranium away from the cranial bone to expose an area for implant placement. Drill a new pilot guide hole through the cranium, and "instrument" the deep portion of the guide hole to ascertain the possible presence of dural contact and lack of sigmoid sinus exposure. Deepen the pilot hole, if necessary. Widen the final guide hole with spiral drilling to achieve a larger opening to receive the implant. Install the implanted fixture in the cranial bone to very specific torque settings. Secure the implanted fixture to the transcutaneous abutment. Thin the overlying flap and surrounding soft tissues to a maximal thickness to allow for transcutaneous attachment to the processor. Make a separate incision in the overlying skin of the flap to allow the percutaneous abutment to extend through the soft tissue flap. Irrigate the wound and obtain hemostasis. Close the wound in a layered fashion. Create a small bolster immediately surrounding the abutment and fix a locking cap to the abutment to keep the small abutment bolster in place and with appropriate pressure.

## Clinical Example (69719)

A 59-year-old female with right mixed-hearing loss had previous placement of a magnetic transcutaneous bone-anchored implant. It worked well, but she has developed discomfort at the device site. The device is removed, and a new device is placed at a different site.

## Description of Procedure (69719)

Make an incision and meticulously dissect through the pericranium. Dissect subpericranially and remove the previous implant. Thoroughly inspect the wound for the cause of the patient's original complication related to the implant. Create a subpericranial pocket for the implant coil and magnet. Identify and mark the area for the transducer using the template on the outer table of the skull. Drill surgical guide and fixation holes, taking care not to penetrate the dura overlying the temporal lobe of the brain. Measure this area for appropriate depth to accommodate the fixation screw. Drill the skull to create a well in the bone to accommodate the transducer device, again staying just superficial to the dura. Place the entire device, including the coil, magnet, and transducer portions, and then fix the device to the skull using the fixation screw to a specific torque setting. Carefully measure the thickness of the flap overlying the magnet and coil portion of the device and then trim it to a specific thickness to allow for transcutaneous transmission. Irrigate the wound and obtain hemostasis. Close the wound in a layered fashion.

## Clinical Example (69726)

A 59-year-old female with a right mixed-hearing loss had previous placement of a percutaneous bone-anchored implant. It worked well, but she has developed discomfort at the device site. The device is removed without replacement.

## Description of Procedure (69726)

Make an incision and meticulously dissect through the pericranium. Dissect subpericranially and expose the previous implant. Drill the cranial bone surrounding the osseointegrated titanium fixture in the patient's skull around the implant. Thoroughly inspect the wound for the cause of the patient's original complication related to the implant. Irrigate the wound and obtain hemostasis. Debride the wound where the external abutment of the implant is debrided and closed, followed by closure of the linear incision anterior to the implant site in a layered fashion.

## Clinical Example (69727)

A 62-year-old male with right mixed-hearing loss had previous placement of a magnetic transcutaneous bone-anchored implant that worked well but has now become infected. The device is removed without replacement.

## Description of Procedure (69727)

Make an incision and meticulously dissect through the pericranium. Dissect subpericranially and expose the previous implant. Drill out the cranial bone surrounding the osseointegrated titanium transducer and the respective fixture screws in the patient's skull to free the implant. Thoroughly inspect the wound for the cause of the patient's original complication related to the implant. Irrigate the wound and obtain hemostasis. Close the wound in a layered fashion.

## Other Procedures

| | |
|---|---|
| 69714 | Code is out of numerical sequence. See 69670-69705 |
| 69716 | Code is out of numerical sequence. See 69670-69705 |
| 69717 | Code is out of numerical sequence. See 69670-69705 |
| 69719 | Code is out of numerical sequence. See 69670-69705 |
| **69720** | Decompression facial nerve, intratemporal; lateral to geniculate ganglion |
| **69725** | including medial to geniculate ganglion |
| 69726 | Code is out of numerical sequence. See 69670-69705 |
| 69727 | Code is out of numerical sequence. See 69670-69705 |

★ = Telemedicine   ✚ = Add-on code   𝗡 = FDA approval pending   # = Resequenced code   ⊘ = Modifier 51 exempt

# Radiology

## Summary of Additions, Deletions, and Revisions

The summary of changes shows the actual changes that have been made to the code descriptors.

New codes appear with a bullet (●) and are indicated as "Code added." Revised codes are preceded with a triangle (▲). Within revised codes, or if a code symbol has been deleted, the deleted language and code symbol appear with a ~~strikethrough~~, while new text appears underlined.

The ⚡ symbol is used to identify codes for vaccines that are pending FDA approval. The # symbol is used to identify codes that have been resequenced. CPT add-on codes are annotated by the ✚ symbol. The ⊘ symbol is used to identify codes that are exempt from the use of modifier 51. The ★ symbol is used to identify codes that may be used for reporting telemedicine services. The ⋈ symbol is used to identify a proprietary laboratory analyses (PLA) test that has an identical descriptor as another PLA test. A PLA code that satisfies Category I code criteria and has been accepted by the CPT Editorial Panel is annotated with the ⇅ symbol.

| Code | Description |
|---|---|
| ~~72275~~ | ~~Epidurography, radiological supervision and interpretation~~ |
| ▲75573 | Computed tomography, heart, with contrast material, for evaluation of cardiac structure and morphology in the setting of congenital heart disease (including 3D image postprocessing, assessment of left ventricular [LV] cardiac function, right ventricular [RV] structure and function and evaluation of ~~venous~~vascular structures, if performed) |
| ~~76101~~ | ~~Radiologic examination, complex motion (ie, hypercycloidal) body section (eg, mastoid polytomography), other than with urography; unilateral~~ |
| ~~76102~~ | ~~bilateral~~ |
| ●77089 | Code added |
| ●77090 | Code added |
| ●77091 | Code added |
| ●77092 | Code added |

# Radiology Guidelines (Including Nuclear Medicine and Diagnostic Ultrasound)

## Written Report(s)

A written report (eg, handwritten or electronic) signed by the interpreting individual should be considered an integral part of a radiologic procedure or interpretation.

With regard to CPT descriptors for imaging services, "images" must contain anatomic information unique to the patient for which the imaging service is provided. "Images" refer to those acquired in either an analog (ie, film) or digital (ie, electronic) manner.

## ►Foreign Body/Implant Definition◄

►An object intentionally placed by a physician or other qualified health care professional for any purpose (eg, diagnostic or therapeutic) is considered an implant. An object that is unintentionally placed (eg, trauma or ingestion) is considered a foreign body. If an implant (or part thereof) has moved from its original position or is structurally broken and no longer serves its intended purpose or presents a hazard to the patient, it qualifies as a foreign body for coding purposes, unless CPT coding instructions direct otherwise or a specific CPT code exists to describe the removal of that broken/moved implant.◄

### Rationale

The introductory language in the Radiology Guidelines section in the CPT code set has been updated to include a new heading and definition of "foreign body" and "implant." The definition clarifies the difference between an implant and a foreign body. It also specifies other conditions that qualify an implant as a foreign body for coding purposes. In addition, the definition provides guidance if other instructions or a specific CPT code exists to describe the removal of a broken or moved implant.

★ = Telemedicine   ✚ = Add-on code   ✚ = FDA approval pending   # = Resequenced code   ⊘ = Modifier 51 exempt

# Radiology

## Diagnostic Radiology (Diagnostic Imaging)

### Head and Neck

**70496**    Computed tomographic angiography, head, with contrast material(s), including noncontrast images, if performed, and image postprocessing

▶(For noninvasive arterial plaque analysis using software processing of data from computerized tomography angiography to quantify structure and composition of the vessel wall, including assessment for lipid-rich necrotic core plaque, see 0710T, 0711T, 0712T, 0713T)◀

**70498**    Computed tomographic angiography, neck, with contrast material(s), including noncontrast images, if performed, and image postprocessing

▶(For noninvasive arterial plaque analysis using software processing of data from computerized tomography angiography to quantify structure and composition of the vessel wall, including assessment for lipid-rich necrotic core plaque, see 0710T, 0711T, 0712T, 0713T)◀

### Rationale

In accordance with the establishment of Category III codes 0710T-0713T to report noninvasive arterial plaque analysis, cross-reference parenthetical notes have been added following codes 70496 and 70498 to direct users to the appropriate codes when reporting noninvasive arterial plaque analysis.

Refer to the codebook and the Rationale for Category III codes 0710T-0713T for a full discussion of these changes.

### Spine and Pelvis

**72191**    Computed tomographic angiography, pelvis, with contrast material(s), including noncontrast images, if performed, and image postprocessing

(Do not report 72191 in conjunction with 73706 or 75635. For CTA aorto-iliofemoral runoff, use 75635)

(Do not report 72191 in conjunction with 74175. For a combined computed tomographic angiography abdomen and pelvis study, use 74174)

▶(For noninvasive arterial plaque analysis using software processing of data from computerized tomography angiography to quantify structure and composition of the vessel wall, including assessment for lipid-rich necrotic core plaque, see 0710T, 0711T, 0712T, 0713T)◀

### Rationale

In accordance with the establishment of Category III codes 0710T-0713T to report noninvasive arterial plaque analysis, a cross-reference parenthetical note has been added following code 72191 to direct users to the appropriate code when reporting noninvasive arterial plaque analysis.

Refer to the codebook and the Rationale for Category III codes 0710T-0713T for a full discussion of these changes.

▶(72275 has been deleted. To report epidurography, radiological supervision and interpretation, see 62281, 62282, 62321, 62323, 62325, 62327, 64479, 64480, 64483, 64484)◀

**72285**    Discography, cervical or thoracic, radiological supervision and interpretation

### Rationale

To reflect current clinical practice, epidurography code 72275 and all related references to the code have been deleted from the CPT 2022 code set. Code 72275 was identified on an AMA/Specialty Society Relative Value Scale (RVS) Update Committee (RUC) Relativity Assessment Workgroup (RAW) high-volume growth screen. More recently, the utilization information from the AMA RVS database had indicated that radiology is no longer the dominant reporting provider. It is believed that the physician work originally represented by code 72275, when originally created, is now encompassed in other codes, and current use of code 72275 appears to be related to miscoding. For these reasons, code 72275 has been deleted.

To accommodate accurate reporting, several parenthetical notes have been added and revised to support the deletion of code 72275. A cross-reference parenthetical note now lists the appropriate codes (62281, 62282, 62321, 62323, 62325, 62327, 64479, 64480, 64483, 64484) to report epidurography and radiological supervision and interpretation. In addition, the exclusionary parenthetical note following code 22586 in the Anterior or Anterolateral Approach Technique subsection in the Spine (Vertebral Column) section has been revised to remove deleted code 72275.

Finally, the injection, drainage, or aspiration guidelines and parenthetical notes following codes 62263 and 62264 have been updated by removing reference to code 72275 for epidurography.

## Lower Extremities

**73706** Computed tomographic angiography, lower extremity, with contrast material(s), including noncontrast images, if performed, and image postprocessing

(For CTA aorto-iliofemoral runoff, use 75635)

▶(For noninvasive arterial plaque analysis using software processing of data from computerized tomography angiography to quantify structure and composition of the vessel wall, including assessment for lipid-rich necrotic core plaque, see 0710T, 0711T, 0712T, 0713T)◀

### Rationale

In accordance with the establishment of Category III codes 0710T-0713T to report noninvasive arterial plaque analysis, a cross-reference parenthetical note has been added following code 73706 to direct users to the appropriate code when reporting noninvasive arterial plaque analysis.

Refer to the codebook and the Rationale for Category III codes 0710T-0713T for a full discussion of these changes.

## Abdomen

**74175** Computed tomographic angiography, abdomen, with contrast material(s), including noncontrast images, if performed, and image postprocessing

(Do not report 74175 in conjunction with 73706 or 75635. For CTA aorto-iliofemoral runoff, use 75635)

(Do not report 74175 in conjunction with 72191. For a combined computed tomographic angiography abdomen and pelvis study, use 74174)

▶(For noninvasive arterial plaque analysis using software processing of data from computerized tomography angiography to quantify structure and composition of the vessel wall, including assessment for lipid-rich necrotic core plaque, see 0710T, 0711T, 0712T, 0713T)◀

### Rationale

In accordance with the establishment of Category III codes 0710T-0713T to report noninvasive arterial plaque analysis, a cross-reference parenthetical note has been added following code 74175 to direct users to the appropriate code when reporting noninvasive arterial plaque analysis.

Refer to the codebook and the Rationale for Category III codes 0710T-0713T for a full discussion of these changes.

## Heart

▲ **75573** Computed tomography, heart, with contrast material, for evaluation of cardiac structure and morphology in the setting of congenital heart disease (including 3D image postprocessing, assessment of left ventricular [LV] cardiac function, right ventricular [RV] structure and function and evaluation of vascular structures, if performed)

### Rationale

Code 75573 has been editorially revised with the removal of the term "venous" and the addition of the term "vascular" to the code descriptor. This change provides more clarity when any vascular evaluation is included, if performed. In addition, the terms "left ventricular" and "right ventricular" have been spelled out per CPT convention.

## Vascular Procedures

### Aorta and Arteries

**75635** Computed tomographic angiography, abdominal aorta and bilateral iliofemoral lower extremity runoff, with contrast material(s), including noncontrast images, if performed, and image postprocessing

(Do not report 75635 in conjunction with 72191, 73706, 74174 or 74175)

▶(For noninvasive arterial plaque analysis using software processing of data from computerized tomography angiography to quantify structure and composition of the vessel wall, including assessment for lipid-rich necrotic core plaque, see 0710T, 0711T, 0712T, 0713T)◀

## Rationale

In accordance with the establishment of Category III codes 0710T-0713T to report noninvasive arterial plaque analysis, a cross-reference parenthetical note has been added following code 75635 to direct users to the appropriate code when reporting noninvasive arterial plaque analysis.

Refer to the codebook and the Rationale for Category III codes 0710T-0713T for a full discussion of these changes.

**+ 75774**  Angiography, selective, each additional vessel studied after basic examination, radiological supervision and interpretation (List separately in addition to code for primary procedure)

(Use 75774 in addition to code for specific initial vessel studied)

(Do not report 75774 as part of diagnostic angiography of the extracranial and intracranial cervicocerebral vessels. It may be appropriate to report 75774 for diagnostic angiography of upper extremities and other vascular beds performed in the same session)

(For angiography, see 75600-75756)

(For catheterizations, see codes 36215-36248)

▶(For cardiac catheterization procedures, see 93452-93462, 93563-93568, 93593, 93594, 93595, 93596, 93597)◀

(For radiological supervision and interpretation of dialysis circuit angiography performed through existing access[es] or catheter-based arterial access, use 36901 with modifier 52)

## Rationale

In accordance with the deletion of codes 93531-93533 and the establishment of codes 93593-93597, the cross-reference parenthetical note following code 75774 has been revised to reflect these changes.

Refer to the codebook and the Rationale for codes 93593-93597 for a full discussion of these changes.

## Other Procedures

**76098**  Radiological examination, surgical specimen

▶(Do not report 76098 in conjunction with 19081-19086, 0694T)◀

▶(For 3-dimensional volumetric specimen imaging, use 0694T)◀

## Rationale

In accordance with the establishment of Category III code 0694T, a cross-reference parenthetical note has been added following code 76098 directing users to code 0694T for three dimensional (3D) volumetric specimen imaging. The exclusionary parenthetical note following code 76098 has also been revised with the addition of code 0694T.

Refer to the codebook and the Rationale for code 0694T for a full description of these changes.

▶(76101, 76102 have been deleted)◀

(For panoramic X-ray, use 70355)

(For nephrotomography, use 74415)

## Rationale

Codes 76101, *Radiologic examination, complex motion (ie, hypercycloidal) body section (eg, mastoid polytomography), other than with urography; unilateral,* and 76102, *Radiologic examination, complex motion (ie, hypercycloidal) body section (eg, mastoid polytomography), other than with urography; bilateral,* have been deleted due to low utilization. A parenthetical note has been added to indicate these deletions.

**76376**  3D rendering with interpretation and reporting of computed tomography, magnetic resonance imaging, ultrasound, or other tomographic modality with image postprocessing under concurrent supervision; not requiring image postprocessing on an independent workstation

(Use 76376 in conjunction with code[s] for base imaging procedure[s])

▶(Do not report 76376 in conjunction with 31627, 34839, 70496, 70498, 70544, 70545, 70546, 70547, 70548, 70549, 71275, 71555, 72159, 72191, 72198, 73206, 73225, 73706, 73725, 74174, 74175, 74185, 74261, 74262, 74263, 75557, 75559, 75561, 75563, 75565, 75571, 75572, 75573, 75574, 75635, 76377, 77046, 77047, 77048, 77049, 77061, 77062, 77063, 78012-78999, 93319, 93355, 0523T, 0559T, 0560T, 0561T, 0562T, 0623T, 0624T, 0625T, 0626T, 0633T, 0634T, 0635T, 0636T, 0637T, 0638T, 0710T, 0711T, 0712T, 0713T)◀

▶(For noninvasive arterial plaque analysis using software processing of data from computerized tomography angiography to quantify structure and composition of the vessel wall, including assessment for lipid-rich necrotic core plaque, see 0710T, 0711T, 0712T, 0713T)◀

Radiology 70010-79999

**76377**    requiring image postprocessing on an independent
workstation

(Use 76377 in conjunction with code[s] for base imaging
procedure[s])

▶(Do not report 76377 in conjunction with 34839, 70496,
70498, 70544, 70545, 70546, 70547, 70548, 70549,
71275, 71555, 72159, 72191, 72198, 73206, 73225,
73706, 73725, 74174, 74175, 74185, 74261, 74262,
74263, 75557, 75559, 75561, 75563, 75565, 75571,
75572, 75573, 75574, 75635, 76376, 77046, 77047,
77048, 77049, 77061, 77062, 77063, 78012-78999,
93319, 93355, 0523T, 0559T, 0560T, 0561T, 0562T, 0623T,
0624T, 0625T, 0626T, 0633T, 0634T, 0635T, 0636T, 0637T,
0638T, 0710T, 0711T, 0712T, 0713T)◀

(76376, 76377 require concurrent supervision of image
postprocessing 3D manipulation of volumetric data set
and image rendering)

▶(For noninvasive arterial plaque analysis using
software processing of data from computerized
tomography angiography to quantify structure and
composition of the vessel wall, including assessment for
lipid-rich necrotic core plaque, see 0710T, 0711T, 0712T,
0713T)◀

## Rationale

In accordance with the establishment of code 93319 for
reporting 3D imaging for the assessment of cardiac
structure and Category III codes 0710T-0713T to report
noninvasive arterial plaque analysis, the exclusionary
parenthetical notes following codes 76376 and 76377
have been revised and updated to include these new
codes. In addition, two cross-reference parenthetical
notes have been added following codes 76376 and 76377
to direct users to the appropriate codes when reporting
noninvasive arterial plaque analysis.

Refer to the codebook and the Rationale for codes 93319
and 0710T-0713T for a full discussion of these changes.

# Diagnostic Ultrasound

## Other Procedures

**76981**    Ultrasound, elastography; parenchyma (eg, organ)

**76982**    first target lesion

**+ 76983**    each additional target lesion (List separately in
addition to code for primary procedure)

(Use 76983 in conjunction with 76982)

(Report 76981 only once per session for evaluation of the
same parenchymal organ)

(To report shear wave liver elastography without imaging
use 91200)

(For evaluation of a parenchymal organ and lesion[s] in
the same parenchymal organ at the same session, report
only 76981)

▶(Do not report 76981, 76982, 76983 in conjunction with
0689T)◀

(Do not report 76983 more than two times per organ)

## Rationale

In accordance with the change in reporting non-
elastographic quantitative ultrasound tissue
characterization obtained without (0689T) and with
(0690T) diagnostic ultrasound examination of the same
anatomy, an exclusionary parenthetical note has been
added following code 76983.

Refer to the codebook and the Rationale for codes 0689T
and 0690T for a full discussion of these changes.

# Bone/Joint Studies

**77084**    Magnetic resonance (eg, proton) imaging, bone marrow
blood supply

**77085**    Code is out of numerical sequence. See 77080-77261

**77086**    Code is out of numerical sequence. See 77080-77261

● **77089**    Trabecular bone score (TBS), structural condition of the
bone microarchitecture; using dual X-ray absorptiometry
(DXA) or other imaging data on gray-scale variogram,
calculation, with interpretation and report on fracture-risk

▶(Do not report 77089 in conjunction with 77090, 77091,
77092)◀

● **77090**    technical preparation and transmission of data for
analysis to be performed elsewhere

● **77091**    technical calculation only

● **77092**    interpretation and report on fracture-risk only by other
qualified health care professional

▶(Do not report 77090, 77091, 77092 in conjunction with
77089)◀

★ = Telemedicine   ✚ = Add-on code   ✗ = FDA approval pending   # = Resequenced code   ⊘ = Modifier 51 exempt

## Rationale

Four new codes (77089-77092) have been established to report trabecular bone score (TBS) procedures. In addition, new parenthetical notes have been added to guide users in the appropriate reporting for these services.

TBS is a measurement of the structural condition of the bone microarchitecture. A high TBS value means the microarchitecture of the bone is dense, well-connected with little spaces between trabeculae, and fairly homogenously distributed. A low TBS value means the microarchitecture of the bone is incomplete and poorly connected with wide spaces between trabeculae and heterogeneously distributed. TBS can predict the risk of major osteoporotic fracture independently of bone mineral density (BMD) and clinical risk factors.

Code 77089 is used to report the TBS procedure. This comprehensive global code also includes using dual X-ray absorptiometry (DXA) or other imaging data on gray-scale variogram, calculation, and interpretation and report on fracture risk. Code 77090 is reported when the technical preparation and transmission of data for analysis is to be performed elsewhere. Code 77091 is reported for the technical calculation only. Code 77092 is reported for the interpretation and report on the fracture risk only by another qualified health care professional (QHP).

To assist in the appropriate reporting of this new series of codes, two exclusionary parenthetical notes have been added following codes 77089 and 77092. The first parenthetical note restricts reporting code 77089 with codes 77090-77092. The second parenthetical note restricts reporting codes 77090-77092 with code 77089.

## Clinical Example (77089)

A 69-year-old female, who had a previous bone-density study, presents with demonstrated osteopenia.

## Description of Procedure (77089)

Verify the previously acquired images (eg, dual-energy X-ray absorptiometry [DEXA], etc) are appropriate for trabecular bone score (TBS) analysis by ensuring the quality and that no anatomy or artifact is excluded. Open the images in the TBS software, separate from the picture archive and communication system (PACS), and verify that those images have transferred appropriately. Identify the appropriate population reference control. Review the images to determine the region to be included in calculations. Interpret the TBS data and compare the data to established norms, including risk analysis to determine if fracture risk analysis (reported separately) is indicated. Compare the results to previous studies. Compare the reported values to population standards. Transfer the TBS images to PACS. Dictate a report.

## Clinical Example (77090)

A 54-year-old female, who is postmenopausal, presents with current tobacco use, a family history of osteoporosis, and a suspicion of Type II diabetes.

## Description of Procedure (77090)

N/A

## Clinical Example (77091)

A 75-year-old male, who has a history of corticosteroids use, presents with bilateral knee osteoarthritis.

## Description of Procedure (77091)

The technologist prepares and manipulates the images for physician interpretation. The technologist performs a quality control check on the images in PACS and checks all images. In addition, the technologist may review the examination with the interpreting physician. The technologist scans the examination documents into PACS and completes the examination in the radiological information system to populate the images into the work queue.

## Clinical Example (77092)

A 60-year-old female presents with a history of breast cancer treated with anti-aromatase inhibitors.

## Description of Procedure (77092)

Verify the previously acquired images (eg, DEXA, etc) are appropriate for TBS analysis by ensuring the quality and that no anatomy or artifact is excluded. Open the images in the TBS software, separate from PACS, and verify that the images have transferred appropriately. Identify the appropriate population reference control. Review the images to determine the region to be included in calculations. Interpret the TBS data and compare the data to established norms, including risk analysis to determine if fracture risk analysis (reported separately) is indicated. Compare the results to previous studies. Compare the reported values to population standards. Transfer the TBS images to PACS. Dictate a report.

# Notes

# Pathology and Laboratory

## Summary of Additions, Deletions, and Revisions

The summary of changes shows the actual changes that have been made to the code descriptors.

New codes appear with a bullet (●) and are indicated as "Code added." Revised codes are preceded with a triangle (▲). Within revised codes, or if a code symbol has been deleted, the deleted language and code symbol appear with a ~~strikethrough~~, while new text appears <u>underlined</u>.

The ✗ symbol is used to identify codes for vaccines that are pending FDA approval. The # symbol is used to identify codes that have been resequenced. CPT add-on codes are annotated by the + symbol. The ⊘ symbol is used to identify codes that are exempt from the use of modifier 51. The ★ symbol is used to identify codes that may be used for reporting telemedicine services. The ✕ symbol is used to identify a proprietary laboratory analyses (PLA) test that has an identical descriptor as another PLA test. A PLA code that satisfies Category I code criteria and has been accepted by the CPT Editorial Panel is annotated with the ↑↓ symbol.

| Code | Description |
|---|---|
| #●80220 | Code added |
| 80500 | ~~Clinical pathology consultation; limited, without review of patient's history and medical records~~ |
| 80502 | ~~comprehensive, for a complex diagnostic problem, with review of patient's history and medical records~~ |
| ●80503 | Code added |
| ●80504 | Code added |
| ●80505 | Code added |
| +●80506 | Code added |
| ▲81228 | Cytogenomic ~~constitutional~~ (genome-wide) ~~microarray~~ analysis <u>for constitutional chromosomal abnormalities</u>; interrogation of genomic regions for copy number variants<u>,</u> ~~(eg, bacterial artificial chromosome [BAC] or oligo-based comparative genomic hybridization ([CGH]) microarray analysis)~~ |
| ▲81229 | interrogation of genomic regions for copy number and single nucleotide polymorphism (SNP) variants<u>,</u> ~~for chromosomal abnormalities~~ <u>comparative genomic hybridization (CGH) microarray analysis</u> |
| #●81349 | Code added |
| ▲81405 | Molecular pathology procedure, Level 6 (eg, analysis of 6-10 exons by DNA sequence analysis, mutation scanning or duplication/deletion variants of 11-25 exons, regionally targeted cytogenomic array analysis) |
| | Cytogenomic constitutional targeted microarray analysis of chromosome 22q13 by interrogation of genomic regions for copy number and single nucleotide polymorphism (SNP) variants for chromosomal abnormalities |
| | (When performing ~~genome-wide~~ cytogenomic ~~constitutional microarray~~ <u>[genome-wide]</u> analysis <u>for constitutional chromosomal abnormalities</u>, see 81228, 81229<u>, 81349</u>) |
| ●81523 | Code added |
| ●81560 | Code added |
| ▲82656 | Elastase, pancreatic (EL-1), fecal~~, qualitative or semi-quantitative~~; <u>qualitative or semi-quantitative</u> |
| #●82653 | Code added |

| Code | Description |
|---|---|
| ●83521 | Code added |
| #●83529 | Code added |
| #●86015 | Code added |
| ●86036 | Code added |
| ●86037 | Code added |
| #●86051 | Code added |
| #●86052 | Code added |
| #●86053 | Code added |
| ●86231 | Code added |
| ●86258 | Code added |
| #●86362 | Code added |
| #●86363 | Code added |
| #●86364 | Code added |
| ●86381 | Code added |
| #●86408 | Code added |
| #●86409 | Code added |
| #●86413 | Code added |
| ●86596 | Code added |
| #●87154 | Code added |
| ▲87301 | Infectious agent antigen detection by immunoassay technique; (eg, enzyme immunoassay [EIA], enzyme-linked immunosorbent assay [ELISA], <u>fluorescence immunoassay [FIA]</u>, immunochemiluminometric assay [IMCA])<u>,</u> qualitative or semiquantitative<u>, multiple-step method</u>; adenovirus enteric types 40/41 |
| ▲87305 | Aspergillus |
| ▲87320 | Chlamydia trachomatis |
| ▲87324 | Clostridium difficile toxin(s) |
| ▲87327 | Cryptococcus neoformans |
| ▲87328 | cryptosporidium |
| ▲87329 | giardia |
| ▲87332 | cytomegalovirus |
| ▲87335 | Escherichia coli 0157 |
| ▲87336 | Entamoeba histolytica dispar group |
| ▲87337 | Entamoeba histolytica group |

★ = Telemedicine   ✚ = Add-on code   ✎ = FDA approval pending   # = Resequenced code   ⊘ = Modifier 51 exempt

| Code | Description |
|---|---|
| ▲87338 | Helicobacter pylori, stool |
| ▲87339 | Helicobacter pylori |
| ▲87340 | hepatitis B surface antigen (HBsAg) |
| ▲87341 | hepatitis B surface antigen (HBsAg) neutralization |
| ▲87350 | hepatitis Be antigen (HBeAg) |
| ▲87380 | hepatitis, delta agent |
| ▲87385 | Histoplasma capsulatum |
| ▲87389 | HIV-1 antigen(s), with HIV-1 and HIV-2 antibodies, single result |
| ▲87390 | HIV-1 |
| ▲87391 | HIV-2 |
| ▲87400 | Influenza, A or B, each |
| ▲87420 | respiratory syncytial virus |
| ▲87425 | rotavirus |
| ▲87426 | severe acute respiratory syndrome coronavirus (eg, SARS-CoV, SARS-CoV-2 [COVID-19]) |
| #●87428 | Code added |
| ▲87427 | Shiga-like toxin |
| ▲87430 | Streptococcus, group A |
| ▲87449 | ~~Infectious agent antigen detection by immunoassay technique, (eg, enzyme immunoassay [EIA], enzyme linked immunosorbent assay [ELISA], immunochemiluminometric assay [IMCA]), qualitative or semiquantitative; multiple-step method,~~ not otherwise specified, each organism |
| 87450 | ~~Infectious agent antigen detection by immunoassay technique, (eg, enzyme immunoassay [EIA], enzyme linked immunosorbent assay [ELISA], immunochemiluminometric assay [IMCA]), qualitative or semiquantitative; single-step method, not otherwise specified, each organism~~ |
| ▲87451 | ~~multiple-step method,~~ polyvalent for multiple organisms, each polyvalent antiserum |
| ●87636 | Code added |
| ●87637 | Code added |
| ▲87802 | Infectious agent antigen detection by immunoassay with direct optical (ie, visual) observation; Streptococcus, group B |
| ▲87803 | Clostridium difficile toxin A |
| #▲87806 | HIV-1 antigen(s), with HIV-1 and HIV-2 antibodies |
| ▲87804 | Influenza |
| ▲87807 | respiratory syncytial virus |
| #●87811 | Code added |

Pathology and Laboratory 80047-89398, 0001U-0284U

| Code | Description |
|---|---|
| ▲87808 | Trichomonas vaginalis |
| ▲87809 | adenovirus |
| ▲87810 | Chlamydia trachomatis |
| ▲87850 | Neisseria gonorrhoeae |
| ▲87880 | Streptococcus, group A |
| ▲87899 | not otherwise specified |
| ▲0051U | Prescription drug monitoring, evaluation of drugs present by <u>liquid chromatography tandem mass spectrometry (LC-MS/MS)</u>, urine <u>or blood</u>, 31 drug panel, reported as quantitative results, detected or not detected, per date of service |
| 0098U | ~~Respiratory pathogen, multiplex reverse transcription and multiplex amplified probe technique, multiple types or subtypes, 14 targets (adenovirus, coronavirus, human metapneumovirus, influenza A, influenza A subtype H1, influenza A subtype H3, influenza A subtype H1-2009, influenza B, parainfluenza virus, human rhinovirus/enterovirus, respiratory syncytial virus, Bordetella pertussis, Chlamydophila pneumoniae, Mycoplasma pneumoniae)~~ |
| 0099U | ~~Respiratory pathogen, multiplex reverse transcription and multiplex amplified probe technique, multiple types or subtypes, 20 targets (adenovirus, coronavirus 229E, coronavirus HKU1, coronavirus, coronavirus OC43, human metapneumovirus, influenza A, influenza A subtype, influenza A subtype H3, influenza A subtype H1-2009, influenza, parainfluenza virus, parainfluenza virus 2, parainfluenza virus 3, parainfluenza virus 4, human rhinovirus/enterovirus, respiratory syncytial virus, Bordetella pertussis, Chlamydophila pneumonia, Mycoplasma pneumoniae)~~ |
| 0100U | ~~Respiratory pathogen, multiplex reverse transcription and multiplex amplified probe technique, multiple types or subtypes, 21 targets (adenovirus, coronavirus 229E, coronavirus HKU1, coronavirus NL63, coronavirus OC43, human metapneumovirus, human rhinovirus/enterovirus, influenza A, including subtypes H1, H1-2009, and H3, influenza B, parainfluenza virus 1, parainfluenza virus 2, parainfluenza virus 3, parainfluenza virus 4, respiratory syncytial virus, Bordetella parapertussis [IS1001], Bordetella pertussis [ptxP], Chlamydia pneumoniae, Mycoplasma pneumoniae)~~ |
| 0139U | ~~Neurology (autism spectrum disorder [ASD]), quantitative measurements of 6 central carbon metabolites (ie, α-ketoglutarate, alanine, lactate, phenylalanine, pyruvate, and succinate), LC-MS/MS, plasma, algorithmic analysis with result reported as negative or positive (with metabolic subtypes of ASD)~~ |
| ▲0152U | Infectious disease (bacteria, fungi, parasites, and DNA viruses), <u>microbial cell-free</u> DNA, ~~PCR and~~ <u>plasma, untargeted</u> next-generation sequencing, ~~plasma, detection of >1,000 potential microbial organisms~~ <u>report</u> for significant positive pathogens |
| 0168U | ~~Fetal aneuploidy (trisomy 21, 18, and 13) DNA sequence analysis of selected regions using maternal plasma without fetal fraction cutoff, algorithm reported as a risk score for each trisomy~~ |
| #●0223U | Code added |
| ●0224U | Code added |
| ●0225U | Code added |
| ●0226U | Code added |
| ●0227U | Code added |
| ●0228U | Code added |
| ●0229U | Code added |
| ●0230U | Code added |
| ●0231U | Code added |

★ = Telemedicine   ✦ = Add-on code   𝑁 = FDA approval pending   # = Resequenced code   ⦸ = Modifier 51 exempt

| Code | Description |
|---|---|
| ●0232U | Code added |
| ●0233U | Code added |
| ●0234U | Code added |
| ●0235U | Code added |
| ●0236U | Code added |
| ●0237U | Code added |
| ●0238U | Code added |
| ●0239U | Code added |
| ●0240U | Code added |
| ●0241U | Code added |
| ●0242U | Code added |
| ●0243U | Code added |
| ●0244U | Code added |
| ●0245U | Code added |
| ●0246U | Code added |
| ●0247U | Code added |
| ●0248U | Code added |
| ●0249U | Code added |
| ●0250U | Code added |
| ●0251U | Code added |
| ●0252U | Code added |
| ●0253U | Code added |
| ●0254U | Code added |
| ●0255U | Code added |
| ●0256U | Code added |
| ●0257U | Code added |
| ●0258U | Code added |
| ●0259U | Code added |
| ✕●0260U | Code added |
| ●0261U | Code added |
| ●0262U | Code added |
| ●0263U | Code added |
| ✕●0264U | Code added |

| Code | Description |
|---|---|
| ●0265U | Code added |
| ●0266U | Code added |
| ●0267U | Code added |
| ●0268U | Code added |
| ●0269U | Code added |
| ●0270U | Code added |
| ●0271U | Code added |
| ●0272U | Code added |
| ●0273U | Code added |
| ●0274U | Code added |
| ●0275U | Code added |
| ●0276U | Code added |
| ●0277U | Code added |
| ●0278U | Code added |
| ●0279U | Code added |
| ●0280U | Code added |
| ●0281U | Code added |
| ●0282U | Code added |
| ●0283U | Code added |
| ●0284U | Code added |

★=Telemedicine    ✚=Add-on code    ✗=FDA approval pending    #=Resequenced code    ⊘=Modifier 51 exempt

# Pathology and Laboratory

## Drug Assay

### DEFINITIONS AND ACRONYM CONVERSION LISTING

| Drug Testing Term/Acronym | Definition |
| --- | --- |
| 6-MAM | Acronym for the heroin drug metabolite 6-monacetylmorphine |
| Acid | Descriptor for classifying drug/drug metabolite molecules based upon chemical ionization properties. Laboratory procedures for drug isolation and identification may include acid, base, or neutral groupings. |
| AM | A category of synthetic marijuana drugs discovered by and named after Alexandros Makriyannis at Northeastern University |
| Analog | A structural derivative of a parent chemical compound that often differs from it by a single element |
| Analyte | The substance or chemical constituent that is of interest in an analytical procedure |
| Base | Descriptor for classifying drug/drug metabolite molecules based upon chemical ionization properties. Laboratory procedures for drug isolation and identification may include acid, base, or neutral groupings. |
| Card(s) | Multiplexed presumptive drug class(es) immunoassay product that is read by visual observation, including instrumented when performed |
| Cassette(s) | Multiplexed presumptive drug class immunoassay product(s) that is read by visual observation, including instrumented when performed |
| CEDIA | Acronym for Cloned-Enzyme-Donor-Immuno-Assay. CEDIA immunoassay is a competitive antibody binding procedure that utilizes enzyme donor fragment-labeled antigens (drugs) to compete for antigens (drugs) contained in the patient sample. Recombination of enzyme donor fragment and enzyme acceptor fragment produces a functional enzyme. CEDIA immunoassay enzyme activity is proportional to concentration of drug(s) detected. |
| Chromatography | An analytical technique used to separate components of a mixture. See thin layer chromatography, gas chromatography, and high performance chromatography. |
| Confirmatory | Term used to describe definitive identification/quantitation procedures that are secondary to presumptive screening methods |
| DART | Acronym for Direct-Analysis-in-Real-Time. DART is an atmospheric pressure ionization method for mass spectrometry analysis |
| Definitive Drug Procedure | A procedure that provides specific identification of individual drugs and drug metabolites |
| DESI | Acronym for Desorption-ElectroSpray-Ionization. DESI is a combination of electrospray ionization and desorption ionization methods for mass spectrometry analysis. |
| Dipstick | A multiplexed presumptive drug class immunoassay product that is read by visual observation, including instrumented when performed |
| Drug test cup | A multiplexed presumptive drug class immunoassay product that is read by visual observation, including instrumented when performed |
| EDDP | Acronym for the methadone drug metabolite 2-ethylidene-1,5-dimethyl-3,3-diphenylpyrrolidine |
| EIA | Acronym for Enzyme Immuno-Assay. Enzyme immunoassay is a competitive antibody binding procedure that utilizes enzyme-labeled antigens (drugs) to compete for antigens (drugs) contained in the patient sample. Enzyme immunoassay enzyme activity is proportional to concentration of drug(s) detected |
| ELISA | Acronym for Enzyme-Linked Immunosorbent Assay. ELISA is a competitive binding immunoassay that is designed to measure antigens (drugs) or antibodies. ELISA immunoassay results are proportional to concentration of drug(s) detected. |

## DEFINITIONS AND ACRONYM CONVERSION LISTING

| Drug Testing Term/Acronym | Definition |
|---|---|
| EMIT | Acronym for Enzyme-Multiplied-Immunoassay-Test. EMIT is a trade name for a type of enzyme immunoassay (EIA). |
| FPIA | Acronym for Fluorescence Polarization Immuno-Assay. FPIA is a competitive binding immunoassay that utilizes fluorescein-labeled antigens (drugs) to compete for antigens (drugs) contained in the patient sample. The measure of polarized light emission is inversely proportional to the concentration of drug(s) detected. |
| Gas chromatography | Gas chromatography is a chromatography technique in which patient sample preparations are vaporized into a gas (mobile phase) which flows through a tubular column (containing a stationary phase) and into a detector. The retention time of a drug on the column is determined by partitioning characteristics of the drug into the mobile and stationary phases. Chromatography column detectors may be non-specific (eg, flame ionization) or specific (eg, mass spectrometry). The combination of column retention time and specific detector response provides a definitive identification of the drug or drug metabolite. |
| GC | Acronym for gas chromatography |
| GC-MS | Acronym for gas chromatography mass spectrometry |
| GC-MS/MS | Acronym for gas chromatography mass spectrometry/mass spectrometry |
| High performance liquid chromatography | High performance liquid chromatography is a chromatography technique in which patient sample preparations are injected into a liquid (mobile phase) which flows through a tubular column (containing a stationary phase) and into a detector. The retention time of a drug on the column is determined by partitioning characteristics of the drug into the mobile and stationary phases. Chromatography column detectors may be non-specific (eg, ultra-violet spectrophotometry) or specific (eg, mass spectrometry). The combination of column retention time and specific detector response provides a definitive identification of the drug or drug metabolite. High performance liquid chromatography is also called high pressure liquid chromatography. |
| HPLC | Acronym for high performance liquid chromatography |
| HU | A category of synthetic marijuana drugs discovered by and named after Raphael Mechoulam at Hebrew University |
| IA | Acronym for immunoassay |
| Immunoassay | Antigen-antibody binding procedures utilized to detect antigens (eg, drugs and/or drug metabolites) in patient samples. Immunoassay designs include competitive or non-competitive with various mechanisms for detection. |
| Isobaric | In mass spectrometry, ions with the same mass |
| Isomers | Compounds that have the same molecular formula but differ in structural formula |
| JWH | A category of synthetic marijuana drugs discovered by and named after John W. Huffman at Clemson University. |
| KIMS | Acronym for kinetic interaction of microparticles in solution. KIMS immunoassay is a competitive antibody binding procedure that utilizes microparticle-labeled antigens (drugs) to compete for antigens (drugs) contained in the patient sample. Microparticle immunoassay absorbance increase is inversely proportional to concentration of drug(s) detected. |
| LC-MS | Acronym for liquid chromatography mass spectrometry |
| LC-MS/MS | Acronym for liquid chromatography mass spectrometry/mass spectrometry |
| LDTD | Acronym for laser diode thermal desorption. LDTD is a combination of atmospheric pressure chemical ionization and laser diode thermal desorption methods for mass spectrometry analysis. |
| MALDI | Acronym for matrix assisted laser desorption/ionization mass spectrometry. MALDI is a soft ionization technique that reduces molecular fragmentation. |
| MDA | Acronym for the drug 3,4-methylenedioxyamphetamine. MDA is also a drug metabolite of MDMA. |
| MDEA | Acronym for the drug 3,4-methylenedioxy-N-ethylamphetamine |
| MDMA | Acronym for the drug 3,4-methylenedioxy-N-methylamphetamine |
| MDPV | Acronym for the drug methylenedioxypyrovalerone |

## DEFINITIONS AND ACRONYM CONVERSION LISTING

| Drug Testing Term/Acronym | Definition |
|---|---|
| MS | Acronym for mass spectrometry. MS is an identification technique that measures the charge-to-mass ratio of charged particles. There are several types of mass spectrometry instruments, such as magnetic sectoring, time of flight, quadrupole mass filter, ion traps, and Fourier transformation. Mass spectrometry is used as part of the process to assign definitive identification of drugs and drug metabolites. |
| MS/MS | Acronym for mass spectrometry/mass spectrometry. MS/MS instruments combine multiple units of mass spectrometry filters into a single instrument. MS/MS is also called tandem mass spectrometry. |
| MS-TOF | Acronym for mass spectrometry time of flight. Time of flight is a mass spectrometry identification technique that utilizes ion velocity to determine the mass-to-charge ratio. |
| Multiplexed | Descriptor for a multiple component test device that simultaneously measures multiple analytes (drug classes) in a single analysis. |
| Neutral | Descriptor for classifying drug/drug metabolite molecules based upon chemical ionization properties. Laboratory procedures for drug isolation and identification may include acid, base, or neutral groupings. |
| ng/mL | Unit of measure for weight per volume calculated as nanograms per milliliter. The ng/mL unit of measure is equivalent to the ug/L unit of measure. |
| Optical observation | Optical observation refers to procedure results that are interpreted visually with or without instrumentation assistance. |
| Opiate | Medicinal category of narcotic alkaloid drugs that are natural products in the opium poppy plant Papaver somniferum. This immunoassay class of drugs typically includes detection of codeine, dihydrocodeine, hydrocodone, hydromorphone, and morphine. |
| Opioids | A category of medicinal synthetic or semi-synthetic narcotic alkaloid opioid receptor stimulating drugs including butorphanol, desomorphine, dextromethorphan, dextrorphan, levorphanol, meperidine, naloxone, naltrexone, normeperidine, and pentazocine. |
| Presumptive | Drug test results that indicate possible, but not definitive, presence of drugs and/or drug metabolites |
| QTOF | Acronym for quadrupole-time of flight mass spectrometry. QTOF is a hybrid mass spectrometry identification technique that combines ion velocity with tandem quadrupole mass spectrometry (MS or MS/MS) to determine the mass-to-charge ratio. |
| RCS | A category of synthetic marijuana drugs that are analogs of JHW compounds. See JWH. |
| RIA | Acronym for radio-immuno-assay. Radioimmunoassay is a competitive antibody binding procedure that utilizes radioactive-labeled antigens (drugs) to compete for antigens (drugs) contained in the patient sample. The measure of radioactivity is inversely proportional to concentration of drug(s) detected. |
| Stereoisomers | Isomeric molecules that have the same molecular formula and sequence of bonded atoms (constitution), but that differ only in the three-dimensional orientations of their atoms in space |
| Substance | A substance is a drug that does not have an established therapeutic use as distinguished from other analytes listed in the Chemistry section (82009-84999). |
| TDM | Acronym for therapeutic drug monitoring |
| THC | Acronym for marijuana active drug ingredient tetrahydrocannabinol |
| Therapeutic Drug Monitoring | Analysis of blood (serum, plasma) drug concentration to monitor clinical response to therapy |
| Time of flight | Time of flight is a mass spectrometry technique that utilizes ion velocity to determine the mass-to-charge ratio |
| TLC | Acronym for thin layer chromatography |
| TOF | Acronym for time of flight |
| ug/L | Unit of measure for mass per volume calculated as micrograms per liter. The ug/L unit of measure is equivalent to the ng/mL unit of measure. |

Pathology and Laboratory 80047-89398, 0001U-0284U

# Therapeutic Drug Assays

| | | |
|---|---|---|
| | **80173** | Haloperidol |
| #● | **80220** | Hydroxychloroquine |
| | 80220 | Code is out of numerical sequence. See 80170-80175 |
| | **80299** | Quantitation of therapeutic drug, not elsewhere specified |

## Rationale

Code 80220 has been established to report therapeutic drug assay testing for hydroxychloroquine.

As noted within the existing therapeutic drug assays guidelines, "therapeutic drug assays are performed to monitor levels of a known, prescribed, or over-the-counter medication." The materials tested may be from whole blood, serum, plasma, and cerebrospinal fluid and are quantitative in nature. Performance of the testing procedure is not limited to a particular method; therefore, the specific method of testing for the noted substance may vary.

## Clinical Example (80220)

A 40-year-old female with systemic lupus erythematosus (SLE) is being treated with hydroxychloroquine. After 6 months of treatment, the patient experiences a flare-up of SLE. A hydroxychloroquine level is ordered.

## Description of Procedure (80220)

Obtain a serum sample and measure the hydroxychloroquine level by liquid chromatography-tandem mass spectrometry (LC-MS/MS). Report the results.

# ►Pathology Clinical Consultations◄

►Physician review of pathology and laboratory findings is frequently performed in the course of providing care to patients. Review of pathology and laboratory test results occurs in conjunction with the provision of an evaluation and management (E/M) service. Considered part of the non-face-to-face time activities associated with the overall E/M service, reviewing pathology and laboratory results is not a separately reportable service. Communicating results to the patient, family, or caregiver of independent interpretation of results (not separately reported) may constitute an E/M service.

Pathology clinical consultation services codes (80503, 80504, 80505, 80506) describe physician pathology clinical consultation services provided at the request of another physician or other qualified health care professional at the same or another facility or institution.

A pathology clinical consultation is a service, including a written report, rendered by the pathologist in response to a request (eg, written request, electronic request, phone request, or face-to-face request) from a physician or other qualified health care professional that is related to clinical assessment, evaluation of pathology and laboratory findings, or other relevant clinical or diagnostic information that requires additional medical interpretive judgment. Reporting pathology and laboratory findings or other relevant clinical or diagnostic information without medical interpretive judgment is not considered a pathology clinical consultation.

The pathology clinical consultation services (80503, 80504, 80505, 80506) may be reported when the following criteria have been met:

■ The pathologist renders a pathology clinical consultation at the request of a physician or other qualified health care professional at the same or another institution.

■ The pathology clinical consultation request is related to pathology and laboratory findings or other relevant clinical or diagnostic information (eg, radiology findings or operative/procedural notes) that require additional medical interpretive judgment.

A pathologist may also render a pathology clinical consultation when mandated by federal or state regulation (eg, Clinical Laboratory Improvement Amendments [CLIA]).◄

# ►Instructions for Selecting a Level of Pathology Clinical Consultation Services◄

►Selection of the appropriate level of pathology clinical consultation services may be based on either the total time for pathology clinical consultation services performed on the date of consultation **or** the level of medical decision making as defined for each service.◄

# ►Medical Decision Making◄

| ►Code | Level of MDM (Based on 2 out of 3 Elements of MDM) | Number and Complexity of Problems Addressed | ►Elements of Medical Decision Making◄ | | Risk of Complications and/or Morbidity or Mortality of Patient Management |
|---|---|---|---|---|---|
| | | | **Amount and/or Complexity of Data to be Reviewed and Analyzed** *Each unique test, order, or document contributes to the combination of 2 or combination of 3 in Category 1 below.* | | |
| 80503 | Low | Low<br>• **1** to **2** laboratory or pathology findings; **or**<br>• **2** or more self-limited problems | Limited<br>*(Must meet the requirements of at least 1 of the 2 categories)*<br>**Category 1: Tests and documents**<br>• **Any combination of 2 from the following:**<br>  ■ Review of prior note(s) from each unique source*;<br>  ■ Review of the result(s) of each unique test*;<br>  ■ Ordering or recommending additional or follow-up testing*<br>**or**<br>**Category 2: Assessment requiring an independent historian(s)**<br>*(For the categories of independent interpretation of tests and discussion of management or test interpretation, see moderate or high)* | | Low risk of morbidity from additional diagnostic testing or treatment |
| 80504 | Moderate | • **Moderate**<br>• **3** to **4** laboratory or pathology findings; or<br>• **1** or more chronic illnesses with exacerbation, progression, or side effects of treatment; **or**<br>• **2** or more stable chronic illnesses; **or**<br>**1** undiagnosed new problem with uncertain prognosis; **or**<br>• **1** acute illness with systemic symptoms | Moderate<br>*(Must meet the requirements of at least 1 out of 3 categories)*<br>**Category 1: Tests, documents, or independent historian(s)**<br>**Any combination of 3 from the following:**<br>  ■ Review of prior note(s) from each unique source*;<br>  ■ Review of the result(s) of each unique test*;<br>  ■ Ordering or recommending additional or follow-up testing*;<br>  ■ Assessment requiring an independent historian(s)<br>**or**<br>**Category 2: Independent interpretation of tests**<br>• Independent interpretation of a test performed by another physician/other qualified health care professional (not separately reported);<br>**or**<br>**Category 3: Discussion of management or test interpretation**<br>• Discussion of management or test interpretation with external physician/other qualified health care professional/appropriate source (not separately reported) | | Moderate risk of morbidity from additional diagnostic testing or treatment<br>*Examples only:*<br>Prescription drug management<br>• Decision regarding minor surgery with identified patient or procedure risk factors<br>• Decision regarding elective major surgery without identified patient or procedure risk factors<br>• Diagnosis or treatment significantly limited by social determinants of health |

*(continued on page 102)*

Pathology and Laboratory  80047-89398, 0001U-0284U

| Code | Level of MDM (Based on 2 out of 3 Elements of MDM) | Number and Complexity of Problems Addressed | ►Elements of Medical Decision Making◄ | Risk of Complications and/or Morbidity or Mortality of Patient Management |
|---|---|---|---|---|
| | | | **Amount and/or Complexity of Data to be Reviewed and Analyzed** *Each unique test, order, or document contributes to the combination of 2 or combination of 3 in Category 1 below.* | |
| 80505 | High | **High** <br> • **5** or more laboratory or pathology findings; <br> **or** <br> • **1** or more chronic illnesses with severe exacerbation, progression, or side effects of treatment; <br> **or** <br> • **1** acute or chronic illness or injury that poses a threat to life or bodily function | **Extensive** *(Must meet the requirements of at least 2 out of 3 categories)* <br> **Category 1: Tests, documents, or independent historian(s)** <br> • **Any combination of 3 from the following:** <br> ■ Review of prior note(s) from each unique source*; <br> ■ Review of the result(s) of each unique test*; <br> ■ Ordering or recommending additional or follow-up testing*; <br> ■ Assessment requiring an independent historian(s) <br> **or** <br> **Category 2: Independent interpretation of tests** <br> • Independent interpretation of a test performed by another physician/other qualified health care professional (not separately reported); <br> **or** <br> **Category 3: Discussion of management or test interpretation** <br> • Discussion of management or test interpretation with external physician/other qualified health care professional/appropriate source (not separately reported) | **High risk of morbidity from additional diagnostic testing or treatment** *Examples only:* <br> • Drug therapy requiring intensive monitoring for toxicity <br> • Decision regarding elective major surgery with identified patient or procedure risk factors <br> • Decision regarding emergency major surgery <br> • Decision regarding hospitalization◄ |

## ►Time◄

►Time alone may be used to select the appropriate code level for the pathology clinical consultation services codes (ie, 80503, 80504, 80505). When time is used to select the appropriate level for pathology clinical consultation codes, time is defined by the service descriptions. When prolonged service time occurs, add-on code 80506 may be reported. The appropriate time should be documented in the medical record when it is used as the basis for code selection.

***Total time on the date of the consultation (pathology clinical consultation services):*** For coding purposes, time for these services is the total time on the date of the consultation. It includes time personally spent by the consultant on the day of the consultation (includes time in activities that require the consultant and does not include time in activities normally performed by clinical staff).

Consultant time includes the following activities, when performed:

■ Review of available medical history, including presenting complaint, signs and symptoms, personal and family history

■ Review of test results

■ Review of all relevant past and current laboratory, pathology, and clinical findings

■ Arriving at a tentative conclusion/differential diagnosis

■ Comparing against previous study reports, including radiographic reports, images as applicable, and results of other clinical testing

■ Ordering or recommending additional or follow-up testing

■ Referring and communicating with other health care professionals (not separately reported)

■ Counseling and educating the clinician or other qualified health care professional

■ Documenting the clinical consultation report in the electronic or other health record◄

►(80500, 80502 have been deleted. To report a clinical pathology consultation, limited or comprehensive, see 80503, 80504, 80505, 80506)◄

★ = Telemedicine     ✚ = Add-on code     ✴ = FDA approval pending     # = Resequenced code     ⊘ = Modifier 51 exempt

● **80503**   Pathology clinical consultation; for a clinical problem, with limited review of patient's history and medical records and straightforward medical decision making

When using time for code selection, 5-20 minutes of total time is spent on the date of the consultation.

►(For consultations involving the examination and evaluation of the patient, see 99241, 99242, 99243, 99244, 99245, 99251, 99252, 99253, 99254, 99255)◄

● **80504**   for a moderately complex clinical problem, with review of patient's history and medical records and moderate level of medical decision making

When using time for code selection, 21-40 minutes of total time is spent on the date of the consultation.

● **80505**   for a highly complex clinical problem, with comprehensive review of patient's history and medical records and high level of medical decision making

When using time for code selection, 41-60 minutes of total time is spent on the date of the consultation.

+● **80506**   prolonged service, each additional 30 minutes (List separately in addition to code for primary procedure)

►(Use 80506 in conjunction with 80505)◄

►(Do not report 80503, 80504, 80505, 80506 in conjunction with 88321, 88323, 88325)◄

►(Prolonged pathology clinical consultation service of less than 15 additional minutes is not reported separately)◄

(For consultations involving the examination and evaluation of the patient, see 99241-99255)

## Rationale

The Pathology Clinical Consultations subsection heading has been revised, subheadings have been added, guidelines have been added and revised, a table that provides instruction regarding identifying the level of medical decision making (MDM) has been added, codes 80500 and 80502 have been deleted, and codes 80503-80506 have been established for reporting pathology clinical consultation for limited, moderately complex, highly complex, and prolonged pathology clinical consultation services.

The AMA/Specialty Society Relative Value Scale (RVS) Update Committee (RUC) Relativity Assessment Workgroup (RAW) recommended a review of codes 80500 and 80502 due to a utilization of over 20,000. As a result, the existing pathology clinical consultation services codes have been deleted, and new codes, guidelines, parenthetical notes, and a table have been added to provide further clarity for defining and reporting pathology

clinical consultation services. Because of many reporting similarities, the added code descriptors, guideline language, parenthetical notes, and table have been patterned after the recently developed changes that were instituted for determining the level of service for evaluation and management (E/M) services.

The added and revised guidelines provide initial reporting instructions and define what constitutes a pathology clinical consultation service and the criteria that must be met for reporting pathology clinical consultations. These guidelines note that review of pathology and laboratory test results that occurs in conjunction with an E/M service is still considered part of the overall E/M service and not separately reported. They also note that reporting pathology and laboratory findings or other relevant clinical or diagnostic information without medical interpretive judgment is not considered a pathology clinical consultation. In addition, communication of pathology laboratory results may constitute an E/M service.

Additional guidelines that provide instruction regarding how to select the level of service for pathology clinical consultations (eg, according to time or level of MDM) have been added. The MDM table breaks down how to review and enumerate the elements for determining level of MDM, which focuses on reviewing the number and complexity of the problems addressed, the amount and/or complexity of data to be reviewed or analyzed, and the complications and/or morbidity or mortality that are at risk for managing the patient's condition. The instructions provided for determining the service level according to time state that the time should be documented and that the total time on the date of the consultation, including time personally spent by the consultant on the day of consultation, are important factors. A listing of important activities for use of time for level determination has also been included.

The Pathology Clinical Consultations subheading has been revised to better emulate terminology that is used for these services today. Two additional subheadings (ie, Medical Decision Making and Time) have been added to assist users in determining the level of service.

Codes 80503-80506 have been added and include specific language that assists users in reporting these services, such as language that identifies choosing a level of service according to the type of MDM provided and a notation regarding the amount of time spent for that level of service. To accommodate the addition of the new, more descriptive codes, codes 80500 and 80502 have been deleted. A parenthetical note has been added to indicate these deletions.

Parenthetical notes associated with the new codes have been added to provide additional instruction, including minimal time reporting requirements and restriction from using the codes in conjunction with other consultation services codes that are already specifically identified within the pathology code section (88321-88325).

## Clinical Example (80503)

A 45-year-old female presents with an abnormal pap smear. A clinicopathologic correlation of the abnormal pap smear with previous pap smears and/or gynecologic biopsies is performed.

## Description of Procedure (80503)

N/A

## Clinical Example (80504)

A 45-year-old female presents with new onset leukocytosis. A pathology clinical consultation is requested.

## Description of Procedure (80504)

N/A

## Clinical Example (80505)

A 41-year-old female presents with acute thrombocytopenia and anemia. A pathology clinical consultation is requested.

## Description of Procedure (80505)

N/A

## Clinical Example (80506)

Assessment of a patient with complex toxicology results. A pathology clinical consultation is requested.

## Description of Procedure (80506)

N/A

# Molecular Pathology

Molecular pathology procedures are medical laboratory procedures involving the analyses of nucleic acid (ie, DNA, RNA) to detect variants in genes that may be indicative of germline (eg, constitutional disorders) or somatic (eg, neoplasia) conditions, or to test for histocompatibility antigens (eg, HLA). Code selection is typically based on the specific gene(s) that is being analyzed. Genes are described using Human Genome

Organization (HUGO) approved gene names and are italicized in the code descriptors. Gene names were taken from tables of the HUGO Gene Nomenclature Committee (HGNC) at the time the CPT codes were developed. For the most part, Human Genome Variation Society (HGVS) recommendations were followed for the names of specific molecular variants. The familiar name is used for some variants because defined criteria were not in place when the variant was first described or because HGVS recommendations were changed over time (eg, intronic variants, processed proteins). When the gene name is represented by an abbreviation, the abbreviation is listed first, followed by the full gene name italicized in parentheses (eg, "F5 *[coagulation Factor V]*"), except for the HLA series of codes. Proteins or diseases commonly associated with the genes are listed as examples in the code descriptors. The examples do not represent all conditions in which testing of the gene may be indicated.

▶***Low-pass sequencing:*** a method of genome sequencing intended for cytogenomic analysis of chromosomal abnormalities, such as that performed for trait mapping or copy number variation, typically performed to an average depth of sequencing ranging from 0.1 to 5X.◀

***Microarray:*** surface(s) on which multiple specific nucleic acid sequences are attached in a known arrangement. Sometimes referred to as a "gene chip." Examples of uses of microarrays include evaluation of a patient specimen for gains or losses of DNA sequences (copy number variants, CNVs), identification of the presence of specific nucleotide sequence variants (also known as single nucleotide polymorphisms, SNPs), mRNA expression levels, or DNA sequence analysis.

## Rationale

In accordance with the addition of code 81349, which is used to report cytogenomic (genome-wide) analysis for constitutional chromosomal abnormalities using low-pass sequencing, a definition has been provided to define "low-pass sequencing" and assist users in understanding how to use the new code.

Refer to the codebook and the Rationale for code 81349 for a full discussion of these changes.

## Tier 1 Molecular Pathology Procedures

81168    Code is out of numerical sequence. See 81215-81220

**# 81231**    *CYP3A5 (cytochrome P450 family 3 subfamily A member 5)*(eg, drug metabolism), gene analysis, common variants (eg, *2, *3, *4, *5, *6, *7)

★ = Telemedicine   ✚ = Add-on code   ✐ = FDA approval pending   # = Resequenced code   ⊘ = Modifier 51 exempt

▲ **81228**   Cytogenomic (genome-wide) analysis for constitutional chromosomal abnormalities; interrogation of genomic regions for copy number variants, comparative genomic hybridization [CGH] microarray analysis

▶(Do not report 81228 in conjunction with 81229, 81349)◀

▲ **81229**   interrogation of genomic regions for copy number and single nucleotide polymorphism (SNP) variants, comparative genomic hybridization (CGH) microarray analysis

▶(Do not report 81229 in conjunction with 81228, 81349)◀

▶(Do not report 88271 when performing cytogenomic [genome-wide] analysis for constitutional chromosomal abnormalities)◀

(For genomic sequencing procedures or other molecular multianalyte assays for copy number analysis using circulating cell-free fetal DNA in maternal blood, see 81420, 81422, 81479)

#● **81349**   interrogation of genomic regions for copy number and loss-of-heterozygosity variants, low-pass sequencing analysis

▶(When performing cytogenomic [genome-wide] analysis for constitutional chromosomal abnormalities that is not genome-wide [ie, regionally targeted], report the specific code for the targeted analysis if available [eg, 81405], or the unlisted molecular pathology code [81479])◀

▶(Do not report 81349 in conjunction with 81228, 81229)◀

▶(Do not report 81349 when analysis for chromosomal abnormalities is performed by sequence analysis included in 81425, 81426)◀

▶(Do not report analyte-specific molecular pathology procedures separately in conjunction with 81228, 81229, 81349, when the specific analytes are included as part of the cytogenomic [genome-wide] analysis for constitutional chromosomal abnormalities)◀

**81346**   *TYMS (thymidylate synthetase)* (eg, 5-fluorouracil/5-FU drug metabolism), gene analysis, common variant(s) (eg, tandem repeat variant)

# Rationale

Codes 81228 and 81229 have been revised to include all common elements of cytogenomic (genome-wide) analysis for constitutional chromosomal abnormalities as part of the parent code (81228) for the family, and to specify use for interrogation of genomic regions for copy number variants, comparative genomic hybridization (CGH) microarray analysis (81228), and copy number and single

nucleotide polymorphism (SNP) variants for comparative genomic hybridization (CGH) microarray analysis (81229).

Code 81349 has been added to report cytogenomic (genome-wide) analysis for constitutional chromosomal abnormalities via interrogation of genomic regions for copy number and loss-of-heterozygosity variants using a low-pass sequencing method.

To accommodate these revisions and the addition of code 81349, parenthetical notes (both instructional and exclusionary) that apply to all codes in this family have been relocated, new parenthetical notes have been added, and other parenthetical notes throughout the code set have been revised or deleted to reflect the changes, restrict reporting where appropriate, and direct users to the appropriate codes to report for each of these services. A definition of the term "low-pass sequencing" has also been included in multiple locations within the code set, and the Molecular Pathology Gene Table has been updated to accommodate these changes.

To clarify the intended use of codes 81228 and 81229 and to accommodate the addition of code 81349 within the family of codes (81228, 81229, and 81349), CPT code convention has been applied to language within the descriptors of codes 81228 and 81229, ie, by moving existing common language embedded within the child portions of these codes into the parent portion of code 81228. Further clarification has also been provided by relocating the term "constitutional" to revise the parent descriptor and more accurately reflect the full procedure that is common to all of the codes within the family: "Cytogenomic (genome-wide) analysis for constitutional chromosomal abnormalities." Clarification of the common elements accommodates the update and addition of code(s) within the code family. This includes revision of code 81228 to eliminate the "eg" reference to "bacterial artificial chromosome/oligo-based" as this example is not necessary for CGH microarray analysis. This also includes the addition of language to code 81229 to reflect that code 81229 is also intended to report "comparative genomic hybridization (CGH) microarray analysis." New code 81349 is intended to identify cytogenomic (genome-wide) analysis for constitutional chromosomal abnormalities that uses interrogation of genomic regions for copy number and loss-of-heterozygosity variants via low-pass sequencing analysis.

To assist in the understanding of how to use code 81349, a definition of "low-pass sequencing" has been added to the Molecular Pathology and Genomic Sequencing Procedure and Other Molecular Multianalyte Assays subsections of the code set.

To accommodate the changes to this family of codes, parenthetical notes have been added or revised throughout the code set to provide instructions regarding procedures that should not be reported together. This includes reporting many mutually excluded services, such as use of the low-pass technique of cytogenomic analysis for constitutional chromosomal abnormalities (81349) in conjunction with sequencing already included in the genome procedures (81425, 81426), or reporting code 81349 in conjunction with code 81228 when the procedure involves interrogation of genomic regions for copy number variants via CGH microarray analysis.

Parenthetical notes previously placed throughout the code set that reference this code family have been updated to reflect the language changes made in this family of codes. In addition, cross-reference parenthetical notes to direct users to code 81349 have been added where appropriate guidance is necessary.

To further consolidate usage instructions for this family of codes, common parenthetical notes that apply to this code family have been moved to the end of the family of codes. This clarifies that the parenthetical notes apply to all codes included within the family. Finally, the Molecular Pathology Gene Table has also been updated to reflect the language changes and addition of code 81349.

## Clinical Example (81349)

A 5-year-old male, who has a history of developmental delay and behavioral problems in preschool, has a neuropsychological evaluation that suggests the possibility of an autism spectrum diagnosis. A test is ordered to assess for constitutional chromosomal abnormalities with cytogenomic low-pass sequencing analysis.

## Description of Procedure (81349)

Extract, purify, and amplify genomic DNA from a patient blood specimen. Perform genomic sequencing at the 0.25X to 0.5X level. Bioinformatic analysis of sequencing data allows for full-chromosomal interrogation, identifying genomic regions with a normal copy number and regions with an abnormal copy number. A pathologist or other qualified health care professional (QHP) reviews the data and reports the results.

## Tier 2 Molecular Pathology Procedures

▲ 81405    Molecular pathology procedure, Level 6 (eg, analysis of 6-10 exons by DNA sequence analysis, mutation scanning or duplication/deletion variants of 11-25 exons, regionally targeted cytogenomic array analysis)

*ABCD1 (ATP-binding cassette, sub-family D [ALD], member 1)* (eg, adrenoleukodystrophy), full gene sequence

*ACADS (acyl-CoA dehydrogenase, C-2 to C-3 short chain)* (eg, short chain acyl-CoA dehydrogenase deficiency), full gene sequence

*ACTA2 (actin, alpha 2, smooth muscle, aorta)* (eg, thoracic aortic aneurysms and aortic dissections), full gene sequence

*ACTC1 (actin, alpha, cardiac muscle 1)* (eg, familial hypertrophic cardiomyopathy), full gene sequence

*ANKRD1 (ankyrin repeat domain 1)* (eg, dilated cardiomyopathy), full gene sequence

*APTX (aprataxin)* (eg, ataxia with oculomotor apraxia 1), full gene sequence

*ARSA (arylsulfatase A)* (eg, arylsulfatase A deficiency), full gene sequence

*BCKDHA (branched chain keto acid dehydrogenase E1, alpha polypeptide)* (eg, maple syrup urine disease, type 1A), full gene sequence

*BCS1L (BCS1-like [S. cerevisiae])* (eg, Leigh syndrome, mitochondrial complex III deficiency, GRACILE syndrome), full gene sequence

*BMPR2 (bone morphogenetic protein receptor, type II [serine/threonine kinase])* (eg, heritable pulmonary arterial hypertension), duplication/deletion analysis

*CASQ2 (calsequestrin 2 [cardiac muscle])* (eg, catecholaminergic polymorphic ventricular tachycardia), full gene sequence

*CASR (calcium-sensing receptor)* (eg, hypocalcemia), full gene sequence

*CDKL5 (cyclin-dependent kinase-like 5)* (eg, early infantile epileptic encephalopathy), duplication/deletion analysis

*CHRNA4 (cholinergic receptor, nicotinic, alpha 4)* (eg, nocturnal frontal lobe epilepsy), full gene sequence

*CHRNB2 (cholinergic receptor, nicotinic, beta 2 [neuronal])* (eg, nocturnal frontal lobe epilepsy), full gene sequence

*COX10 (COX10 homolog, cytochrome c oxidase assembly protein)* (eg, mitochondrial respiratory chain complex IV deficiency), full gene sequence

*COX15 (COX15 homolog, cytochrome c oxidase assembly protein)* (eg, mitochondrial respiratory chain complex IV deficiency), full gene sequence

*CPOX (coproporphyrinogen oxidase)* (eg, hereditary coproporphyria), full gene sequence

*CTRC (chymotrypsin C)* (eg, hereditary pancreatitis), full gene sequence

★ = Telemedicine    ✦ = Add-on code    ⟋ = FDA approval pending    # = Resequenced code    ⊘ = Modifier 51 exempt

*CYP11B1 (cytochrome P450, family 11, subfamily B, polypeptide 1)* (eg, congenital adrenal hyperplasia), full gene sequence

*CYP17A1 (cytochrome P450, family 17, subfamily A, polypeptide 1)* (eg, congenital adrenal hyperplasia), full gene sequence

*CYP21A2 (cytochrome P450, family 21, subfamily A, polypeptide2)* (eg, steroid 21-hydroxylase isoform, congenital adrenal hyperplasia), full gene sequence

Cytogenomic constitutional targeted microarray analysis of chromosome 22q13 by interrogation of genomic regions for copy number and single nucleotide polymorphism (SNP) variants for chromosomal abnormalities

▶(When performing cytogenomic [genome-wide] analysis for constitutional chromosomal abnormalities, see 81228, 81229, 81349)◀

(Do not report analyte-specific molecular pathology procedures separately when the specific analytes are included as part of the microarray analysis of chromosome 22q13)

(Do not report 88271 when performing cytogenomic microarray analysis)

*DBT (dihydrolipoamide branched chain transacylase E2)* (eg, maple syrup urine disease, type 2), duplication/deletion analysis

*DCX (doublecortin)* (eg, X-linked lissencephaly), full gene sequence

*DES (desmin)* (eg, myofibrillar myopathy), full gene sequence

*DFNB59 (deafness, autosomal recessive 59)* (eg, autosomal recessive nonsyndromic hearing impairment), full gene sequence

*DGUOK (deoxyguanosine kinase)* (eg, hepatocerebral mitochondrial DNA depletion syndrome), full gene sequence

*DHCR7 (7-dehydrocholesterol reductase)* (eg, Smith-Lemli-Opitz syndrome), full gene sequence

*EIF2B2 (eukaryotic translation initiation factor 2B, subunit 2 beta, 39kDa)* (eg, leukoencephalopathy with vanishing white matter), full gene sequence

*EMD (emerin)* (eg, Emery-Dreifuss muscular dystrophy), full gene sequence

*ENG (endoglin)* (eg, hereditary hemorrhagic telangiectasia, type 1), duplication/deletion analysis

*EYA1 (eyes absent homolog 1 [Drosophila])* (eg, branchio-oto-renal [BOR] spectrum disorders), duplication/deletion analysis

*FGFR1 (fibroblast growth factor receptor 1)* (eg, Kallmann syndrome 2), full gene sequence

*FH (fumarate hydratase)* (eg, fumarate hydratase deficiency, hereditary leiomyomatosis with renal cell cancer), full gene sequence

*FKTN (fukutin)* (eg, limb-girdle muscular dystrophy [LGMD] type 2M or 2L), full gene sequence

*FTSJ1 (FtsJ RNA methyltransferase homolog 1 [E. coli])* (eg, X-linked mental retardation 9), duplication/deletion analysis

*GABRG2 (gamma-aminobutyric acid [GABA] A receptor, gamma 2)* (eg, generalized epilepsy with febrile seizures), full gene sequence

*GCH1 (GTP cyclohydrolase 1)* (eg, autosomal dominant dopa-responsive dystonia), full gene sequence

*GDAP1 (ganglioside-induced differentiation-associated protein 1)* (eg, Charcot-Marie-Tooth disease), full gene sequence

*GFAP (glial fibrillary acidic protein)* (eg, Alexander disease), full gene sequence

*GHR (growth hormone receptor)* (eg, Laron syndrome), full gene sequence

*GHRHR (growth hormone releasing hormone receptor)* (eg, growth hormone deficiency), full gene sequence

*GLA (galactosidase, alpha)* (eg, Fabry disease), full gene sequence

*HNF1A (HNF1 homeobox A)* (eg, maturity-onset diabetes of the young [MODY]), full gene sequence

*HNF1B (HNF1 homeobox B)* (eg, maturity-onset diabetes of the young [MODY]), full gene sequence

*HTRA1 (HtrA serine peptidase 1)* (eg, macular degeneration), full gene sequence

*IDS (iduronate 2-sulfatase)* (eg, mucopolysacchridosis, type II), full gene sequence

*IL2RG (interleukin 2 receptor, gamma)* (eg, X-linked severe combined immunodeficiency), full gene sequence

*ISPD (isoprenoid synthase domain containing)* (eg, muscle-eye-brain disease, Walker-Warburg syndrome), full gene sequence

*KRAS (Kirsten rat sarcoma viral oncogene homolog)* (eg, Noonan syndrome), full gene sequence

*LAMP2 (lysosomal-associated membrane protein 2)* (eg, Danon disease), full gene sequence

*LDLR (low density lipoprotein receptor)* (eg, familial hypercholesterolemia), duplication/deletion analysis

*MEN1 (multiple endocrine neoplasia I)* (eg, multiple endocrine neoplasia type 1, Wermer syndrome), full gene sequence

*MMAA (methylmalonic aciduria [cobalamine deficiency] type A)* (eg, MMAA-related methylmalonic acidemia), full gene sequence

Pathology and Laboratory 80047-89398, 0001U-0284U

*MMAB (methylmalonic aciduria [cobalamine deficiency] type B)* (eg, MMAA-related methylmalonic acidemia), full gene sequence

*MPI (mannose phosphate isomerase)* (eg, congenital disorder of glycosylation 1b), full gene sequence

*MPV17 (MpV17 mitochondrial inner membrane protein)* (eg, mitochondrial DNA depletion syndrome), full gene sequence

*MPZ (myelin protein zero)* (eg, Charcot-Marie-Tooth), full gene sequence

*MTM1 (myotubularin 1)* (eg, X-linked centronuclear myopathy), duplication/deletion analysis

*MYL2 (myosin, light chain 2, regulatory, cardiac, slow)* (eg, familial hypertrophic cardiomyopathy), full gene sequence

*MYL3 (myosin, light chain 3, alkali, ventricular, skeletal, slow)* (eg, familial hypertrophic cardiomyopathy), full gene sequence

*MYOT (myotilin)* (eg, limb-girdle muscular dystrophy), full gene sequence

*NDUFS7 (NADH dehydrogenase [ubiquinone] Fe-S protein 7, 20kDa [NADH-coenzyme Q reductase])* (eg, Leigh syndrome, mitochondrial complex I deficiency), full gene sequence

*NDUFS8 (NADH dehydrogenase [ubiquinone] Fe-S protein 8, 23kDa [NADH-coenzyme Q reductase])* (eg, Leigh syndrome, mitochondrial complex I deficiency), full gene sequence

*NDUFV1 (NADH dehydrogenase [ubiquinone] flavoprotein 1, 51kDa)* (eg, Leigh syndrome, mitochondrial complex I deficiency), full gene sequence

*NEFL (neurofilament, light polypeptide)* (eg, Charcot-Marie-Tooth), full gene sequence

*NF2 (neurofibromin 2 [merlin])* (eg, neurofibromatosis, type 2), duplication/deletion analysis

*NLGN3 (neuroligin 3)* (eg, autism spectrum disorders), full gene sequence

*NLGN4X (neuroligin 4, X-linked)* (eg, autism spectrum disorders), full gene sequence

*NPHP1 (nephronophthisis 1 [juvenile])* (eg, Joubert syndrome), deletion analysis, and duplication analysis, if performed

*NPHS2 (nephrosis 2, idiopathic, steroid-resistant [podocin])* (eg, steroid-resistant nephrotic syndrome), full gene sequence

*NSD1 (nuclear receptor binding SET domain protein 1)* (eg, Sotos syndrome), duplication/deletion analysis

*OTC (ornithine carbamoyltransferase)* (eg, ornithine transcarbamylase deficiency), full gene sequence

*PAFAH1B1 (platelet-activating factor acetylhydrolase 1b regulatory subunit 1 [45kDa])* (eg, lissencephaly, Miller-Dieker syndrome), duplication/deletion analysis

*PARK2 (Parkinson protein 2, E3 ubiquitin protein ligase [parkin])* (eg, Parkinson disease), duplication/deletion analysis

*PCCA (propionyl CoA carboxylase, alpha polypeptide)* (eg, propionic acidemia, type 1), duplication/deletion analysis

*PCDH19 (protocadherin 19)* (eg, epileptic encephalopathy), full gene sequence

*PDHA1 (pyruvate dehydrogenase [lipoamide] alpha 1)* (eg, lactic acidosis), duplication/deletion analysis

*PDHB (pyruvate dehydrogenase [lipoamide] beta)* (eg, lactic acidosis), full gene sequence

*PINK1 (PTEN induced putative kinase 1)* (eg, Parkinson disease), full gene sequence

*PKLR (pyruvate kinase, liver and RBC)* (eg, pyruvate kinase deficiency), full gene sequence

*PLP1 (proteolipid protein 1)* (eg, Pelizaeus-Merzbacher disease, spastic paraplegia), full gene sequence

*POU1F1 (POU class 1 homeobox 1)* (eg, combined pituitary hormone deficiency), full gene sequence

*PRX (periaxin)* (eg, Charcot-Marie-Tooth disease), full gene sequence

*PQBP1 (polyglutamine binding protein 1)* (eg, Renpenning syndrome), full gene sequence

*PSEN1 (presenilin 1)* (eg, Alzheimer disease), full gene sequence

*RAB7A (RAB7A, member RAS oncogene family)* (eg, Charcot-Marie-Tooth disease), full gene sequence

*RAI1 (retinoic acid induced 1)* (eg, Smith-Magenis syndrome), full gene sequence

*REEP1 (receptor accessory protein 1)* (eg, spastic paraplegia), full gene sequence

*RET (ret proto-oncogene)* (eg, multiple endocrine neoplasia, type 2A and familial medullary thyroid carcinoma), targeted sequence analysis (eg, exons 10, 11 13-16)

*RPS19 (ribosomal protein S19)* (eg, Diamond-Blackfan anemia), full gene sequence

*RRM2B (ribonucleotide reductase M2 B [TP53 inducible])* (eg, mitochondrial DNA depletion), full gene sequence

*SCO1 (SCO cytochrome oxidase deficient homolog 1)* (eg, mitochondrial respiratory chain complex IV deficiency), full gene sequence

*SDHB (succinate dehydrogenase complex, subunit B, iron sulfur)* (eg, hereditary paraganglioma), full gene sequence

★ = Telemedicine  ✚ = Add-on code  𝒩 = FDA approval pending  # = Resequenced code  ⊘ = Modifier 51 exemp

SDHC (succinate dehydrogenase complex, subunit C, integral membrane protein, 15kDa) (eg, hereditary paraganglioma-pheochromocytoma syndrome), full gene sequence

SGCA (sarcoglycan, alpha [50kDa dystrophin-associated glycoprotein]) (eg, limb-girdle muscular dystrophy), full gene sequence

SGCB (sarcoglycan, beta [43kDa dystrophin-associated glycoprotein]) (eg, limb-girdle muscular dystrophy), full gene sequence

SGCD (sarcoglycan, delta [35kDa dystrophin-associated glycoprotein]) (eg, limb-girdle muscular dystrophy), full gene sequence

SGCE (sarcoglycan, epsilon) (eg, myoclonic dystonia), duplication/deletion analysis

SGCG (sarcoglycan, gamma [35kDa dystrophin-associated glycoprotein]) (eg, limb-girdle muscular dystrophy), full gene sequence

SHOC2 (soc-2 suppressor of clear homolog) (eg, Noonan-like syndrome with loose anagen hair), full gene sequence

SHOX (short stature homeobox) (eg, Langer mesomelic dysplasia), full gene sequence

SIL1 (SIL1 homolog, endoplasmic reticulum chaperone [S. cerevisiae]) (eg, ataxia), full gene sequence

SLC2A1 (solute carrier family 2 [facilitated glucose transporter], member 1) (eg, glucose transporter type 1 [GLUT 1] deficiency syndrome), full gene sequence

SLC16A2 (solute carrier family 16, member 2 [thyroid hormone transporter]) (eg, specific thyroid hormone cell transporter deficiency, Allan-Herndon-Dudley syndrome), full gene sequence

SLC22A5 (solute carrier family 22 [organic cation/carnitine transporter], member 5) (eg, systemic primary carnitine deficiency), full gene sequence

SLC25A20 (solute carrier family 25 [carnitine/acylcarnitine translocase], member 20) (eg, carnitine-acylcarnitine translocase deficiency), full gene sequence

SMAD4 (SMAD family member 4) (eg, hemorrhagic telangiectasia syndrome, juvenile polyposis), duplication/deletion analysis

SPAST (spastin) (eg, spastic paraplegia), duplication/deletion analysis

SPG7 (spastic paraplegia 7 [pure and complicated autosomal recessive]) (eg, spastic paraplegia), duplication/deletion analysis

SPRED1 (sprouty-related, EVH1 domain containing 1) (eg, Legius syndrome), full gene sequence

STAT3 (signal transducer and activator of transcription 3 [acute-phase response factor]) (eg, autosomal dominant hyper-IgE syndrome), targeted sequence analysis (eg, exons 12, 13, 14, 16, 17, 20, 21)

STK11 (serine/threonine kinase 11) (eg, Peutz-Jeghers syndrome), full gene sequence

SURF1 (surfeit 1) (eg, mitochondrial respiratory chain complex IV deficiency), full gene sequence

TARDBP (TAR DNA binding protein) (eg, amyotrophic lateral sclerosis), full gene sequence

TBX5 (T-box 5) (eg, Holt-Oram syndrome), full gene sequence

TCF4 (transcription factor 4) (eg, Pitt-Hopkins syndrome), duplication/deletion analysis

TGFBR1 (transforming growth factor, beta receptor 1) (eg, Marfan syndrome), full gene sequence

TGFBR2 (transforming growth factor, beta receptor 2) (eg, Marfan syndrome), full gene sequence

THRB (thyroid hormone receptor, beta) (eg, thyroid hormone resistance, thyroid hormone beta receptor deficiency), full gene sequence or targeted sequence analysis of >5 exons

TK2 (thymidine kinase 2, mitochondrial) (eg, mitochondrial DNA depletion syndrome), full gene sequence

TNNC1 (troponin C type 1 [slow]) (eg, hypertrophic cardiomyopathy or dilated cardiomyopathy), full gene sequence

TNNI3 (troponin I, type 3 [cardiac]) (eg, familial hypertrophic cardiomyopathy), full gene sequence

TPM1 (tropomyosin 1 [alpha]) (eg, familial hypertrophic cardiomyopathy), full gene sequence

TSC1 (tuberous sclerosis 1) (eg, tuberous sclerosis), duplication/deletion analysis

TYMP (thymidine phosphorylase) (eg, mitochondrial DNA depletion syndrome), full gene sequence

VWF (von Willebrand factor) (eg, von Willebrand disease type 2N), targeted sequence analysis (eg, exons 18-20, 23-25)

WT1 (Wilms tumor 1) (eg, Denys-Drash syndrome, familial Wilms tumor), full gene sequence

ZEB2 (zinc finger E-box binding homeobox 2) (eg, Mowat-Wilson syndrome), full gene sequence

## Rationale

In accordance with the changes made to cytogenomic (genome-wide) analysis for constitutional chromosomal abnormalities, the descriptor for code 81405 has been revised with the addition of code 81349 to the list of codes to refer to when performing these services.

Refer to the codebook and the Rationale for code 81349 for a full discussion of these changes.

# Genomic Sequencing Procedures and Other Molecular Multianalyte Assays

Genomic sequencing procedures (GSPs) and other molecular multianalyte assays GSPs are DNA or RNA sequence analysis methods that simultaneously assay multiple genes or genetic regions relevant to a clinical situation. They may target specific combinations of genes or genetic material, or assay the exome or genome. The technology used for genomic sequencing is commonly referred to as next generation sequencing (NGS) or massively parallel sequencing (MPS). GSPs are performed on nucleic acids from germline or neoplastic samples. Examples of applications include aneuploidy analysis of cell-free circulating fetal DNA, gene panels for somatic alterations in neoplasms, and sequence analysis of the exome or genome to determine the cause of developmental delay. The exome and genome procedures are designed to evaluate the genetic material in totality or near totality. Although commonly used to identify sequence (base) changes, they can also be used to identify copy number, structural changes, and abnormal zygosity patterns. Another unique feature of GSPs is the ability to "re-query" or re-evaluate the sequence data (eg, complex phenotype such as developmental delay is reassessed when new genetic knowledge is attained, or for a separate unrelated clinical indication). The analyses listed below represent groups of genes that are often performed by GSPs; however, the analyses may also be performed by other molecular techniques (polymerase chain reaction [PCR] methods and microarrays). These codes should be used when the components of the descriptor(s) are fulfilled regardless of the technique used to provide the analysis, unless specifically noted in the code descriptor. When a GSP assay includes gene(s) that is listed in more than one code descriptor, the code for the most specific test for the primary disorder sought should be reported,

rather than reporting multiple codes for the same gene(s). When all of the components of the descriptor are not performed, use individual Tier 1 codes, Tier 2 codes, or 81479 (Unlisted molecular pathology procedure).

▶*Low-pass sequencing:* a method of genome sequencing intended for cytogenomic analysis of chromosomal abnormalities, such as that performed for trait mapping or copy number variation, typically performed to an average depth of sequencing ranging from 0.1 to 5X.◀

The assays in this section represent discrete genetic values, properties, or characteristics in which the measurement or analysis of each analyte is potentially of independent medical significance or useful in medical management. In contrast to multianalyte assays with algorithmic analyses (MAAAs), the assays in this section do not represent algorithmically combined results to obtain a risk score or other value, which in itself represents a new and distinct medical property that is of independent medical significance relative to the individual, component test results.

▶(For cytogenomic [genome-wide] analysis for constitutional chromosomal abnormalities, see 81228, 81229, 81405, 81406)◀

**81415** Exome (eg, unexplained constitutional or heritable disorder or syndrome); sequence analysis

**+ 81416** sequence analysis, each comparator exome (eg, parents, siblings) (List separately in addition to code for primary procedure)

(Use 81416 in conjunction with 81415)

**81417** re-evaluation of previously obtained exome sequence (eg, updated knowledge or unrelated condition/syndrome)

(Do not report 81417 for incidental findings)

▶(Do not report 81349 when analysis for chromosomal abnormalities is performed by sequence analysis included in 81415, 81416)◀

▶(For cytogenomic [genome-wide] copy number assessment, see 81228, 81229)◀

**81420** Fetal chromosomal aneuploidy (eg, trisomy 21, monosomy X) genomic sequence analysis panel, circulating cell-free fetal DNA in maternal blood, must include analysis of chromosomes 13, 18, and 21

(Do not report 81228, 81229, 88271 when performing genomic sequencing procedures or other molecular multianalyte assays for copy number analysis)

▶(Do not report 81349 when analysis for chromosomal abnormalities is performed by sequence analysis included in 81425, 81426)◀

**81422** Fetal chromosomal microdeletion(s) genomic sequence analysis (eg, DiGeorge syndrome, Cri-du-chat syndrome), circulating cell-free fetal DNA in maternal blood

★ = Telemedicine    ✚ = Add-on code    ✚ = FDA approval pending    # = Resequenced code    ⃠ = Modifier 51 exempt

(Do not report 81228, 81229, 88271 when performing genomic sequencing procedures or other molecular multianalyte assays for copy number analysis)

▶(Do not report 81349 when analysis for chromosomal abnormalities is performed by sequence analysis included in 81425, 81426)◀

**81425** Genome (eg, unexplained constitutional or heritable disorder or syndrome); sequence analysis

**+ 81426** sequence analysis, each comparator genome (eg, parents, siblings) (List separately in addition to code for primary procedure)

(Use 81426 in conjunction with 81425)

**81427** re-evaluation of previously obtained genome sequence (eg, updated knowledge or unrelated condition/syndrome)

(Do not report 81427 for incidental findings)

▶(Do not report 81349 when analysis for chromosomal abnormalities is performed by sequence analysis included in 81425, 81426)◀

▶(For copy number assessment by cytogenomic [genome-wide] analysis for constitutional chromosomal abnormalities, see 81228, 81229)◀

▶(For cytogenomic [genome-wide] analysis for constitutional chromosomal abnormalities interrogation of genomic regions for copy number and loss-of-heterozygosity variants, low-pass sequencing analysis, use 81349)◀

## Rationale

In accordance with the changes made to cytogenomic (genome-wide) analysis for constitutional chromosomal abnormalities and the addition of code 81349 to report low-pass sequencing for these procedures, a definition has been added to the guidelines in the Genomic Sequencing Procedures and Other Molecular Multianalyte Assays subsection to define "low-pass sequencing" and assist users in understanding use of the new code. In addition, parenthetical notes following these guidelines and following codes 81417, 81420, 81422, and 81427 have been added, deleted, or revised to accommodate the changes made to these procedures.

Refer to the codebook and the Rationale for code 81349 for a full discussion of these changes.

# Multianalyte Assays with Algorithmic Analyses

**81507** Fetal aneuploidy (trisomy 21, 18, and 13) DNA sequence analysis of selected regions using maternal plasma, algorithm reported as a risk score for each trisomy

(Do not report 81228, 81229, 88271 when performing genomic sequencing procedures or other molecular multianalyte assays for copy number analysis)

▶(For cytogenomic [genome-wide] analysis for constitutional chromosomal abnormalities interrogation of genomic regions for copy number and loss-of-heterozygosity variants, low-pass sequencing analysis, use 81349)◀

## Rationale

In accordance with the changes made to cytogenomic (genome-wide) analysis for constitutional chromosomal abnormalities and the addition of code 81349 used to report low-pass sequencing for these procedures, a parenthetical note following code 81507 has been added.

Refer to the codebook and the Rationale for code 81349 for a full discussion of these changes.

**81521** Oncology (breast), mRNA, microarray gene expression profiling of 70 content genes and 465 housekeeping genes, utilizing fresh frozen or formalin-fixed paraffin-embedded tissue, algorithm reported as index related to risk of distant metastasis

▶(Do not report 81521 in conjunction with 81523 for the same specimen)◀

**● 81523** Oncology (breast), mRNA, next-generation sequencing gene expression profiling of 70 content genes and 31 housekeeping genes, utilizing formalin-fixed paraffin-embedded tissue, algorithm reported as index related to risk to distant metastasis

▶(Do not report 81523 in conjunction with 81521 for the same specimen)◀

## Rationale

A new Category I multianalyte assay with algorithmic analysis (MAAA) code (81523) has been established to report oncology, mRNA, with next-generation sequencing. An exclusionary parenthetical note has been added following code 81521 to restrict the reporting of code 81523 with code 81521 for the same specimen. A separate listing of this code that includes the proprietary test name has been added to Appendix O of the CPT code set.

## Clinical Example (81523)

A 55-year-old female, who has node-negative stage IIIA breast cancer, discusses adjuvant chemotherapy with her oncologist. The patient is eligible to receive chemotherapy; however, there are no obvious clinical features to inform that decision. A gene expression profiling test is requested.

## Description of Procedure (81523)

Using formalin-fixed paraffin-embedded (FFPE) tissue slides or FFPE tissue blocks, the laboratory prepares hematoxylin and eosin (H&E)–stained slides to assesses the tumor cell percentage. Specimens with a minimum of 30% invasive tumor cells proceed to next-generation sequencing (NGS) analysis. To assess the gene expression, extract total RNA from the tissue. Generate, amplify, and analyze sequencing libraries to determine the expression levels of specific genes. Use the resulting expression profile to calculate an index correlating with low or high risk of tumor metastasis. Return a report to the health care professional.

81554    Pulmonary disease (idiopathic pulmonary fibrosis [IPF]), mRNA, gene expression analysis of 190 genes, utilizing transbronchial biopsies, diagnostic algorithm reported as categorical result (eg, positive or negative for high probability of usual interstitial pneumonia [UIP])

● 81560    Transplantation medicine (allograft rejection, pediatric liver and small bowel), measurement of donor and third-party-induced CD154+T-cytotoxic memory cells, utilizing whole peripheral blood, algorithm reported as a rejection risk score

▶(Do not report 81560 in conjunction with 85032, 86353, 86821, 88184, 88185, 88187, 88230, 88240, 88241, 0018M)◀

### Rationale

A new Category I MAAA code 81560 has been established to report transplantation medicine (ie, measurement of donor and third party–induced CD154+T-cytotoxic memory cells). The descriptor includes language that notes that whole peripheral blood is used for the procedure. In addition, common to MAAA testing, the algorithm is reported as a rejection risk score.

An exclusionary parenthetical note has been included following the code to restrict reporting code 81560 in conjunction with other related laboratory procedures, such as blood counts, lymphocyte transformation or lymphocyte culture, and flow cytometry.

A separate listing of this code that includes the proprietary test name has been added to Appendix O of the CPT code set.

In accordance with the addition of administrative MAAA code 0018M, the exclusionary parenthetical note following code 81560 has been revised with the addition of code 0018M.

## Clinical Example (81560)

A 5-year-old male requires regular surveillance clinic visits to assess the status of his liver transplant (allograft). In addition to other clinical assessments (eg, liver function tests), the patient's physician orders the test to predict whether he is at increased or decreased risk of acute cellular rejection.

## Description of Procedure (81560)

Isolate, count, and assess the viability of peripheral blood leukocytes (PBLs) from the patient's blood sample. Use patient human leukocyte antigen (HLA) information supplied with the sample to identify appropriate cryopreserved PBL stimulators that resemble the donor (donor) or are different (reference). Thaw, count, and assess the viability of these stimulators. Pre-label the recipient PBLs and stimulator PBLs; separately mix the recipient PBLs with each type of stimulator PBL (donor and reference, respectively); add antibodies to CD154; and culture them separately overnight. Enumerate the number of CD154+T-cytotoxic memory cells induced in the donor and reference cultures. Report the test results as a binary risk score for acute cellular rejection (ACR), which is calculated algorithmically by expressing the ratio of donor-induced CD154+CD8-memory cells and those induced by reference. Send the patient report to the ordering physician.

# Chemistry

82642    Dihydrotestosterone (DHT)

(For dihydrotestosterone analysis for anabolic drug testing, see 80327, 80328)

(Dipropylacetic acid, use 80164)

(Dopamine, see 82382-82384)

(Duodenal contents, see individual enzymes; for intubation and collection, see 43756, 43757)

82653    Code is out of numerical sequence. See 82642-82658

▲ 82656    Elastase, pancreatic (EL-1), fecal; qualitative or semi-quantitative

#● 82653        quantitative

★ = Telemedicine   ✚ = Add-on code   ✍ = FDA approval pending   # = Resequenced code   ⊘ = Modifier 51 exempt

## Rationale

Code 82656 has been revised, and code 82653 has been added to the Chemistry subsection.

Code 82653 has been established to report quantitative testing for pancreatic elastase. To accommodate code 82653 as a child code, code 82656 has been revised as a parent code to the newly established child code 82653.

## Clinical Example (82653)

A 25-year-old female presents with chronic diarrhea, bloating, abdominal pain, and unexplained weight loss. Fecal pancreatic elastase quantitative testing is ordered.

## Description of Procedure (82653)

Submit the patient's fecal specimen for immunoassay testing. Determine and report the quantitative results directly from the curve.

| | |
|---|---|
| 83516 | Immunoassay for analyte other than infectious agent antibody or infectious agent antigen; qualitative or semiquantitative, multiple step method |
| 83520 | quantitative, not otherwise specified |
| | (For immunoassays for antibodies to infectious agent antigens, see analyte and method specific codes in the **Immunology** section) |
| | (For immunoassay of tumor antigen not elsewhere specified, use 86316) |
| | (Immunoglobulins, see 82784, 82785) |
| ● 83521 | Immunoglobulin light chains (ie, kappa, lambda), free, each |

## Rationale

Code 83521 has been established in the Chemistry section to report each immunoglobulin light chains tested.

Prior to 2022, there was no specific CPT code to describe testing for kappa and lambda light chains in serum. However, codes 83520, *Immunoassay for analyte other than infectious agent antibody or infectious agent antigen; quantitative, not otherwise specified,* and 83883, *Nephelometry, each analyte not elsewhere specified,* were used to report this testing. Codes 83520 and 83883 are both methodology codes that do not provide specificity of the analytes being tested.

Code 83521 describes testing for kappa and lambda light chains in serum, and it is intended to be used for patients who are clinically suspected of having hematologic diseases based on certain symptoms and/or medical conditions, such as bone pain, bone fractures, normocytic

anemia, kidney disease, and recurrent infections suggestive of an underlying plasma-cell disorder. This procedure is performed using the immunoturbidimetric method. In addition, the kappa and lambda light chains testing may be used to assist in the diagnosis of plasma-cell disorders, such as multiple myeloma, primary amyloidosis, monoclonal gammopathy of unknown significance (MGUS), Waldenström's macroglobulinemia, and related disorders.

## Clinical Example (83521)

A 68-year-old male with a 3-year history of an IgG kappa monoclonal gammopathy of undetermined significance (MGUS) is seen by his medical oncologist. Serum kappa and lambda light chains are ordered.

## Description of Procedure (83521)

Submit the patient's serum sample for testing. Determine free kappa and lambda light chain concentration by measuring antigen-antibody complex formation (eg, immunonephelometry, immunoturbidimetry). Report results.

| | | |
|---|---|---|
| | 83525 | Insulin; total |
| | | (For proinsulin, use 84206) |
| | 83527 | free |
| #● | 83529 | Interleukin-6 (IL-6) |
| | 83528 | Intrinsic factor |
| | | (For intrinsic factor antibodies, use 86340) |
| | 83529 | Code is out of numerical sequence. See 83525-83540 |

## Rationale

A new Category I code (83529) has been established to report interleukin-6 testing for the evaluation of conditions, such as inflammation, diabetes, stroke, or cardiovascular disease, in patients. The addition of this new code will allow for greater specificity by identifying the particular analyte when tested, instead of identifying the method-specific service (ie, quantitative immunoassay).

## Clinical Example (83529)

A 42-year-old male is admitted to the hospital with shortness of breath. Testing for severe acute respiratory syndrome coronavirus 2 (SARS-CoV-2) was positive. Serum level of interleukin-6 is obtained.

## Description of Procedure (83529)

Test patient serum for interleukin-6 concentration using enzyme-linked immunosorbent assay (ELISA). Report quantitative results.

# Immunology

(Acetylcholine receptor antibody, see 83519, 86255, 86256)

#● 86015    Actin (smooth muscle) antibody (ASMA), each

(Actinomyces, antibodies to, use 86602)

(Adrenal cortex antibodies, see 86255, 86256)

### Rationale

Code 86015 has been added to the Immunology subsection to identify testing for antibodies that aid in the diagnosis of autoimmune liver diseases, such as autoimmune hepatitis (AIH) and primary biliary cholangitis (PBC). This code is more specific because the focus is on the analyte (actin antibodies) tested instead of the method used. This code may be reported for each actin (smooth muscle) antibody tested.

To accommodate addition of this code, cross-reference parenthetical notes for smooth-muscle antibody and antibody testing have been revised with the addition of the new code and, where appropriate, deletion of reference to the method-specific codes (86255, 86256) previously used for reporting this service.

### Clinical Example (86015)

A 56-year-old female presents with liver failure. Serum testing for actin (smooth muscle) antibody is ordered to assist in the diagnosis of autoimmune hepatitis.

### Description of Procedure (86015)

Test a serum sample for actin (smooth muscle) antibodies by immunoassay. Report the results.

| | |
|---|---|
| 86015 | Code is out of numerical sequence. See 85810-86001 |
| 86021 | Antibody identification; leukocyte antibodies |
| 86022 | platelet antibodies |
| 86023 | platelet associated immunoglobulin assay |
| ● 86036 | Antineutrophil cytoplasmic antibody (ANCA); screen, each antibody |
| ● 86037 | titer, each antibody |

### Rationale

Two new codes (86036, 86037) have been added to the Immunology subsection to report an antineutrophil cytoplasmic antibody (ANCA) screen and a titer antibody test.

ANCA antibodies are broadly used across a number of autoimmune and inflammatory diseases. Tests for these antibodies were previously reported using method-specific codes 86255 and 86256.

### Clinical Example (86036)

A 40-year-old male presents with relapsing infections of the upper respiratory tract and nasal bleeding for 5 months. Antineutrophil cytoplasmic antibody testing for cytoplasmic stained antineutrophil antibodies (c-ANCA), perinuclear stained antineutrophil antibodies (p-ANCA), and perinuclear stained antineutrophil antibodies (atypical p-ANCA) are ordered.

### Description of Procedure (86036)

Obtain a serum sample and perform an indirect immunofluorescent antibody test for c-ANCA, p-ANCA, and atypical p-ANCA. Report the qualitative results.

### Clinical Example (86037)

A 40-year-old male presents with relapsing infections of the upper respiratory tract and nasal bleeding for 5 months. Antineutrophil cytoplasmic antibody testing for c-ANCA is positive and a c-ANCA titer is ordered.

### Description of Procedure (86037)

Obtain a serum sample and perform an indirect immunofluorescent antibody titer test for c-ANCA. Report the results as a titer.

| | |
|---|---|
| 86038 | Antinuclear antibodies (ANA); |
| 86051 | Code is out of numerical sequence. See 86060-86078 |
| 86052 | Code is out of numerical sequence. See 86060-86078 |
| 86053 | Code is out of numerical sequence. See 86060-86078 |
| #● 86051 | Aquaporin-4 (neuromyelitis optica [NMO]) antibody; enzyme-linked immunosorbent immunoassay (ELISA) |
| #● 86052 | cell-based immunofluorescence assay (CBA), each |
| #● 86053 | flow cytometry (ie, fluorescence-activated cell sorting [FACS]), each |

★=Telemedicine   ✦=Add-on code   ✗=FDA approval pending   #=Resequenced code   ⊘=Modifier 51 exemp

# Rationale

Codes 86051-86053, 86362, and 86363 have been added to the Immunology subsection of the Pathology and Laboratory section to report: (1) neuromyelitis optica (NMO) antibody testing using enzyme-linked immunosorbent immunoassay (ELISA) (86051), (2) NMO testing using cell-based immunofluorescence assay (86052), (3) NMO using flow cytometry (86053), (4) myelin oligodendrocyte glycoprotein (MOG-IgG1) antibody testing using cell-based immunofluorescence assay (86362), and (5) MOG-IgG1 using flow cytometry (86363).

These codes have been established to offer a reporting mechanism that provides more specificity by including the condition tested in addition to noting the method used (ie, NMO spectrum/MOG-IgG1 antibody in conjunction with the ELISA, CBA, and FACS methods of testing). As a result of including language that specifies the antibody tested, use of these codes will allow better differentiation of the testing procedures provided, instead of using the same method-only code multiple times to identify the different conditions tested.

## Clinical Example (86051)

A 25-year-old female with eye pain leading to loss of clear vision in one eye and pain in her back and legs sees her primary health care provider, who orders tests including imaging and blood tests for AQP4-IgG with reflex to MOG-IgG.

## Description of Procedure (86051)

Submit a serum sample for testing. Perform an enzyme-linked immunosorbent immunoassay (ELISA). Report results.

## Clinical Example (86052)

A 25-year-old female with eye pain leading to loss of clear vision in one eye and pain in her back and legs sees her primary health care provider, who orders tests including imaging and blood tests for AQP4-IgG with reflex to MOG-IgG.

## Description of Procedure (86052)

Submit a serum sample for testing. Perform a cell-based assay (CBA) and, if necessary, perform a titration of results. Report results.

## Clinical Example (86053)

A 25-year-old female with eye pain leading to loss of clear vision in one eye and pain in her back and legs sees her primary health care provider, who orders tests including imaging and blood tests for AQP4-IgG with reflex to MOG-IgG.

## Description of Procedure (86053)

Measure serum antibodies using flow cytometry to quantitate human antibodies bound to AQP4 expressing cells, and then titrate if present. Report qualitative results and titer results (semi-quantitative), if performed.

---

| | |
|---|---|
| 86225 | Deoxyribonucleic acid (DNA) antibody; native or double stranded |
| | (Echinococcus, antibodies to, see code for specific method) |
| | (For HIV antibody tests, see 86701-86703) |
| 86226 | single stranded |
| | (Anti D.S., DNA, IFA, eg, using C.Lucilae, see 86255 and 86256) |
| ● 86231 | Endomysial antibody (EMA), each immunoglobulin (Ig) class |

# Rationale

A new code (86231) has been added to the Immunology subsection to report endomysial antibody testing for each immunoglobulin (Ig) class. This code is more specific because the focus is on the analyte (endomysial antibody) tested instead of the method used. Prior to CPT 2022, this service was reported using a method-specific code.

## Clinical Example (86231)

A 29-year-old female presents with worsening abdominal pain. Symptoms are constant, worse before a bowel movement, and with no alleviating factors. Endomysial (EMA), gliadin (DPG), and tissue transglutaminase (tTG) antibody were ordered to evaluate for celiac disease.

## Description of Procedure (86231)

EMA antibody by indirect fluorescent antibody (IFA). Report results.

Pathology and Laboratory 80047-89398, 0001U-0284U

86235    Extractable nuclear antigen, antibody to, any method (eg, nRNP, SS-A, SS-B, Sm, RNP, Sc170, J01), each antibody

86255    Fluorescent noninfectious agent antibody; screen, each antibody

86256        titer, each antibody

(Fluorescent technique for antigen identification in tissue, use 88346; for indirect fluorescence, see 88346, 88350)

(FTA, use 86780)

(Gel [agar] diffusion tests, use 86331)

● 86258    Gliadin (deamidated) (DGP) antibody, each immunoglobulin (Ig) class

## Rationale

A new code (86258) has been added to the Immunology subsection to report gliadin (deamidated) (DGP [deamidated gliadin peptide]) antibody testing for each Ig class.

This code is intended to identify a serum DGP that is measured by immunoassay via, for example, ELISA or automated, multiplex bead assays.

## Clinical Example (86258)

A 29-year-old female presents with worsening abdominal pain. Symptoms are constant, worse before a bowel movement, and with no alleviating factors. EMA, DPG, and tissue transglutaminase (tTG) antibodies were ordered to evaluate for celiac disease.

## Description of Procedure (86258)

Measure serum DGP by immunoassay, (eg, ELISA, multiplexed bead assays). Report results.

86277    Growth hormone, human (HGH), antibody

86317    Immunoassay for infectious agent antibody, quantitative, not otherwise specified

▶(For immunoassay techniques for non-infectious agent antigens, see 83516, 83518, 83519, 83520)◄

(For particle agglutination procedures, use 86403)

▶(For infectious agent antigen detection by immunoassay technique, see 87301-87451. For infectious agent antigen detection by immunoassay technique with direct optical [ie, visual] observation, see 87802-87899)◄

## Rationale

In accordance with the extensive revisions made to the Immunology subsection of the Pathology and Laboratory section, a parenthetical note has been revised and a new parenthetical note has been added following code 86317. These parenthetical notes provide instructions for correct reporting of non-infectious agent antigens and infectious agent antigen detection by immunoassay technique performed with direct optical observation and performed without direct optical observation.

86356    Mononuclear cell antigen, quantitative (eg, flow cytometry), not otherwise specified, each antigen

(Do not report 88187-88189 for interpretation of 86355, 86356, 86357, 86359, 86360, 86361, 86367)

#● 86362    Myelin oligodendrocyte glycoprotein (MOG-IgG1) antibody; cell-based immunofluorescence assay (CBA), each

#● 86363        flow cytometry (ie, fluorescence-activated cell sorting [FACS]), each

## Rationale

Codes 86362 and 86363 have been added to the Immunology subsection of the Pathology and Laboratory section to report MOG-IgG1 antibody testing using cell-based immunofluorescence assay (86362) and MOG-IgG1 using flow cytometry (86363).

Refer to the codebook and the Rationale for codes 86051-86053 for a full discussion of these changes.

## Clinical Example (86362)

A 25-year-old female with eye pain leading to loss of clear vision in one eye and pain in her back and legs sees her primary health care provider, who orders tests including imaging and blood tests for AQP4-IgG with reflex to MOG-IgG.

## Description of Procedure (86362)

Submit a serum sample for testing. Perform a CBA and, if necessary, perform a titration of results. Report results.

## Clinical Example (86363)

A 25-year-old female with eye pain leading to loss of clear vision in one eye and pain in her back and legs sees her primary health care provider, who orders tests including imaging and blood tests for AQP4-IgG with reflex to MOG-IgG.

## Description of Procedure (86363)

Measure serum antibodies using flow cytometry to quantitate human antibodies bound to MOG expressing cells, and then titrate if present. Report qualitative results and titer results (semi-quantitative), if performed.

| | | |
|---|---|---|
| | 86357 | Natural killer (NK) cells, total count |
| #● | 86364 | Tissue transglutaminase, each immunoglobulin (Ig) class |

### Rationale

A new code (86364) has been added to the Immunology subsection to report tissue transglutaminase for each Ig class.

This code is intended to identify a serum tissue transglutaminase that is measured by immunoassay, for example, via ELISA or automated, multiplexed bead assays. Prior to the addition of code 86364, this test was reported with a methodological code.

## Clinical Example (86364)

A 29-year-old female presents with worsening abdominal pain. Symptoms are constant, worse before a bowel movement, and with no alleviating factors. EMA, gliadin DPG, and tTG antibodies were ordered to evaluate for celiac disease.

## Description of Procedure (86364)

Measure serum tTG by immunoassay (eg, ELISA or automated, multiplexed bead assays). Report results.

| | | |
|---|---|---|
| | 86359 | T cells; total count |
| | 86362 | Code is out of numerical sequence. See 86355-86364 |
| | 86363 | Code is out of numerical sequence. See 86355-86364 |
| | 86364 | Code is out of numerical sequence. See 86356-86360 |
| | 86376 | Microsomal antibodies (eg, thyroid or liver-kidney), each |
| ● | 86381 | Mitochondrial antibody (eg, M2), each |

### Rationale

Code 86381 has been added to the Immunology subsection to report each mitochondrial antibody tested because there were no specific codes to describe testing for mitochondrial antibody before 2022. Code 86381 is intended to describe testing for each mitochondrial antibody to detect certain liver disorders.

## Clinical Example (86381)

A 52-year-old female presents with pruritis, fatigue, and a history of rheumatoid arthritis. Her physician requests a mitochondrial antibody test.

## Description of Procedure (86381)

Obtain a serum sample and perform an indirect immunofluorescent antibody test to detect the circulating levels of human mitochondrial antibody. If the test is positive, perform a titer. Report the results.

| | | |
|---|---|---|
| | 86382 | Neutralization test, viral |
| #● | 86408 | Neutralizing antibody, severe acute respiratory syndrome coronavirus 2 (SARS-CoV-2) (coronavirus disease [COVID-19]); screen |
| #● | 86409 | titer |
| #● | 86413 | Severe acute respiratory syndrome coronavirus 2 (SARS-CoV-2) (coronavirus disease [COVID-19]) antibody, quantitative |

### Rationale

Several codes have been added to report testing for severe acute respiratory syndrome coronavirus 2 (SARS-CoV-2) (coronavirus disease [COVID-19]). Codes 86408 and 86409 have been established to report neutralizing antibody testing for COVID-19. Code 86408 describes a screen and code 86409 describes a titer. Code 86413 has been established to report quantitative antibody testing for COVID-19.

## Clinical Example (86408)

A 56-year-old female was discharged from the hospital after a lengthy stay with severe COVID-19, which was confirmed with molecular testing for SARS-CoV-2. Two weeks after her recovery, she presents at a blood donation center for testing to determine eligibility for convalescent plasma donation.

Pathology and Laboratory 80047-89398, 0001U-0284U

## Description of Procedure (86408)

Combine the patient's serum, diluent, and pseudovirion expressing the SARS-CoV-2 spike protein with cultured cells in a multi-well plate. Following incubation period, add substrate, which will luminesce in the presence of viral infection. Measure the signal on a multi-well plate reader. Compare the specimen measurements to the control specimen to generate a qualitative result.

## Clinical Example (86409)

A 56-year-old female was discharged from the hospital after a lengthy stay with severe COVID-19, which was confirmed with molecular testing for SARS-CoV-2. Two weeks after her recovery, she presents at a blood donation center for testing to determine eligibility for convalescent plasma donation.

## Description of Procedure (86409)

Incubate serial dilutions of patient's sera with target cells and pseudovirion expressing the SARS-CoV-2 spike protein. Measure antibody-neutralizing activity using quantitative or semi-quantitative assessment of the changes in the signal activity. Compare the results to the control specimen and interpret and report the results.

## Clinical Example (86413)

A 52-year-old female was discharged from the hospital after a lengthy stay with severe COVID-19, which is confirmed by molecular testing for SARS-CoV-2. Four weeks after her recovery, a blood specimen was submitted for quantitative antibody evaluation to assess her immune response to the virus.

## Description of Procedure (86413)

Incubate and wash patient serum and diluent added to a SARS-CoV-2 spike protein receptor binding domain (RBD)-complexed solid-phase surface, followed by adding antihuman-signal antibodies to detect bound anti-RBD antibodies. The relative amount of signal measured is directly proportional to the anti-RBD antibody concentration in the specimen and is interpreted using a standards-generated calibration curve with results reported in quantitative units.

| | |
|---|---|
| 86408 | Code is out of numerical sequence. See 86376-86386 |
| 86409 | Code is out of numerical sequence. See 86376-86386 |
| 86413 | Code is out of numerical sequence. See 86376-86386 |
| **86485** | Skin test; candida |
| | (For antibody, candida, use 86628) |
| **86486** | unlisted antigen, each |

| | |
|---|---|
| **86490** | coccidioidomycosis |
| **86510** | histoplasmosis |
| | (For histoplasma, antibody, use 86698) |
| **86580** | tuberculosis, intradermal |
| | (For tuberculosis test, cell mediated immunity measurement of gamma interferon antigen response, use 86480) |
| | (For skin tests for allergy, see 95012-95199) |
| | ▶(Smooth muscle antibody, use 86015)◄ |

## Rationale

To accommodate the addition of code 86015, a cross-reference parenthetical note for smooth-muscle antibody testing has been revised with the addition of code 86015 to direct users to this code, instead of the method-specific codes for antibody screening.

Refer to the codebook and the Rationale for code 86015 for a full discussion of these changes.

| | |
|---|---|
| | (Sporothrix, antibodies to, see code for specific method) |
| **86593** | quantitative |
| | (For antibodies to infectious agents, see 86602-86804) |
| | (Tetanus antibody, use 86774) |
| | (Thyroglobulin antibody, use 86800) |
| | (Thyroglobulin, use 84432) |
| | (Thyroid microsomal antibody, use 86376) |
| | (For toxoplasma antibody, see 86777-86778) |
| ● **86596** | Voltage-gated calcium channel antibody, each |

## Rationale

Code 86596 has been established to report voltage-gated calcium channel antibody testing. The test identifies a particular type of antibody that exhibits a neurological autoimmune response to voltage-gated calcium channels. Testing for the presence of these antibodies aids in the diagnosis of autoimmune responses to neuropathology in patients with a history of cancer. Code 86596 may be reported for each antibody tested.

## Clinical Example (86596)

A 50-year-old male with progressive muscle weakness of his lower extremities and gait disturbance is seen by his physician. Serum testing for voltage-gated calcium channel P/Q antibody level is ordered.

★ = Telemedicine   ✚ = Add-on code   ⬧ = FDA approval pending   # = Resequenced code   ⊘ = Modifier 51 exempt

## Description of Procedure (86596)

Test a serum sample using an immunoassay method to detect voltage-gated calcium channel P/Q antibody Report the results.

---

The following codes (86602-86804) are qualitative or semiquantitative immunoassays performed by multiple-step methods for the detection of antibodies to infectious agents. For immunoassays by single-step method (eg, reagent strips), see codes 86318, 86328. Procedures for the identification of antibodies should be coded as precisely as possible. For example, an antibody to a virus could be coded with increasing specificity for virus, family, genus, species, or type. In some cases, further precision may be added to codes by specifying the class of immunoglobulin being detected. When multiple tests are done to detect antibodies to organisms classified more precisely than the specificity allowed by available codes, it is appropriate to code each as a separate service. For example, a test for antibody to an enterovirus is coded as 86658. Coxsackie viruses are enteroviruses, but there are no codes for the individual species of enterovirus. If assays are performed for antibodies to coxsackie A and B species, each assay should be separately coded. Similarly, if multiple assays are performed for antibodies of different immunoglobulin classes, each assay should be coded separately. When a coding option exists for reporting IgM specific antibodies (eg, 86632), the corresponding nonspecific code (eg, 86631) may be reported for performance of either an antibody analysis not specific for a particular immunoglobulin class or for an IgG analysis.

▶(For the detection of antibodies other than those to infectious agents, see specific antibody [eg, 86015, 86021-86023, 86376, 86800, 86850-86870] or specific method [eg, 83516, 86255, 86256])◀

(For infectious agent/antigen detection, see 87260-87899)

**86602**    Antibody; actinomyces

### Rationale

To accommodate the addition of code 86015, a cross-reference parenthetical note for antibody testing has been revised with the addition of code 86015 to direct users to this specific code for actin (smooth muscle) antibody testing.

Refer to the codebook and the Rationale for code 86015 for a full discussion of these changes.

# Microbiology

**87140**    Culture, typing; immunofluorescent method, each antiserum

**87149**        identification by nucleic acid (DNA or RNA) probe, direct probe technique, per culture or isolate, each organism probed

(Do not report 87149 in conjunction with 81161, 81200-81408)

**87150**        identification by nucleic acid (DNA or RNA) probe, amplified probe technique, per culture or isolate, each organism probed

(Do not report 87150 in conjunction with 81161, 81200-81408)

#● **87154**        identification of blood pathogen and resistance typing, when performed, by nucleic acid (DNA or RNA) probe, multiplexed amplified probe technique including multiplex reverse transcription, when performed, per culture or isolate, 6 or more targets

### Rationale

Child code 87154 has been added to the culture, typing family of codes (87140, 87149, 87150) in the Microbiology subsection.

Code 87154 specifically identifies blood pathogen and resistance typing. This test is performed by nucleic acid (DNA or RNA) probe, multiplexed amplified probe technique, including multiplex reverse transcription, per culture or isolate, for 6 or more targets.

## Clinical Example (87154)

An 85-year-old male presents with a fever, chills, rigors, confusion, and difficulty breathing. A blood culture is ordered. The blood culture returns positive with gram-stain revealing gram-negative rods and is submitted for blood-culture pathogen identification.

## Description of Procedure (87154)

Isolate a sample from the positive blood culture and subject the sample to multiplex nucleic acid amplification. Review and report the results.

---

**87154**    Code is out of numerical sequence. See 87149-87153

**87250**    Virus isolation; inoculation of embryonated eggs, or small animal, includes observation and dissection

**87255**        including identification by non-immunologic method, other than by cytopathic effect (eg, virus specific enzymatic activity)

▶These codes are intended for primary source only. For similar studies on culture material, refer to codes 87140-87158. Infectious agents by antigen detection, immunofluorescence microscopy, or nucleic acid probe techniques should be reported as precisely as possible. The molecular pathology procedures codes (81161, 81200-81408) are not to be used in combination with or instead of the procedures represented by 87471-87801. The most specific code possible should be reported. If there is no specific agent code, the general methodology code (eg, 87299, 87449, 87797, 87798, 87799, 87899) should be used. For identification of antibodies to many of the listed infectious agents, see 86602-86804. When separate results are reported for different species or strain of organisms, each result should be coded separately. Use modifier 59 when separate results are reported for different species or strains that are described by the same code.

When identifying infectious agents on primary-source specimens (eg, tissue, smear) microscopically by direct/indirect immunofluorescent assay [IFA] techniques, see 87260-87300. When identifying infectious agents on primary-source specimens or derivatives via non-microscopic immunochemical techniques with fluorescence detection (ie, fluorescence immunoassay [FIA]), see 87301-87451, 87802-87899. When identifying infectious agents on primary-source specimens using antigen detection by immunoassay with direct optical (ie, visual) observation, see 87802-87899.◀

## Rationale

Extensive revisions have been made to the Microbiology subsection of the Pathology and Laboratory section of the CPT 2022 code set. These revisions were the result of the rapid, ongoing reporting needs for proper reporting of diagnostic testing for SARS-CoV-2 (COVID-19). As a result of these dynamic needs, the code set has been updated to clarify existing areas that have caused confusion.

Historically, multiple methods have been available for the detection and measurement of infectious disease agents. When the primary-source infectious agent codes were created, it was essentially split into four sections based on methodology: immunofluorescent technique, immunoassay technique, detection by nucleic acid (DNA or RNA), and immunoassay with direct optical observation. Over time, confusion arose over the definition of "direct optical observation." In contrast to the differentiation between the two methods that are based on detection (ie, by immunofluorescence and other immunologic techniques), the direct optical observation codes used a different paradigm to separate these methodologies based on how a physician observes the results.

Additional consideration was made to the definition of "single step" vs "multi-step" methodologies for immunoassays. Although these codes were generally well understood at the time of their creation, the differentiation between the two methodologies over time has become difficult with the advent of automation and matrix processes (eg, lateral flow), which allow multiple steps to occur within the analysis, even though the operator had a single touch point.

Based on this historical understanding, the following revisions have been made to the code set:

■ Introductory guidelines have been added to the Microbiology subsection to provide instruction on correct reporting of infectious agent antigen primary-source studies using microscopic direct or indirect IFA techniques vs immunoassay with direct optical (ie, visual) observation, and primary-source specimen or derivative studies using non-microscopic immunochemical techniques with fluorescence detection.

■ Twenty-nine codes (87301-87451) have been revised to add "fluorescence immunoassay [FIA]" and remove the phrase "multiple-step method" from the code descriptors and code 87450 for single step has been deleted. Revisions have also been made to codes 87802-87899 to clarify the definition of direct optical observation by adding "(ie, visual)."

| | | |
|---|---|---|
| 87260 | | Infectious agent antigen detection by immunofluorescent technique; adenovirus |
| ▲ 87301 | | Infectious agent antigen detection by immunoassay technique (eg, enzyme immunoassay [EIA], enzyme-linked immunosorbent assay [ELISA], fluorescence immunoassay [FIA], immunochemiluminometric assay [IMCA]), qualitative or semiquantitative; adenovirus enteric types 40/41 |
| ▲ 87305 | | Aspergillus |
| ▲ 87320 | | Chlamydia trachomatis |
| ▲ 87324 | | Clostridium difficile toxin(s) |
| ▲ 87327 | | Cryptococcus neoformans |
| | | (For Cryptococcus latex agglutination, use 86403) |
| ▲ 87328 | | cryptosporidium |
| ▲ 87329 | | giardia |
| ▲ 87332 | | cytomegalovirus |
| ▲ 87335 | | Escherichia coli 0157 |
| | | (For giardia antigen, use 87329) |
| ▲ 87336 | | Entamoeba histolytica dispar group |

★ = Telemedicine  ✚ = Add-on code  ⊘ = FDA approval pending  # = Resequenced code  ⊘ = Modifier 51 exempt

▲ **87337**     Entamoeba histolytica group

▲ **87338**     Helicobacter pylori, stool

▲ **87339**     Helicobacter pylori

(For H. pylori, stool, use 87338. For H. pylori, breath and blood by mass spectrometry, see 83013, 83014. For H. pylori, liquid scintillation counter, see 78267, 78268)

▲ **87340**     hepatitis B surface antigen (HBsAg)

▲ **87341**     hepatitis B surface antigen (HBsAg) neutralization

▲ **87350**     hepatitis Be antigen (HBeAg)

▲ **87380**     hepatitis, delta agent

▲ **87385**     Histoplasma capsulatum

▲ **87389**     HIV-1 antigen(s), with HIV-1 and HIV-2 antibodies, single result

▲ **87390**     HIV-1

▲ **87391**     HIV-2

▲ **87400**     Influenza, A or B, each

▲ **87420**     respiratory syncytial virus

▲ **87425**     rotavirus

▲ **87426**     severe acute respiratory syndrome coronavirus (eg, SARS-CoV, SARS-CoV-2 [COVID-19])

#●  **87428**     severe acute respiratory syndrome coronavirus (eg, SARS-CoV, SARS-CoV-2 [COVID-19]) and influenza virus types A and B

▲ **87427**     Shiga-like toxin

**87428**     Code is out of numerical sequence. See 87425-87430

▲ **87430**     Streptococcus, group A

▲ **87449**     not otherwise specified, each organism

▶(87450 has been deleted. For infectious agent antigen detection by immunoassay technique, see 87301-87451. For infectious agent antigen detection by immunoassay technique with direct optical [ie, visual] observation, see 87802-87899)◀

▲ **87451**     polyvalent for multiple organisms, each polyvalent antiserum

## Rationale

Codes 87301-87451 have been revised with the removal of the phrase "multiple-step method" and the addition of the phrase "fluorescence immunoassay (FIA)." The revision is before the semicolon in the descriptor of parent code 87301, which means the revision applies to all child codes of code 87301.

Code 87428 has been established as a child code of code 87301 to report infectious agent antigen detection by immunoassay technique (eg, enzyme immunoassay [EIA], enzyme-linked immunosorbent assay [ELISA], FIA, immunochemiluminometric assay [IMCA]), qualitative or semiquantitative for testing for COVID-19 and influenza virus types A and B.

Code 87450 has been deleted and a parenthetical note has been added directing users to codes 87301-87451 for infectious agent antigen detection by immunoassay technique and to codes 87802-87899 for infectious agent antigen detection by immunoassay technique with direct optical (ie, visual) observation.

Code 87449 has been revised with removal of the phrase "multiple-step method" to be consistent with the revision of code 87301.

## Clinical Example (87428)

A 50-year-old female presents with fever, cough, and shortness of breath. A nasopharyngeal swab is collected for SARS CoV-2, influenza A, and influenza B antigen testing.

## Description of Procedure (87428)

Place the swab and swirl it in a supplied reagent tube to disrupt and release viral nucleoprotein antigens; transfer an aliquot of that sample to the test cassette sample well; and place it in the analyzer. Report the qualitative results to the ordering health care professional.

**87471**     Infectious agent detection by nucleic acid (DNA or RNA); Bartonella henselae and Bartonella quintana, amplified probe technique

●  **87636**     severe acute respiratory syndrome coronavirus 2 (SARS-CoV-2) (coronavirus disease [COVID-19]) and influenza virus types A and B, multiplex amplified probe technique

●  **87637**     severe acute respiratory syndrome coronavirus 2 (SARS-CoV-2) (coronavirus disease [COVID-19]), influenza virus types A and B, and respiratory syncytial virus, multiplex amplified probe technique

▶(For nucleic acid detection of multiple respiratory infectious agents, not including severe acute respiratory syndrome coronavirus 2 [SARS-CoV-2] [coronavirus disease {COVID-19}], see 87631, 87632, 87633)◀

▶(For nucleic acid detection of multiple respiratory infectious agents, including severe acute respiratory syndrome coronavirus 2 [SARS-CoV-2] [coronavirus disease {COVID-19}] in conjunction with additional target[s] beyond influenza virus types A and B and respiratory syncytial virus, see 87631, 87632, 87633)◀

## Rationale

Codes 87636 and 87637 have been established to report infectious agent detection by nucleic acid (DNA or RNA) for testing for COVID-19 with other viruses. Code 87636 describes testing for COVID-19 and influenza virus types A and B. Code 87637 describes testing for COVID-19, influenza virus types A and B, and respiratory syncytial virus. The tests described in both codes use a multiplex amplified probe technique.

Two cross-reference parenthetical notes have been added following codes 87636 and 87637 to direct users to codes 87631-87633 for nucleic acid detection of multiple respiratory infectious agents.

## Clinical Example (87636)

A 25-year-old female calls her health care professional's health line after 2 days of fever, coughing, runny nose, and muscle aches. The health care professional recommends collecting a nasal swab to test for influenza and COVID-19 because of the overlapping symptoms.

## Description of Procedure (87636)

Perform a multiplex reverse transcription polymerase chain reaction (RT-PCR) assay for the simultaneous qualitative detection and differentiation of SARS-CoV-2, influenza A, and influenza B using a sample of the collected specimen. Provide the results to the health care professional.

## Clinical Example (87637)

A mother calls her health care professional's health line after her 2-year-old child has been having 2 days of fever, coughing, runny nose, and muscle aches. The health care professional recommends collecting a nasal swab to test for influenza A, influenza B, respiratory syncytial virus (RSV), and COVID-19 because of the overlapping symptoms.

## Description of Procedure (87637)

Perform a multiplex RT-PCR assay for the simultaneous qualitative detection and differentiation of SARS-CoV-2, influenza A, influenza B, and RSV using a sample of the collected specimen. Provide the results to the health care professional.

▲ 87802    Infectious agent antigen detection by immunoassay with direct optical (ie, visual) observation; Streptococcus, group B

▲ 87803    Clostridium difficile toxin A

#▲ 87806    HIV-1 antigen(s), with HIV-1 and HIV-2 antibodies

▲ 87804    Influenza

▲ 87807    respiratory syncytial virus

#● 87811    severe acute respiratory syndrome coronavirus 2 (SARS-CoV-2) (coronavirus disease [COVID-19])

▲ 87808    Trichomonas vaginalis

▲ 87809    adenovirus

▲ 87810    Chlamydia trachomatis

87811    Code is out of numerical sequence. See 87804-87809

▲ 87850    Neisseria gonorrhoeae

▲ 87880    Streptococcus, group A

▲ 87899    not otherwise specified

## Rationale

Codes 87802-87899 have been revised to clarify that direct optical observation specifically means visual observation with the addition of the phrase "ie, visual" placed in parentheses. The revision is before the semicolon in the descriptor of parent code 87802, which means the revision applies to all child codes of code 87802.

Code 87811 has been established to report infectious agent antigen detection by immunoassay with direct optical observation for testing for COVID-19.

## Clinical Example (87811)

A 25-year-old female calls her health care professional's health line after 2 days of fever, coughing, runny nose, and muscle aches. The health care professional recommends collecting a nasal swab to test for COVID-19.

## Description of Procedure (87811)

Following the manufacturer's instructions, add a nasal swab specimen from the patient to a lateral flow test system to detect SARS-CoV-2 antigen using an immunochromatographic immunoassay. The operator who visually inspects the test cartridge reads the result, noting the internal control and patient result. Report the qualitative result to the ordering health care professional.

# Cytogenetic Studies

88271    Molecular cytogenetics; DNA probe, each (eg, FISH)

▶(For cytogenomic [genome-wide] analysis for constitutional chromosomal abnormalities, see 81228, 81229, 81349, 81405, 81406, 81479)◀

★ = Telemedicine    ✚ = Add-on code    ✔ = FDA approval pending    # = Resequenced code    ⊘ = Modifier 51 exempt

(For genomic sequencing procedures or other molecular multianalyte assays for copy number analysis using circulating cell-free fetal DNA in maternal blood, see 81420, 81422, 81479)

## Rationale

In accordance with the changes made to cytogenomic (genome-wide) analysis for constitutional chromosomal abnormalities and the addition of code 81349 to report low-pass sequencing for these procedures, a parenthetical note following code 88271 has been revised.

Refer to the codebook and the Rationale for code 81349 for a full discussion of these changes.

# Proprietary Laboratory Analyses

▲ **0051U** Prescription drug monitoring, evaluation of drugs present by liquid chromatography tandem mass spectrometry (LC-MS/MS), urine or blood, 31 drug panel, reported as quantitative results, detected or not detected, per date of service

▶(0098U has been deleted)◀

▶(0099U has been deleted)◀

▶(0100U has been deleted)◀

**0120U** Oncology (B-cell lymphoma classification), mRNA, gene expression profiling by fluorescent probe hybridization of 58 genes (45 content and 13 housekeeping genes), formalin-fixed paraffin-embedded tissue, algorithm reported as likelihood for primary mediastinal B-cell lymphoma (PMBCL) and diffuse large B-cell lymphoma (DLBCL) with cell of origin subtyping in the latter

▶(Do not report 0120U in conjunction with 0017M)◀

▶(0139U has been deleted)◀

▲ **0152U** Infectious disease (bacteria, fungi, parasites, and DNA viruses), microbial cell-free DNA, plasma, untargeted next-generation sequencing, report for significant positive pathogens

▶(0168U has been deleted)◀

**0178U** Peanut allergen-specific quantitative assessment of multiple epitopes using enzyme-linked immunosorbent assay (ELISA), blood, report of minimum eliciting exposure for a clinical reaction

⋇ **0202U** Infectious disease (bacterial or viral respiratory tract infection), pathogen-specific nucleic acid (DNA or RNA), 22 targets including severe acute respiratory syndrome

coronavirus 2 (SARS-CoV-2), qualitative RT-PCR, nasopharyngeal swab, each pathogen reported as detected or not detected

▶(For additional PLA code with identical clinical descriptor, see 0223U. See Appendix O or the most current listing on the AMA CPT website to determine appropriate code assignment)◀

**0222U** Red cell antigen (RH blood group) genotyping (RHD and RHCE), gene analysis, next-generation sequencing, RH proximal promoter, exons 1-10, portions of introns 2-3

⋇● **0223U** Infectious disease (bacterial or viral respiratory tract infection), pathogen-specific nucleic acid (DNA or RNA), 22 targets including severe acute respiratory syndrome coronavirus 2 (SARS-CoV-2), qualitative RT-PCR, nasopharyngeal swab, each pathogen reported as detected or not detected

▶(For additional PLA code with identical clinical descriptor, see 0202U. See Appendix O or the most current listing on the AMA CPT website to determine appropriate code assignment)◀

● **0224U** Antibody, severe acute respiratory syndrome coronavirus 2 (SARS-CoV-2) (coronavirus disease [COVID-19]), includes titer(s), when performed

▶(Do not report 0224U in conjunction with 86769)◀

● **0225U** Infectious disease (bacterial or viral respiratory tract infection) pathogen-specific DNA and RNA, 21 targets, including severe acute respiratory syndrome coronavirus 2 (SARS-CoV-2), amplified probe technique, including multiplex reverse transcription for RNA targets, each analyte reported as detected or not detected

● **0226U** Surrogate viral neutralization test (sVNT), severe acute respiratory syndrome coronavirus 2 (SARS-CoV-2) (coronavirus disease [COVID-19]), ELISA, plasma, serum

● **0227U** Drug assay, presumptive, 30 or more drugs or metabolites, urine, liquid chromatography with tandem mass spectrometry (LC-MS/MS) using multiple reaction monitoring (MRM), with drug or metabolite description, includes sample validation

● **0228U** Oncology (prostate), multianalyte molecular profile by photometric detection of macromolecules adsorbed on nanosponge array slides with machine learning, utilizing first morning voided urine, algorithm reported as likelihood of prostate cancer

● **0229U** *BCAT1 (Branched chain amino acid transaminase 1)* or *IKZF1 (IKAROS family zinc finger 1)* (eg, colorectal cancer) promoter methylation analysis

● **0230U** *AR (androgen receptor)* (eg, spinal and bulbar muscular atrophy, Kennedy disease, X chromosome inactivation), full sequence analysis, including small sequence changes in exonic and intronic regions, deletions, duplications, short tandem repeat (STR) expansions, mobile element insertions, and variants in non-uniquely mappable regions

● **0231U**  *CACNA1A (calcium voltage-gated channel subunit alpha 1A)* (eg, spinocerebellar ataxia), full gene analysis, including small sequence changes in exonic and intronic regions, deletions, duplications, short tandem repeat (STR) gene expansions, mobile element insertions, and variants in non-uniquely mappable regions

● **0232U**  *CSTB (cystatin B)* (eg, progressive myoclonic epilepsy type 1A, Unverricht-Lundborg disease), full gene analysis, including small sequence changes in exonic and intronic regions, deletions, duplications, short tandem repeat (STR) expansions, mobile element insertions, and variants in non-uniquely mappable regions

● **0233U**  *FXN (frataxin)* (eg, Friedreich ataxia), gene analysis, including small sequence changes in exonic and intronic regions, deletions, duplications, short tandem repeat (STR) expansions, mobile element insertions, and variants in non-uniquely mappable regions

● **0234U**  *MECP2 (methyl CpG binding protein 2)* (eg, Rett syndrome), full gene analysis, including small sequence changes in exonic and intronic regions, deletions, duplications, mobile element insertions, and variants in non-uniquely mappable regions

● **0235U**  *PTEN (phosphatase and tensin homolog)* (eg, Cowden syndrome, PTEN hamartoma tumor syndrome), full gene analysis, including small sequence changes in exonic and intronic regions, deletions, duplications, mobile element insertions, and variants in non-uniquely mappable regions

● **0236U**  *SMN1 (survival of motor neuron 1, telomeric)* and *SMN2 (survival of motor neuron 2, centromeric)* (eg, spinal muscular atrophy) full gene analysis, including small sequence changes in exonic and intronic regions, duplications, deletions, and mobile element insertions

● **0237U**  Cardiac ion channelopathies (eg, Brugada syndrome, long QT syndrome, short QT syndrome, catecholaminergic polymorphic ventricular tachycardia), genomic sequence analysis panel including *ANK2, CASQ2, CAV3, KCNE1, KCNE2, KCNH2, KCNJ2, KCNQ1, RYR2,* and *SCN5A,* including small sequence changes in exonic and intronic regions, deletions, duplications, mobile element insertions, and variants in non-uniquely mappable regions

● **0238U**  Oncology (Lynch syndrome), genomic DNA sequence analysis of *MLH1, MSH2, MSH6, PMS2,* and *EPCAM,* including small sequence changes in exonic and intronic regions, deletions, duplications, mobile element insertions, and variants in non-uniquely mappable regions

● **0239U**  Targeted genomic sequence analysis panel, solid organ neoplasm, cell-free DNA, analysis of 311 or more genes, interrogation for sequence variants, including substitutions, insertions, deletions, select rearrangements, and copy number variations

● **0240U**  Infectious disease (viral respiratory tract infection), pathogen-specific RNA, 3 targets (severe acute respiratory syndrome coronavirus 2 [SARS-CoV-2], influenza A, influenza B), upper respiratory specimen, each pathogen reported as detected or not detected

● **0241U**  Infectious disease (viral respiratory tract infection), pathogen-specific RNA, 4 targets (severe acute respiratory syndrome coronavirus 2 [SARS-CoV-2], influenza A, influenza B, respiratory syncytial virus [RSV]), upper respiratory specimen, each pathogen reported as detected or not detected

● **0242U**  Targeted genomic sequence analysis panel, solid organ neoplasm, cell-free circulating DNA analysis of 55-74 genes, interrogation for sequence variants, gene copy number amplifications, and gene rearrangements

● **0243U**  Obstetrics (preeclampsia), biochemical assay of placental-growth factor, time-resolved fluorescence immunoassay, maternal serum, predictive algorithm reported as a risk score for preeclampsia

● **0244U**  Oncology (solid organ), DNA, comprehensive genomic profiling, 257 genes, interrogation for single-nucleotide variants, insertions/deletions, copy number alterations, gene rearrangements, tumor-mutational burden and microsatellite instability, utilizing formalin-fixed paraffin-embedded tumor tissue

● **0245U**  Oncology (thyroid), mutation analysis of 10 genes and 37 RNA fusions and expression of 4 mRNA markers using next-generation sequencing, fine needle aspirate, report includes associated risk of malignancy expressed as a percentage

● **0246U**  Red blood cell antigen typing, DNA, genotyping of at least 16 blood groups with phenotype prediction of at least 51 red blood cell antigens

● **0247U**  Obstetrics (preterm birth), insulin-like growth factor–binding protein 4 (IBP4), sex hormone–binding globulin (SHBG), quantitative measurement by LC-MS/MS, utilizing maternal serum, combined with clinical data, reported as predictive-risk stratification for spontaneous preterm birth

● **0248U**  Oncology (brain), spheroid cell culture in a 3D microenvironment, 12 drug panel, tumor-response prediction for each drug

● **0249U**  Oncology (breast), semiquantitative analysis of 32 phosphoproteins and protein analytes, includes laser capture microdissection, with algorithmic analysis and interpretative report

● **0250U**  Oncology (solid organ neoplasm), targeted genomic sequence DNA analysis of 505 genes, interrogation for somatic alterations (SNVs [single nucleotide variant], small insertions and deletions, one amplification, and four translocations), microsatellite instability and tumor-mutation burden

★ = Telemedicine   ✛ = Add-on code   ✳ = FDA approval pending   # = Resequenced code   ⊘ = Modifier 51 exempt

● **0251U** Hepcidin-25, enzyme-linked immunosorbent assay (ELISA), serum or plasma

● **0252U** Fetal aneuploidy short tandem—repeat comparative analysis, fetal DNA from products of conception, reported as normal (euploidy), monosomy, trisomy, or partial deletion/duplication, mosaicism, and segmental aneuploidy

● **0253U** Reproductive medicine (endometrial receptivity analysis), RNA gene expression profile, 238 genes by next-generation sequencing, endometrial tissue, predictive algorithm reported as endometrial window of implantation (eg, pre-receptive, receptive, post-receptive)

● **0254U** Reproductive medicine (preimplantation genetic assessment), analysis of 24 chromosomes using embryonic DNA genomic sequence analysis for aneuploidy, and a mitochondrial DNA score in euploid embryos, results reported as normal (euploidy), monosomy, trisomy, or partial deletion/duplication, mosaicism, and segmental aneuploidy, per embryo tested

● **0255U** Andrology (infertility), sperm-capacitation assessment of ganglioside GM1 distribution patterns, fluorescence microscopy, fresh or frozen specimen, reported as percentage of capacitated sperm and probability of generating a pregnancy score

● **0256U** Trimethylamine/trimethylamine N-oxide (TMA/TMAO) profile, tandem mass spectrometry (MS/MS), urine, with algorithmic analysis and interpretive report

● **0257U** Very long chain acyl-coenzyme A (CoA) dehydrogenase (VLCAD), leukocyte enzyme activity, whole blood

● **0258U** Autoimmune (psoriasis), mRNA, next-generation sequencing, gene expression profiling of 50-100 genes, skin-surface collection using adhesive patch, algorithm reported as likelihood of response to psoriasis biologics

● **0259U** Nephrology (chronic kidney disease), nuclear magnetic resonance spectroscopy measurement of myo-inositol, valine, and creatinine, algorithmically combined with cystatin C (by immunoassay) and demographic data to determine estimated glomerular filtration rate (GFR), serum, quantitative

⌘● **0260U** Rare diseases (constitutional/heritable disorders), identification of copy number variations, inversions, insertions, translocations, and other structural variants by optical genome mapping

▶(For additional PLA code with identical clinical descriptor, see 0264U. See Appendix O or the most current listing on the AMA CPT website to determine appropriate code assignment)◀

● **0261U** Oncology (colorectal cancer), image analysis with artificial intelligence assessment of 4 histologic and immunohistochemical features (CD3 and CD8 within tumor-stroma border and tumor core), tissue, reported as immune response and recurrence-risk score

● **0262U** Oncology (solid tumor), gene expression profiling by real-time RT-PCR of 7 gene pathways *(ER, AR, PI3K, MAPK, HH, TGFB,* Notch), formalin-fixed paraffin-embedded (FFPE), algorithm reported as gene pathway activity score

● **0263U** Neurology (autism spectrum disorder [ASD]), quantitative measurements of 16 central carbon metabolites (ie, $\alpha$-ketoglutarate, alanine, lactate, phenylalanine, pyruvate, succinate, carnitine, citrate, fumarate, hypoxanthine, inosine, malate, S-sulfocysteine, taurine, urate, and xanthine), liquid chromatography tandem mass spectrometry (LC-MS/MS), plasma, algorithmic analysis with result reported as negative or positive (with metabolic subtypes of ASD)

⌘● **0264U** Rare diseases (constitutional/heritable disorders), identification of copy number variations, inversions, insertions, translocations, and other structural variants by optical genome mapping

▶(For additional PLA code with identical clinical descriptor, see 0260U. See Appendix O or the most current listing on the AMA CPT website to determine appropriate code assignment)◀

● **0265U** Rare constitutional and other heritable disorders, whole genome and mitochondrial DNA sequence analysis, blood, frozen and formalin-fixed paraffin-embedded (FFPE) tissue, saliva, buccal swabs or cell lines, identification of single nucleotide and copy number variants

● **0266U** Unexplained constitutional or other heritable disorders or syndromes, tissue-specific gene expression by whole-transcriptome and next-generation sequencing, blood, formalin-fixed paraffin-embedded (FFPE) tissue or fresh frozen tissue, reported as presence or absence of splicing or expression changes

● **0267U** Rare constitutional and other heritable disorders, identification of copy number variations, inversions, insertions, translocations, and other structural variants by optical genome mapping and whole genome sequencing

● **0268U** Hematology (atypical hemolytic uremic syndrome [aHUS]), genomic sequence analysis of 15 genes, blood, buccal swab, or amniotic fluid

● **0269U** Hematology (autosomal dominant congenital thrombocytopenia), genomic sequence analysis of 14 genes, blood, buccal swab, or amniotic fluid

● **0270U** Hematology (congenital coagulation disorders), genomic sequence analysis of 20 genes, blood, buccal swab, or amniotic fluid

● **0271U** Hematology (congenital neutropenia), genomic sequence analysis of 23 genes, blood, buccal swab, or amniotic fluid

● **0272U** Hematology (genetic bleeding disorders), genomic sequence analysis of 51 genes, blood, buccal swab, or amniotic fluid, comprehensive

Pathology and Laboratory  80047-89398, 0001U-0284U

Pathology and Laboratory 80047-89398, 0001U-0284U

- **0273U**  Hematology (genetic hyperfibrinolysis, delayed bleeding), genomic sequence analysis of 8 genes *(F13A1, F13B, FGA, FGB, FGG, SERPINA1, SERPINE1, SERPINF2, PLAU)*, blood, buccal swab, or amniotic fluid

- **0274U**  Hematology (genetic platelet disorders), genomic sequence analysis of 43 genes, blood, buccal swab, or amniotic fluid

- **0275U**  Hematology (heparin-induced thrombocytopenia), platelet antibody reactivity by flow cytometry, serum

- **0276U**  Hematology (inherited thrombocytopenia), genomic sequence analysis of 23 genes, blood, buccal swab, or amniotic fluid

- **0277U**  Hematology (genetic platelet function disorder), genomic sequence analysis of 31 genes, blood, buccal swab, or amniotic fluid

- **0278U**  Hematology (genetic thrombosis), genomic sequence analysis of 12 genes, blood, buccal swab, or amniotic fluid

- **0279U**  Hematology (von Willebrand disease [VWD]), von Willebrand factor (VWF) and collagen III binding by enzyme-linked immunosorbent assays (ELISA), plasma, report of collagen III binding

- **0280U**  Hematology (von Willebrand disease [VWD]), von Willebrand factor (VWF) and collagen IV binding by enzyme-linked immunosorbent assays (ELISA), plasma, report of collagen IV binding

- **0281U**  Hematology (von Willebrand disease [VWD]), von Willebrand propeptide, enzyme-linked immunosorbent assays (ELISA), plasma, diagnostic report of von Willebrand factor (VWF) propeptide antigen level

- **0282U**  Red blood cell antigen typing, DNA, genotyping of 12 blood group system genes to predict 44 red blood cell antigen phenotypes

- **0283U**  von Willebrand factor (VWF), type 2B, platelet-binding evaluation, radioimmunoassay, plasma

- **0284U**  von Willebrand factor (VWF), type 2N, factor VIII and VWF binding evaluation, enzyme-linked immunosorbent assays (ELISA), plasma

### Rationale

A total of 62 new proprietary laboratory analyses (PLA) codes have been established for the CPT 2022 code set. PLA test codes are released and posted online at https://www.ama-assn.org/practice-management/cpt/cpt-pla-codes on a quarterly basis (Fall, Winter, Spring, and Summer).

New codes are effective the quarter following their publication online. Other changes include the deletion of five codes (0098U-0100U, 0139U, 0168U), the revision of two codes (0051U, 0152U), the addition of two exclusionary parenthetical notes to instruct proper reporting of codes 0120U and 0224U, the revision of a test name only (0178U), and the addition of parenthetical notes to inform users of PLA codes with identical clinical descriptors (0202U, 0223U, 0260U, 0264U).

Refer to the codebook and the Rationale for code 0017M for a full discussion of the new parenthetical note following code 0120U.

## Clinical Example (0223U)

A 62-year-old male presents to the emergency department (ED) with fever (103.4°F), shortness of breath, and headache for the past 24 hours, as well as a dry cough and muscle pain for a week. The clinician orders a molecular syndromic respiratory panel.

## Description of Procedure (0223U)

Obtain a nasopharyngeal swab specimen and elute the specimen in a universal transport medium (UTM). Transfer an aliquot from the UTM to a ready-to-use cartridge and place it in the QIAstat-Dx Analyzer, which performs a fully automated sample preparation and multiplex real-time (RT) polymerase chain reaction (PCR). The instrument generates a report that includes cycle threshold (CT) values and amplification curves for each pathogen detected and internal control (IC) to aid in the diagnosis of coinfections or to identify contaminants. Communicate the results to the appropriate health care professional.

## Clinical Example (0224U)

A 68-year-old male, who has a history of coronary artery disease, aortic valve replacement, and lymphoma, presents to the ED with a 6-day history of malaise, a nonproductive cough, and low-grade fevers (eg, 100.4°F/38°C). A severe acute respiratory syndrome coronavirus 2 (SARS-CoV-2) (coronavirus disease [COVID-19]) IgG antibody test was ordered to inform diagnosis of a recent past infection (within 10 to 14 days) or convalescent phase of COVID-19. Serum or plasma is collected from the patient for testing.

## Description of Procedure (0224U)

Perform an enzyme-linked immunosorbent assay (ELISA) for both the qualitative and quantitative detection of human IgG antibodies in serum or plasma to SARS-CoV-2 receptor-binding domain and spike-protein antigens. Report results as negative or positive using a defined threshold for both IgG antibody concentrations.

★ = Telemedicine   ✛ = Add-on code   ✗ = FDA approval pending   # = Resequenced code   ⊘ = Modifier 51 exempt

## Clinical Example (0225U)

A 77-year-old female, who has hypertension and diabetes, presents with worsening fevers, cough, and respiratory distress. A respiratory pathogen panel is ordered to determine possible infectious causes for her findings.

## Description of Procedure (0225U)

Load a sample of a nasopharyngeal swab specimen into the ePlex RP2 Panel cartridge and insert it into the instrument, which provides a result of detected or not detected for 22 pathogens.

## Clinical Example (0226U)

A 45-year-old male presented to his physician with flu-like symptoms a few months ago. He did not get a PCR viral test for SARS-CoV-2 but thinks he had COVID-19. He is concerned about future exposure to the SARS-CoV-2 virus and wants to know if he has immunity. Plasma is submitted to assess the patient's viral neutralization capacity to SARS-CoV-2.

## Description of Procedure (0226U)

Subject a plasma specimen to a multistep-blocking ELISA. The laboratory professional reads the absorbance. interprets the findings, and sends a report specifying the patient's inhibition capacity to SARS-CoV-2 to the ordering provider.

## Clinical Example (0227U)

A 34-year-old male is in a treatment center 7 days post-heroin overdose. His physician orders a comprehensive drug screen to detect recent drug use.

## Description of Procedure (0227U)

Subject a urine specimen to drug analysis by liquid chromatography–tandem mass spectrometry (LC-MS/MS) and sample validation. The pathologist or other qualified health care professional (QHP) analyzes the data against the test order's list of prescribed drugs and generates a report.

## Clinical Example (0228U)

A 55-year-old male presents with an elevated prostate-specific antigen (PSA) level and abnormal digital rectal examination. The urologist orders testing for the risk of prostate cancer prior to biopsy.

## Description of Procedure (0228U)

Apply a first morning-voided urine sample to nanosponge array slides. Digitally scan the treated slides to a cloud-based machine learning system that performs analysis. A QHP reviews and reports the results.

## Clinical Example (0229U)

A 65-year-old male is diagnosed with stage II colon cancer. A colorectal surgeon resects the primary tumor. Following this curative intent surgery, the colorectal surgeon orders specific gene promotor methylation studies to assess whether the patient has residual disease.

## Description of Procedure (0229U)

Isolate and subject high-quality genomic DNA from plasma to a quantitative methylation-specific PCR (qPCR) assay of the BCAT1 and/or IKZF1 genes. The pathologist or other QHP analyzes the data and composes a report.

## Clinical Example (0230U)

A neonate presents with ambiguous genitalia. His mother reports that her younger brother has gynecomastia and infertility. No other abnormalities were identified. Blood is submitted for analysis given suspicion of an androgen receptor (AR) disorder.

## Description of Procedure (0230U)

Isolate and sequence genomic DNA from blood or saliva. The laboratory professional examines deviations or variants in the AR gene sequence and evaluates them for potential impact on protein function and pathogenicity based on American College of Medical Genetics (ACMG) guidelines. Compose the report. The laboratory director reviews the report and sends it to the ordering provider.

## Clinical Example (0231U)

A 5-year-old male presents with generalized seizures, global developmental delay, moderate intellectual disability, and autism spectrum disorder. Blood is submitted for CACNA1A analysis given suspicion of a CACNA1A-related disorder.

## Description of Procedure (0231U)

Isolate and sequence genomic DNA from blood or saliva. The laboratory professional examines deviations or variants in the CACNA1A gene sequence and evaluates them for potential impact on protein function and pathogenicity based on ACMG guidelines. Compose the report. The laboratory director reviews the report and sends it to the ordering provider.

## Clinical Example (0232U)

An 11-year-old female presents with ataxia and incoordination. She has had intractable epilepsy since the age of 5. There is no family history of epilepsy or ataxia. A blood sample is submitted for analysis given suspicion of Unverricht-Lundborg disease.

## Description of Procedure (0232U)

Isolate and sequence genomic DNA from blood or saliva. The laboratory professional examines deviations or variants in the CSTB gene and evaluates them for potential effect on protein function and pathogenicity based on ACMG guidelines. Compose the report. The laboratory director reviews the report and sends it to the ordering provider.

## Clinical Example (0233U)

A 12-year-old male presents with progressive loss of coordination. A blood sample was submitted for analysis given suspicion of an FXN-related disorder.

## Description of Procedure (0233U)

Isolate and sequence genomic DNA from blood or saliva. The laboratory professional examines deviations or variants in the FXN gene sequence and evaluates them for potential impact on protein function and pathogenicity based on ACMG guidelines. Compose the report. The laboratory director reviews the report and sends it to the ordering provider.

## Clinical Example (0234U)

A 2-year-old female presents with regression in language and motor skills after meeting developmental milestones in her first year. Her mother reports stereotypic hand movements and fits of screaming. Blood is submitted for MECP2 analysis given suspicion of an MECP2-related disorder.

## Description of Procedure (0234U)

Isolate and sequence genomic DNA from blood or saliva. The laboratory professional examines deviations or variants in the MECP2 gene sequence and evaluates them for potential effect on protein function and pathogenicity based on ACMG guidelines. Compose the report. The laboratory director reviews the report and sends it to the ordering provider.

## Clinical Example (0235U)

A 30-year-old female, who has a history of osteosarcoma of the left tibia, presents with a benign breast mass. Her family history includes several maternal relatives with bladder, ovarian, brain, breast, colon, and thyroid cancers. A blood sample was submitted for PTEN analysis given suspicion of a PTEN-related disorder.

## Description of Procedure (0235U)

Isolate and sequence genomic DNA from blood or saliva. The laboratory professional examines deviations or variants in the PTEN gene sequence and evaluates them

for potential effect on protein function and pathogenicity based on ACMG guidelines. Compose the report. The laboratory director reviews the report and sends it to the ordering provider.

## Clinical Example (0236U)

A 15-year-old female presents to her physician with moderate muscle weakness, tremors, and mild breathing problems. SMN1/2 testing was ordered.

## Description of Procedure (0236U)

Isolate and sequence genomic DNA from blood or saliva. The laboratory professional examines deviations or variants in the SMN1 and SMN2 gene sequences and evaluates them for potential effect on protein function and pathogenicity based on ACMG guidelines. Compose the report. The laboratory director reviews the report and sends it to the ordering provider.

## Clinical Example (0237U)

A 30-year-old female presents with syncope, dizziness, and exercise intolerance. Her family history includes a daughter who died at 5 months from sudden infant death syndrome (SIDS). Blood is submitted for cardiac ion channelopathy gene analysis given suspicion of a genetic cardiac ion channelopathy.

## Description of Procedure (0237U)

Isolate and sequence genomic DNA from blood or saliva. The laboratory professional examines deviations or variants in the cardiac ion channelopathy genes and evaluates them for potential effect on protein function and pathogenicity based on ACMG guidelines. Compose the report. The laboratory director reviews the report and sends it to the ordering provider.

## Clinical Example (0238U)

A 40-year-old male presents with a strong family history of colorectal cancer. Blood is submitted for Lynch syndrome analysis given suspicion of Lynch syndrome.

## Description of Procedure (0238U)

Isolate and sequence genomic DNA from blood or saliva. The laboratory professional examines deviations or variants in the Lynch syndrome–related genes and evaluates them for potential effect on protein function and pathogenicity based on ACMG guidelines. Compose the report. The laboratory director reviews the report and sends it to the ordering provider.

★ = Telemedicine   ✚ = Add-on code   ✐ = FDA approval pending   # = Resequenced code   ⦸ = Modifier 51 exempt

## Clinical Example (0239U)

A 70-year-old female presents with shortness of breath and hemoptysis. A chest X ray reveals several lung lesions. Subsequent biopsy and computed tomography (CT) scan reveal stage IV non-small cell lung cancer (NSCLC). A blood sample is submitted for FoundationOne® Liquid CDx.

## Description of Procedure (0239U)

Extract circulating cell-free DNA from plasma and subject the sample to hybridization capture-based next-generation sequencing (NGS). Process the sequenced data using a customized analysis pipeline designed to detect four classes of genomic alterations and analyze genomic signatures. The automated software annotates and merges the results with patient demographics and any additional information provided. Issue a report to the ordering provider.

## Clinical Example (0240U)

A 14-year-old female presents with a 2-day history of fever, sore throat, and fatigue and no underlying conditions. The physician collects a nasopharyngeal swab and submits it for simultaneous evaluation of SARS-CoV-2, influenza A, and influenza B.

## Description of Procedure (0240U)

Add a sample of the nasopharyngeal specimen to the test cartridge and load the cartridge onto the instrument for the RT-PCR detection of viral RNA from SARS-CoV-2, influenza A, and influenza B, if present. Report positive and negative results for each pathogen to the ordering provider.

## Clinical Example (0241U)

A 14-year-old female presents with a 2-day history of fever, sore throat, and fatigue. The physician collects a nasopharyngeal swab and orders testing for simultaneous evaluation of SARS-CoV-2, influenza A, influenza B, and RSV.

## Description of Procedure (0241U)

Add a sample of the collected specimen to a test cartridge and load the cartridge onto the automated instrument for the RT-PCR detection of viral RNA from SARS-CoV-2, influenza A, influenza B, and RSV, if present. Report the qualitative results for the four targets to the ordering provider.

## Clinical Example (0242U)

A 65-year-old female with advanced lung adenocarcinoma consults her oncologist. Blood is submitted to examine the patient's tumor genomic makeup to provide therapeutic options.

## Description of Procedure (0242U)

Isolate and subject high-quality cell-free DNA from whole blood to hybridization capture-based NGS of 55 to 74 genes for nucleotide substitutions, indels, copy number amplifications, and genomic fusions or rearrangements. The pathologist or other QHP analyzes the data and composes a report.

## Clinical Example (0243U)

A 28-year-old female presents for routine first trimester pregnancy care. A test is ordered to identify possible increased risk of preeclampsia during the second or third trimesters.

## Description of Procedure (0243U)

Test maternal serum by fluoroimmunometric sandwich assay. Use the placental growth factor concentration and maternal history to calculate the reported predictive risk for preeclampsia.

## Clinical Example (0244U)

A 65-year-old male presents with recently diagnosed metastatic lung cancer. FFPE tissue is submitted for comprehensive tumor profiling to assess the patient's suitability for treatment with targeted therapies.

## Description of Procedure (0244U)

Isolate and prepare tumor DNA from an FFPE sample for NGS to identify genetic alterations (SNV, CNA, indel, fusions) among 257 genes. Compute genomic signatures (eg, tumor mutational burden, microsatellite instability). A qualified laboratory professional prepares a report specifying identified biomarkers and associated drug-therapy options and sends it to the ordering provider.

## Clinical Example (0245U)

A 67-year-old presents with a 2.2-cm thyroid nodule with microcalcifications. A fine-needle aspiration (FNA) biopsy is performed, and one aspirate sample is placed in a proprietary preservative. Based on indeterminate or uncertain cytology, the physician orders molecular analysis on the preserved specimen.

## Description of Procedure (0245U)

Extract nucleic acid from the sample of aspirated thyroid material. Perform DNA and RNA sequencing using NGS with analysis of specific DNA mutations and detection of mRNA fusions, which are used in a pre-defined reporting protocol to assign a risk of malignancy. A pathologist or other QHP composes a report that is communicated to the ordering provider.

## Clinical Example (0246U)

A 46-year-old male presents with acute pancreatitis, sepsis, and renal failure. He was recently transfused and has a positive antibody screen. The antibody identification (ID) panel reacted with all serologically treated cells. NGS was ordered with phenotype prediction to guide transfusion.

## Description of Procedure (0246U)

Isolate and subject DNA from whole blood to NGS for the detection of a minimum of 51 human erythrocyte antigens from a minimum of 16 blood groups. The transfusion medicine professional reviews the NGS results and issues a report listing each detected antigen and associated blood group.

## Clinical Example (0247U)

A 31-year-old patient presents with a 17-week gestation age singleton pregnancy with no signs of preterm labor. Maternal serum is submitted to determine her risk for preterm birth.

## Description of Procedure (0247U)

Process and evaluate maternal serum for proteotypic peptides of insulin-like growth factor binding protein 4 (IBP4) and sex hormone binding globulin (SHBG). Measure relative levels of IBP4 and SHBG peptides by liquid chromatography-multiple reaction monitoring-mass spectrometry (LC-MRM-MS). Combine the findings with the patient's clinical data and issue a report detailing the risk of spontaneous preterm birth.

## Clinical Example (0248U)

A 65-year-old male, who has a high-grade glioma, has fresh tissue from the tumor submitted to assess the tumor's response to drug therapies.

## Description of Procedure (0248U)

Grow cells isolated from the tumor specimens in cell culture as spheroids. Expose the specimens to potential therapeutic agents and assess them for cell viability via luminescence. A qualified laboratory professional reviews the data and issues a report indicating tumor-specific drug responses.

## Clinical Example (0249U)

A 51-year-old premenopausal female presents with estrogen receptor (ER)–positive, ERBB2 (HER2)–negative breast cancer that has progressed from first-line therapy. Tissue is submitted to provide a more definitive biomarker status to guide treatment.

## Description of Procedure (0249U)

Isolate tumor cells by laser-capture microdissection. Print protein extracts on multiple nitrocellulose slides for reverse phase protein array (RPPA) analysis of specific proteins and phosphoproteins. Score signal intensities and put them into an algorithm. A qualified laboratory professional issues a report.

## Clinical Example (0250U)

A 44-year-old male presents with late-stage colorectal adenocarcinoma. FFPE tumor tissue is submitted to assess for targeted mutations relevant to therapy, mismatch repair status, and tumor mutational burden.

## Description of Procedure (0250U)

Isolate and analyze genomic DNA from FFPE tissue by hybridization capture–based NGS to identify genomic alterations in 505 targeted genes, and to determine mismatch repair status and tumor mutational burden. Report a summary of the alterations found.

## Clinical Example (0251U)

A 45-year-old male presents with severe iron deficiency anemia that has not improved on oral supplements. Blood is submitted to assess the plasma or serum concentration of hepcidin-25.

## Description of Procedure (0251U)

Analyze patient serum or plasma by ELISA for hepcidin-25 and report the result in ng/mL.

## Clinical Example (0252U)

A 31-year-old female contacts her obstetrician following a third spontaneous-pregnancy loss in the first trimester. Products of conception and blood are submitted for analysis to determine if chromosomal aneuploidy is present.

## Description of Procedure (0252U)

Extract DNA from the products of conception and from a maternal specimen for short tandem repeat analysis. Perform NGS to detect chromosomal abnormalities and generate a karyogram. A qualified laboratory professional reviews the karyogram and reports the results.

★ = Telemedicine   ✚ = Add-on code   ✔ = FDA approval pending   # = Resequenced code   ⊘ = Modifier 51 exempt

## Clinical Example (0253U)

A 36-year-old female continues to pursue in vitro fertilization after a previous failed implantation cycle. Endometrial tissue was submitted for endometrial receptivity analysis to evaluate endometrial receptivity and the window of implantation.

## Description of Procedure (0253U)

Extract and sequence RNA from endometrial tissue by NGS and analyze it for 238 genes. Using gene expression values in an algorithm, determine endometrial receptivity status. A qualified laboratory professional reviews the findings and issues a report.

## Clinical Example (0254U)

A 37-year-old female with recurrent pregnancy loss elects in vitro fertilization. Genetic counseling recommends pre-implantation genetic testing; a trophectoderm biopsy of each embryo is submitted for aneuploidy evaluation.

## Description of Procedure (0254U)

Extract DNA from blastocyst biopsies and analyze by whole-genome amplification. Perform aneuploidy analysis on each embryo and determine a mitochondrial DNA score for each euploid embryo. A qualified laboratory professional prepares and communicates the report to the ordering provider.

## Clinical Example (0255U)

A 32-year-old male presents to evaluate conception failure. There is no history of testicular injury, libido issues, or erectile dysfunction issues. A semen sample is submitted to assess the patient's capacitated sperm percentage and the probability of generating a pregnancy (PGP).

## Description of Procedure (0255U)

Isolate sperm from seminal plasma and incubate the sperm for capacitation. Fix and label the sperm to determine ganglioside GM1 localization patterns by fluorescence microscopy. A laboratory professional evaluates at least 100 sperm and reports a score reflecting the percentage of capacitation-competent sperm and PGP.

## Clinical Example (0256U)

A 33-year-old female presents with a concern regarding a "rotten fish odor." She feels socially ostracized due to this smell. A frozen urine specimen is submitted for LC-MS trimethylamine (TMA) analysis testing.

## Description of Procedure (0256U)

Use tandem mass spectrometry (MS/MS) to calculate TMA and trimethylamine N-oxide (TMAO) present. Calculate results in micromoles/millimole creatinine. Calculate the TMAO percentage and issue a report to the ordering provider.

## Clinical Example (0257U)

A newborn is seen following a positive newborn screen showing a C14:1 elevation. A request for evaluation of very long chain aycl-CoA dehydrogenase (VLCAD) leukocyte enzyme activity is requested to evaluate the infant for this inborn error of metabolism.

## Description of Procedure (0257U)

Analyze a whole-blood sample for VLCAD leukocyte enzyme activity using a fluorescence-based assay. The results reported may indicate deficiency in VLCAD enzyme activity. Issue a report to the ordering provider.

## Clinical Example (0258U)

A 57-year-old patient, who presents with moderate to severe plaque psoriasis, is considered for biologic therapy. Skin-surface collection is submitted to determine the optimal class of psoriasis biologics (eg, TNFa, IL-17 and IL-23 inhibitors).

## Description of Procedure (0258U)

Elute and evaluate RNA from the skin surface–collection patch using NGS. Evaluate the results using an algorithm that generates a report predicting the patient's response to classes of psoriasis biologics. A qualified laboratory professional reviews and submits the report to the ordering provider.

## Clinical Example (0259U)

A 65-year-old female, who has a history of chronic kidney disease, presents with recent loss of appetite and peripheral edema. Serum is sent for nuclear magnetic resonance (NMR) spectroscopy estimation of glomerular filtration rate (GFR).

## Description of Procedure (0259U)

Analyze a serum sample using NMR spectroscopy to measure creatinine, valine, and myo-inositol. Combine these findings together algorithmically with cystatin C, age, and sex to derive an estimated GFR.

## Clinical Example (0260U)

An 18-month-old male presents with hypotonia, delayed motor milestones, and features concerning for autism. A blood sample is submitted for genetic evaluation for inherited conditions.

## Description of Procedure (0260U)

Isolate and evaluate DNA from blood or cells using optical whole-genome mapping to detect structural variants, including copy number variants associated with genetic syndromes. A QHP interprets and reports the results to the ordering provider.

## Clinical Example (0261U)

A 70-year-old female is referred following hemicolectomy for a pT4a N0 M0 ascending colon tumor. The oncologist considers prescribing adjuvant chemotherapy and requests evaluation of the FFPE surgical specimen to predict recurrence risk and inform treatment selection.

## Description of Procedure (0261U)

Stain FFPE tumor slides for CD3+ and CD8+ T-lymphocytes. Evaluate digital slide images using a computer algorithm that automatically identifies positive cells, defines the invasive margin via an AI-based algorithm, and uses the measured values as part of a proprietary scoring algorithm to create a recurrence risk. A qualified laboratory professional reviews and reports the findings to the ordering provider.

## Clinical Example (0262U)

A 65-year-old female presents with a recent diagnosis of breast cancer. An FFPE sample is submitted for abnormal signaling pathway activity to better direct treatment.

## Description of Procedure (0262U)

Perform reverse transcription (RT)-qPCR on the isolated tumor RNA for seven signal pathways (ER, AR, PI3K, MAPK, HH, TGFB, Notch). Analyze the data and report an activity score.

## Clinical Example (0263U)

An 18-month-old male is brought to see his pediatrician. The pediatrician administers the Modified Checklist for Autism in Toddlers (MCHAT) to assess the patient's development. The patient scores well below expected developmental milestones. Based on this and other information from the mother, the pediatrician suspects the child may have autism. The pediatrician submits a fasting blood plasma sample from the child for analysis and algorithmic comparisons of his energy production and central carbon metabolite levels.

## Description of Procedure (0263U)

Subject plasma to tandem mass spectrometry (MS/MS) analysis to measure the levels of the energy production and central carbon metabolites. Perform algorithmic analysis to compare the levels to the metabolic subtypes associated with autism spectrum disorder (ASD). Report the quantitative measurement of the metabolites and the presence of any metabolic imbalance identified through algorithmic analysis. a qualified laboratory professional reviews and reports the findings to the ordering provider.

## Clinical Example (0264U)

A 5-year-old male presents with delayed motor development, muscle weakness, and abnormal gait. Following a negative whole exome–sequence analysis for Duchenne muscular dystrophy, the geneticist orders optical genome mapping.

## Description of Procedure (0264U)

Isolate and evaluate DNA from blood or cells using optical whole-genome mapping to detect structural variants, including copy number variants associated with genetic syndromes. A QHP interprets and reports the results to the ordering provider.

## Clinical Example (0265U)

A 5-year-old male presents with delayed motor development, muscle weakness, and abnormal gait. Following a negative whole exome–sequencing study, the geneticist requests additional sequencing, including splice-site variants.

## Description of Procedure (0265U)

Isolate high-quality genomic DNA from whole blood, tissue, or other sources and subject it to NGS. The pathologist or other QHP analyzes the data and composes a report, including repeat size estimates, single nucleotide variants, and copy number variants in the nuclear and mitochondrial genome.

## Clinical Example (0266U)

A 5-year-old female presents with ASD, global developmental delay, strabismus, and a unilateral preauricular ear tag. Whole-genome sequencing produced a heterozygous single nucleotide variant in an associated gene believed to be related to the presentation. The geneticist orders a transcriptome test to further evaluate the findings.

## Description of Procedure (0266U)

Extract RNA from blood, a tissue biopsy, or cell lines. Perform whole-transcriptome analysis. A QHP reviews the findings and issues a report identifying the transcript level or processing changes related to the clinical presentation and detailing the functional consequences of DNA mutations previously identified.

## Clinical Example (0267U)

A 12-year-old male presents with anxiety, depression, and elevated inflammatory markers. He was diagnosed with amplified musculoskeletal pain syndrome (AMPS) and benign joint hypermobility syndrome and whole-exome sequencing is negative. The geneticist orders whole-genome sequencing and optical genome to further evaluate the genetic basis for the patient's findings.

## Description of Procedure (0267U)

Isolate and evaluate DNA from blood or cells using optical whole-genome mapping and whole-genome sequencing to detect structural variants, including copy number variants associated with genetic syndromes. A QHP interprets and reports the results to the ordering provider.

## Clinical Example (0268U)

A 24-year-old female, who is at 36 weeks gestation, presents with abdominal pain, hypertension, anemia, and thrombocytopenia. With a diagnosis of HELLP (hemolysis, elevated liver enzymes, low platelet count) syndrome, emergent cesarian section was performed. The differential diagnosis included atypical hemolytic uremic syndrome. A genetic panel is ordered.

## Description of Procedure (0268U)

Isolate and subject high-quality genomic DNA to NGS of 15 genes (ADAMTS13, C3, C4BPA, C4BPB, CFB, CFH, CFHR1, CFHR3, CFHR4, CFHR5, CFI, DGKE, LMNA, MCP, THBD). The pathologist or QHP analyzes the data and composes a report.

## Clinical Example (0269U)

A 14-year-old healthy male, who has a personal and family history of mild chronic thrombocytopenia, is evaluated by a hematologist. Genetic testing is ordered for possible inherited thrombocytopenia with autosomal dominant inheritance.

## Description of Procedure (0269U)

Isolate and subject high-quality genomic DNA to NGS of 14 genes (ACTN1, ANKRD26, CYCS, ETV6, FLI1, GFI1B, GP1BA, GP1BB, GP9, ITGA2B, ITGB3, MYH9, RUNX1, TUBB1). The pathologist or other QHP analyzes the data and composes a report.

## Clinical Example (0270U)

A 21-year-old male, who has a family and personal history of easy bruisability, developed knee hemarthrosis after minimal trauma. Commonly ordered diagnostic tests were not informative. The hematologist ordered a genetic panel to look for variants associated with congenitally abnormal coagulation.

## Description of Procedure (0270U)

Isolate and subject high-quality genomic DNA to NGS of 20 genes (F10, F11, F13A1, F13B, F2, F5, F7, F8, F9, FGA, FGB, FGG, GGCX, LMAN1, MCFD2, SERPINA1, SERPINE1, SERPINF2, VKORC1, VWF). The pathologist or other QHP analyzes the data and composes a report.

## Clinical Example (0271U)

A 14-year-old female with short stature, skin hypopigmentation, and nail dyskeratosis was noted to have lifelong mild or moderate isolated neutropenia. A younger brother has similar skin findings. A congenital neutropenia panel is ordered to evaluate her for a possible genetic cause of the findings.

## Description of Procedure (0271U)

Isolate and subject high-quality genomic DNA to NGS of 23 genes (AP3B1, CSF3R, CXCR4, ELANE, G6PC3, GATA1, GATA2, GFI1, HAX1, JAGN1, LAMTOR2, LYST, RAB27A, RAC2, SBDS, SLC37A4, TAZ, TCIRG1, USB1, VPS13B, VPS45, WAS, WIPF1). The pathologist or other QHP analyzes the data and composes a report.

## Clinical Example (0272U)

A 45-year-old female presents with lifelong bleeding and impaired wound healing. Based on conventional studies, a combined coagulation factor deficiency and platelet function disorder is suspected. A comprehensive bleeding disorder panel is ordered.

## Description of Procedure (0272U)

Isolate and subject high-quality genomic DNA to NGS of 51 genes (ANO6, AP3B1, BLOC1S3, BLOCK1S6, DTNBP1, F10, F11, F13A1, F13B, F2, F5, F7, F8, F9, FERMT3, FGA, FGB, FGG, FLI1, GATA1, GFI1B, GGCX, GP1BA, GP1BB, GP6, GP9, HPS1, HPS3, HPS4, HPS5, HPS6, ITGA2B, ITGB3, LMAN1, LYST, MCFD2, NBEAL2, P2RY12, PLA2G4A, PRKACG, RASGRP2, RUNX1, SERPINA1, SERPINE1, SERPINF2, STIM1, TBXA2R, VIPAS39, VKORC1, VPS33B, VWF). The pathologist or other QHP analyzes the data and composes a report.

## Clinical Example (0273U)

A 32-year-old female presents for preconception counseling with a personal and family history of menorrhagia, delayed wound healing, and bleeding after dental procedures. Genetic testing to evaluate for a fibrinolytic disorder is ordered.

## Description of Procedure (0273U)

Isolate and subject high-quality genomic DNA to full NGS of eight genes (F13A1, F13B, FGA, FGB, FGG, SERPINA1, SERPINE1, SERPINF2) and array comparative genomic hybridization for plasminogen activator, urokinase (PLAU). The pathologist or other QHP analyzes the data and composes a report.

## Clinical Example (0274U)

A 9-year-old male presents with recurrent epistaxis and thrombocytopenia since birth. The bleeding is out of proportion to the degree of thrombocytopenia. A comprehensive genetic platelet disorder panel is ordered to determine if there is an inherited disorder of platelet number and function.

## Description of Procedure (0274U)

Isolate and subject high-quality genomic DNA to NGS of 43 genes (ACTN1, ANKRD26, ANO6, AP3B1, BLOC1S3, BLOC1S6, CYCS, DTNBP1, ETV6, FERMT3, FLI1, GATA1, GFI1B, GP1BA, GP1BB, GP6, GP9, HOXA11, HPS1, HPS3, HPS4, HPS5, HPS6, ITGA2B, ITGB3, LYST, MPL, MYH9, NBEAL2, P2RY12, PLA2G4A, PRKACG, RASGRP2, RBM8A, RUNX1, STIM1, STXBP2, TBXA2R, TUBB1, VIPAS39, VPS33B, WAS, WIPF1). The pathologist or other QHP analyzes the data and composes a report.

## Clinical Example (0275U)

A 70-year-old male, who had a routine orthopedic procedure, received heparin thromboprophylaxis. One week later, he develops thrombocytopenia. After evaluation, heparin-induced thrombocytopenia (HIT) is suspected. Blood is submitted for functional confirmation of HIT.

## Description of Procedure (0275U)

Incubate patient serum with Group O donor platelets. After incubation, add labeled anti-human IgG antibody and labeled anti-GPIIb antibody. Acquire platelet GPIIb positivity and anti-human IgG fluorescein median fluorescence intensity by flow cytometry. Analyze and report the results to the ordering provider.

## Clinical Example (0276U)

A 2-month-old Ashkenazi Jewish male, who has severe thrombocytopenia requiring multiple platelet transfusions and who was unresponsive to intravenous Ig, presents to the pediatric hematologist. There is no family history of thrombocytopenia. Inherited thrombocytopenia is suspected, and a genetic panel is ordered.

## Description of Procedure (0276U)

Isolate and subject high-quality genomic DNA to NGS of 23 genes (ACTN1, ANKRD26, CYCS, ETV6, FLI1, GATA1, GFI1B, GP1BA, GP1BB, GP9, HOXA11, ITGA2B, ITGB3, MPL, MYH9, NBEAL2, PRKACG, RBM8A, RUNX1, STXBP2, TUBB1, WAS, WIPF1). The pathologist or other QHP analyzes the data and composes a report.

## Clinical Example (0277U)

A 3-year-old male has recurrent serious bleeding leading to anemia. Coagulation factors, platelet electron microscopy, and flow cytometry are normal, but platelet aggregation is abnormal with adenosine 5'-diphosphate (ADP) and arachidonic acid. Inherited platelet dysfunction is suspected, and genetic testing is ordered.

## Description of Procedure (0277U)

Isolate and subject high-quality genomic DNA to NGS of 31 genes (ANO6, AP3B1, BLOC1S3, BLOC1S6, DTNBP1, FERMT3, FLI1, GFI1B, GP1BA, GP1BB, GP6, GP9, HPS1, HPS3, HPS4, HPS5, HPS6, ITGA2B, ITGB3, LYST, NBEAL2, P2RY12, PLA2G4A, PLAU, PRKACG, RASGRP2, RUNX1, STIM1, TBXA2R, VIPAS39, VPS33B). The pathologist or other QHP analyzes the data and composes a report.

## Clinical Example (0278U)

A 32-year-old male presents with an unprovoked pulmonary embolus and bilateral deep vein thrombosis (DVT). He developed recurrent thrombosis despite anticoagulation. Antithrombin activity was normal. Antiphospholipid syndrome antibody, paroxysmal nocturnal hemoglobinuria, and JAK2 were negative. Protein C and S decreased at presentation and cannot be rechecked because the patient is on warfarin. An inherited hypercoagulopathy panel is ordered.

## Description of Procedure (0278U)

Isolate and subject high-quality genomic DNA to NGS of 12 genes (ADAMTS13, F2, F5, FGA, FGB, FGG, HRG, KNG1, PROC, PROS1, SERPINC1, THBD). The pathologist or other QHP analyzes the data and composes a report.

★ = Telemedicine   ✚ = Add-on code   ✔ = FDA approval pending   # = Resequenced code   ⊘ = Modifier 51 exempt

## Clinical Example (0279U)

A 35-year-old female presents with a history of occasional bleeding and heavy menstrual bleeding. Initial coagulation studies are normal. A comprehensive von Willebrand disease (VWD) evaluation is ordered, including assessment of possible collagen-binding abnormalities.

## Description of Procedure (0279U)

Analyze patient serum or plasma by ELISA for human type III collagen for a minimum of two dilutions for each sample. Use a combination of two anti-von Willebrand factor (VWF) monoclonal antibodies to detect bound VWF. Analyze and report the results to the ordering provider.

## Clinical Example (0280U)

A 35-year-old female presents with a history of occasional bleeding and heavy menstrual bleeding. Initial coagulation studies are normal. A comprehensive VWD evaluation is ordered, including assessment of possible collagen-binding abnormalities.

## Description of Procedure (0280U)

Analyze patient serum or plasma by ELISA for human type IV collagen for a minimum of two dilutions for each sample. Use a combination of two anti-VWF monoclonal antibodies to detect bound VWF. Analyze and report the results to the ordering provider.

## Clinical Example (0281U)

A 3-year-old male, who has seizures, easy bruising, and recurrent epistaxis, presents with an abnormal thrombophilia evaluation (VWF antigen = 20%, VWF activity = 12%, Factor VIII = 20%). The hematologist ordered VWF antigen and VWF propeptide antigen assay to determine the VWFpp/VWF:Ag ratio.

## Description of Procedure (0281U)

Analyze patient serum or plasma by ELISA for the VWF propeptide antigen. Analyze and report the results to the ordering provider.

## Clinical Example (0282U)

A 15-year-old male presents with known sickle cell disease. He recently had an immune reaction after transfusion. A peripheral blood sample is submitted for genotyping to assess the patient's red cell antigen status.

## Description of Procedure (0282U)

Isolate and subject high-quality genomic DNA to PCR and hybridization of Rh, Kell, Duffy, Kidd, MNS, Lutheran, Dombrock, Colton, Cromer, Yt, Diego, and Vel blood group system genes and identify the following variant RHCE alleles: ceMO, ceBI, ceAR, ceEK, ceS, ce(48C), ce(733G), ceAG, ceTI, ceJAL, and ceCF. The pathologist or other QHP analyzes the data and composes a report.

## Clinical Example (0283U)

A 4-year-old female with recurrent epistaxis and thrombocytopenia has laboratory findings suggesting type 2 VWD (VWF antigen = 35%, VWF activity = 20%, and Factor VIII = 67%). The hematologist wishes to determine if the patient has type 2A, 2B, or platelet-type VWD, but the platelet count is too low to do a low-dose ristocetin-induced platelet aggregation test. A type 2B binding assay is ordered.

## Description of Procedure (0283U)

Evaluate the ability of plasma VWF to bind to formalin-fixed platelets in the presence of low-dose ristocetin using a VWD-specific monoclonal antibody. After incubation, measure bound and unbound VWF by radioimmunoassay. Perform VWF multimer analysis to assist with interpretation. A qualified laboratory professional reviews the binding assay and multimer profile and issues a report.

## Clinical Example (0284U)

A 13-year-old male has excessive bruising. Coagulation studies show Factor VIII (FVIII) of 13%, VWF antigen of 75%, and VWF activity of 72%. There is no family history of hemophilia A. To determine if the patient has mild hemophilia A or type 2N VWD, the hematologist orders a type 2N binding assay.

## Description of Procedure (0284U)

Incubate citrated patient plasma with monoclonal anti-VWF attached to the surface of a microtiter plate to capture patient-derived VWF. Remove endogenous VWF-bound FVIII by thrombin cleavage, then add and quantify recombinant FVIII using a chromogenic assay. Quantify VWF using ELISA. Report the results as the ratio of FVIII to VWF. A qualified laboratory professional reviews the results and issues a report.

# Notes

# Medicine

## Summary of Additions, Deletions, and Revisions

The summary of changes shows the actual changes that have been made to the code descriptors.

New codes appear with a bullet (●) and are indicated as "Code added." Revised codes are preceded with a triangle (▲). Within revised codes, or if a code symbol has been deleted, the deleted language and code symbol appear with a ~~strikethrough~~, while new text appears <u>underlined</u>.

The ✗ symbol is used to identify codes for vaccines that are pending FDA approval. The # symbol is used to identify codes that have been resequenced. CPT add-on codes are annotated by the ✚ symbol. The ⊘ symbol is used to identify codes that are exempt from the use of modifier 51. The ★ symbol is used to identify codes that may be used for reporting telemedicine services. The ✕ symbol is used to identify a proprietary laboratory analyses (PLA) test that has an identical descriptor as another PLA test. A PLA code that satisfies Category I code criteria and has been accepted by the CPT Editorial Panel is annotated with the ↑↓ symbol.

| Code | Description |
|---|---|
| ●0001A | Code added |
| ●0002A | Code added |
| ●0011A | Code added |
| ●0012A | Code added |
| ●0021A | Code added |
| ●0022A | Code added |
| ●0031A | Code added |
| ●0041A | Code added |
| ●0042A | Code added |
| #●91300 | Code added |
| #●91301 | Code added |
| #✗●91302 | Code added |
| #●91303 | Code added |
| #✗●91304 | Code added |
| ✗●90671 | Code added |
| #●90677 | Code added |
| #✗●90626 | Code added |
| #✗●90627 | Code added |
| #✗●90759 | Code added |

Medicine 90281-99607

| Code | Description |
|------|-------------|
| #●90758 | Code added |
| #●91113 | Code added |
| ▲92065 | Orthoptic ~~and/or pleoptic~~ training~~, with continuing medical direction and evaluation~~ |
| 92559 | ~~Audiometric testing of groups~~ |
| 92560 | ~~Bekesy audiometry; screening~~ |
| 92561 | ~~diagnostic~~ |
| 92564 | ~~Short increment sensitivity index (SISI)~~ |
| #+●93319 | Code added |
| 93530 | ~~Right heart catheterization, for congenital cardiac anomalies~~ |
| 93531 | ~~Combined right heart catheterization and retrograde left heart catheterization, for congenital cardiac anomalies~~ |
| 93532 | ~~Combined right heart catheterization and transseptal left heart catheterization through intact septum with or without retrograde left heart catheterization, for congenital cardiac anomalies~~ |
| 93533 | ~~Combined right heart catheterization and transseptal left heart catheterization through existing septal opening, with or without retrograde left heart catheterization, for congenital cardiac anomalies~~ |
| 93561 | ~~Indicator dilution studies such as dye or thermodilution, including arterial and/or venous catheterization; with cardiac output measurement (separate procedure)~~ |
| 93562 | ~~subsequent measurement of cardiac output~~ |
| ●93593 | Code added |
| ●93594 | Code added |
| ●93595 | Code added |
| ●93596 | Code added |
| ●93597 | Code added |
| +●93598 | Code added |
| ▲93653 | Comprehensive electrophysiologic evaluation ~~including~~ <u>with</u> insertion and repositioning of multiple electrode catheters<u>,</u> ~~with~~ induction or attempted induction of an arrhythmia with right atrial pacing and recording <u>and catheter ablation of arrhythmogenic focus, including intracardiac electrophysiologic 3-dimensional mapping</u>, right ventricular pacing and recording ~~(when necessary)~~<u>, left atrial pacing and recording from coronary sinus or left atrium,</u> and His bundle recording<u>, when performed</u> ~~(when necessary) with intracardiac catheter ablation of arrhythmogenic focus~~; with treatment of supraventricular tachycardia by ablation of fast or slow atrioventricular pathway, accessory atrioventricular connection, cavo-tricuspid isthmus or other single atrial focus or source of atrial re-entry |
| ▲93654 | with treatment of ventricular tachycardia or focus of ventricular ectopy including ~~intracardiac electrophysiologic 3D mapping, when performed, and~~ left ventricular pacing and recording, when performed |
| ▲93656 | Comprehensive electrophysiologic evaluation including transseptal catheterizations, insertion and repositioning of multiple electrode catheters with <u>intracardiac catheter ablation of atrial fibrillation by pulmonary vein isolation, including intracardiac electrophysiologic 3-dimensional mapping, intracardiac echocardiography including imaging supervision and interpretation,</u> induction or attempted induction of an arrhythmia including left or right atrial pacing/recording ~~when necessary~~, right ventricular pacing/recording ~~when necessary~~, and His bundle recording<u>,</u> ~~when necessary~~ <u>when performed</u>~~with intracardiac catheter ablation of atrial fibrillation by pulmonary vein isolation~~ |

| Code | Description |
|---|---|
| ●**94625** | Code added |
| ●**94626** | Code added |
| **95943** | ~~Simultaneous, independent, quantitative measures of both parasympathetic function and sympathetic function, based on time-frequency analysis of heart rate variability concurrent with time-frequency analysis of continuous respiratory activity, with mean heart rate and blood pressure measures, during rest, paced (deep) breathing, Valsalva maneuvers, and head-up postural change~~ |
| ●**98975** | Code added |
| ●**98976** | Code added |
| ●**98977** | Code added |
| ●**98980** | Code added |
| ✚●**98981** | Code added |
| ●**99072** | Code added |

▲ = Revised code    ● = New code    ▶ ◀ = Contains new or revised text    ✕ = Duplicate PLA test    ↑↓ = Category I PLA    American Medical Association    **139**

Medicine 90281-99607

# Medicine Guidelines

## Supplied Materials

Supplies and materials (eg, trays, drug supplies, and materials) over and above those usually included with the procedure(s) rendered are reported separately using code 99070 or a specific supply code.

## ►Foreign Body/Implant Definition◄

►An object intentionally placed by a physician or other qualified health care professional for any purpose (eg, diagnostic or therapeutic) is considered an implant. An object that is unintentionally placed (eg, trauma or ingestion) is considered a foreign body. If an implant (or part thereof) has moved from its original position or is structurally broken and no longer serves its intended purpose or presents a hazard to the patient, it qualifies as a foreign body for coding purposes, unless CPT coding instructions direct otherwise or a specific CPT code exists to describe the removal of that broken/moved implant.◄

### Rationale

The introductory language in the Medicine Guidelines section of the CPT code set has been updated to include a new heading and a definition of "foreign body" and "implant." The definition clarifies the difference between an implant and a foreign body. It also specifies other conditions that qualify an implant as a foreign body for coding purposes. In addition, the definition provides guidance if other instructions or a specific CPT code exists to describe the removal of a broken or moved implant.

★ =Telemedicine   + =Add-on code   ✐ =FDA approval pending   # =Resequenced code   ⊘ =Modifier 51 exemp

# Medicine

## Immunization Administration for Vaccines/Toxoids

▶Report vaccine immunization administration codes (90460, 90461, 90471-90474, 0001A, 0002A, 0011A, 0012A, 0021A, 0022A, 0031A, 0041A, 0042A) in addition to the vaccine and toxoid code(s) (90476-90759, 91300, 91301, 91302, 91303, 91304).

Report codes 90460 and 90461 only when the physician or other qualified health care professional provides face-to-face counseling of the patient/family during the administration of a vaccine other than when performed for severe acute respiratory syndrome coronavirus 2 (SARS-CoV-2) (coronavirus disease [COVID-19]) vaccines. For immunization administration of any vaccine, other than SARS-CoV-2 (coronavirus disease [COVID-19]) vaccines, that is not accompanied by face-to-face physician or other qualified health care professional counseling to the patient/family/guardian or for administration of vaccines to patients over 18 years of age, report codes 90471-90474. (See also **Instructions for Use of the CPT Codebook** for definition of reporting qualifications.)

Report 0001A, 0002A, 0011A, 0012A, 0021A, 0022A, 0031A, 0041A, 0042A for immunization administration of SARS-CoV-2 (coronavirus disease [COVID-19]) vaccines only. Each administration code is specific to each individual vaccine product (eg, 91300, 91301, 91302, 91303, 91304), the dosage schedule (eg, first dose, second dose), and counseling, when performed. The appropriate administration code is chosen based on the type of vaccine and the specific dose number the patient receives in the schedule. For example, 0012A is reported for the second dose of vaccine 91301. Do not report 90460-90474 for the administration of SARS-CoV-2 (coronavirus disease [COVID-19]) vaccines. Codes related to SARS-CoV-2 (coronavirus disease [COVID-19]) vaccine administration are listed in Appendix Q, with their associated vaccine code descriptors, vaccine administration codes, vaccine manufacturer, vaccine name(s), National Drug Code (NDC) Labeler Product ID, and interval between doses. In order to report these codes, the vaccine must fulfill the code descriptor and must be the vaccine represented by the manufacturer and vaccine name listed in Appendix Q.◀

If a significant separately identifiable evaluation and management service (eg, new or established patient office or other outpatient services [99202-99215], office or other outpatient consultations [99241-99245], emergency department services [99281-99285], preventive medicine services [99381-99429]) is performed, the appropriate E/M service code should be reported in addition to the vaccine and toxoid administration codes.

A component refers to all antigens in a vaccine that prevent disease(s) caused by one organism (90460 and 90461). Multi-valent antigens or multiple serotypes of antigens against a single organism are considered a single component of vaccines. Combination vaccines are those vaccines that contain multiple vaccine components. Conjugates or adjuvants contained in vaccines are not considered to be component parts of the vaccine as defined above.

(For allergy testing, see 95004 et seq)

(For skin testing of bacterial, viral, fungal extracts, see 86485-86580)

(For therapeutic or diagnostic injections, see 96372-96379)

**90460** Immunization administration through 18 years of age via any route of administration, with counseling by physician or other qualified health care professional; first or only component of each vaccine or toxoid administered

**+ 90461** each additional vaccine or toxoid component administered (List separately in addition to code for primary procedure)

(Use 90460 for each vaccine administered. For vaccines with multiple components [combination vaccines], report 90460 in conjunction with 90461 for each additional component in a given vaccine)

▶(Do not report 90460, 90461 in conjunction with 91300, 91301, 91302, 91303, 91304, unless both a severe acute respiratory syndrome coronavirus 2 [SARS-CoV-2] [coronavirus disease {COVID-19}] vaccine/toxoid product and at least one vaccine/toxoid product from 90476-90759 are administered at the same encounter)◀

**90471** Immunization administration (includes percutaneous, intradermal, subcutaneous, or intramuscular injections); 1 vaccine (single or combination vaccine/toxoid)

(Do not report 90471 in conjunction with 90473)

**+ 90472** each additional vaccine (single or combination vaccine/toxoid) (List separately in addition to code for primary procedure)

(Use 90472 in conjunction with 90460, 90471, 90473)

▶(Do not report 90471, 90472 in conjunction with 91300, 91301, 91302, 91303, 91304, unless both a severe acute respiratory syndrome coronavirus 2 [SARS-CoV-2] [coronavirus disease {COVID-19}] vaccine/toxoid product and at least one vaccine/toxoid product from 90476-90759 are administered at the same encounter)◀

(For immune globulins, see 90281-90399. For administration of immune globulins, see 96365, 96366, 96367, 96368, 96369, 96370, 96371, 96374)

(For intravesical administration of BCG vaccine, see 51720, 90586)

**90473**  Immunization administration by intranasal or oral route; 1 vaccine (single or combination vaccine/toxoid)

(Do not report 90473 in conjunction with 90471)

**+ 90474**  each additional vaccine (single or combination vaccine/toxoid) (List separately in addition to code for primary procedure)

(Use 90474 in conjunction with 90460, 90471, 90473)

▶(Do not report 90473, 90474 in conjunction with 91300, 91301, 91302, 91303, 91304, unless both a severe acute respiratory syndrome coronavirus 2 [SARS-CoV-2] [coronavirus disease {COVID-19}] vaccine/toxoid product and at least one vaccine/toxoid product from 90476-90759 are administered at the same encounter)◀

● **0001A**  Immunization administration by intramuscular injection of severe acute respiratory syndrome coronavirus 2 (SARS-CoV-2) (coronavirus disease [COVID-19]) vaccine, mRNA-LNP, spike protein, preservative free, 30 mcg/0.3 mL dosage, diluent reconstituted; first dose

● **0002A**  second dose

▶(Report 0001A, 0002A for the administration of vaccine 91300)◀

● **0011A**  Immunization administration by intramuscular injection of severe acute respiratory syndrome coronavirus 2 (SARS-CoV-2) (coronavirus disease [COVID-19]) vaccine, mRNA-LNP, spike protein, preservative free, 100 mcg/0.5 mL dosage; first dose

● **0012A**  second dose

▶(Report 0011A, 0012A for the administration of vaccine 91301)◀

● **0021A**  Immunization administration by intramuscular injection of severe acute respiratory syndrome coronavirus 2 (SARS-CoV-2) (coronavirus disease [COVID-19]) vaccine, DNA, spike protein, chimpanzee adenovirus Oxford 1 (ChAdOx1) vector, preservative free, 5x10$^{10}$ viral particles/0.5 mL dosage; first dose

● **0022A**  second dose

▶(Report 0021A, 0022A for the administration of vaccine 91302)◀

● **0031A**  Immunization administration by intramuscular injection of severe acute respiratory syndrome coronavirus 2 (SARS-CoV-2) (coronavirus disease [COVID-19]) vaccine, DNA, spike protein, adenovirus type 26 (Ad26) vector, preservative free, 5x10$^{10}$ viral particles/0.5 mL dosage, single dose

▶(Report 0031A for the administration of vaccine 91303)◀

● **0041A**  Immunization administration by intramuscular injection o severe acute respiratory syndrome coronavirus 2 (SARS-CoV-2) (coronavirus disease [COVID-19]) vaccine, recombinant spike protein nanoparticle, saponin-based adjuvant, preservative free, 5 mcg/0.5 mL dosage; first dose

● **0042A**  second dose

▶(Report 0041A, 0042A for the administration of vaccine 91304)◀

## Rationale

New vaccine product and administration codes (0001A-0042A) and a new appendix (Appendix Q) have been established for reporting severe acute respiratory syndrome coronavirus 2 (SARS-CoV-2) (coronavirus disease [COVID-19]) vaccine products and administrations. In addition, updates have been made to existing guidelines and parenthetical notes and new parenthetical notes have been added throughout the code set to accommodate the changes and additions.

To address the urgent health care need and facilitate the curtailing of the rapid pandemic spread of the COVID-19 virus throughout the United States, Emergency Use Authorization (EUA) was provided by the Food and Drug Administration (FDA). This allows more rapid development of vaccine codes from multiple manufacturers and makes COVID vaccine products available earlier for code development.

As a result, new codes have been included within the Vaccine, Toxoids subsection to allow: (1) reporting of separate COVID-19 vaccine product codes according to manufacturer; and (2) reporting of specific administration codes that are unique to the various COVID-19 vaccine products. This is exemplified by the inclusion of five codes for COVID vaccine products (91300-91304), as well as nine COVID-19 vaccine administration codes (0001A-0042A) that are only reported according to the COVID-19 vaccine product administered.

CPT code convention typically uses common language within a code descriptor to better specify identification of the procedure or vaccine and removes focus from proprietary language that may be specific to a particular manufacturer. However, due to the unique needs of these products, separate codes have been assigned for COVID-19 vaccine products that would ordinarily be assigned a single code. The differentiation is exemplified within the code descriptor according to elements that would not ordinarily be used. Use of components such as notation of use of spike protein in the compilation and indication of the type of vector used (eg, chimpanzee adenovirus Oxford 1 [ChAdOx1]) provide differentiation that is not ordinarily included within a vaccine product code. As a result, each

★ = Telemedicine  + = Add-on code  ✗ = FDA approval pending  # = Resequenced code  ⊘ = Modifier 51 exemp

COVID-19 vaccine product code includes language within its descriptor that is different from other COVID vaccines.

Use of separate codes for the administration of COVID-19 vaccine products is unique to COVID-19 vaccine reporting. To eliminate confusion, instructions have been included throughout the code set wherever vaccine administrations are discussed. This includes instruction within the Evaluation and Management (E/M) and Medicine sections that direct use of the special COVID-19 administration codes only for the specific COVID-19 product for which it was created. These instructions also restrict the use of non-COVID-19 administration codes (90460-90474) in conjunction with COVID-19 vaccine product codes unless both a COVID vaccine/toxoid product and at least one vaccine/toxoid product from 90476-90759 are administered at the same encounter.

To further assist users in the appropriate reporting of COVID-19 vaccine services, guidelines and parenthetical notes throughout the code set have been updated or added to accommodate the addition of the new codes, provide instructions regarding codes that may or may not be reported together, direct users to appropriate codes for non-COVID vaccine administrations, and provide instruction regarding the appropriate codes to use for COVID-19 vaccine products and administrations. In addition, the new Appendix Q has been added to further assist users in differentiating and selecting the appropriate vaccine product codes and the associated administration code(s).

The table in Appendix Q consists of the individual COVID-19 vaccine product codes (91300-91304) and their associated immunization administration codes (0001A, 0002A, 0011A, 0012A, 0021A, 0022A, 0031A, 0041A, 0042A), manufacturer name, vaccine name(s), 10- and 11-digit National Drug Code (NDC) Labeler Product ID, and interval between doses. This table allows easy visualization of all information related to a particular COVID vaccine product and administration code.

Finally, on the AMA's COVID-19 CPT® Coding and Guidance webpage (https://www.ama-assn.org/practice-management/cpt/covid-19-cpt-vaccine-and-immunization-codes), a built-in tool has also been included to assist vaccine product code and administration code selection. The AMA COVID-19 webpage should be consulted for frequent updates to CPT codes for COVID-19 vaccines and services.

## Clinical Example (0001A)

A 33-year-old individual seeks immunization against SARS-CoV-2 to decrease the risk of contracting this disease, consistent with evidence-supported guidelines. The individual is offered and accepts an intramuscular injection of SARS-CoV-2 vaccine for this purpose.

## Description of Procedure (0001A)

The physician or other qualified health care professional (QHP) reviews the patient's chart to confirm that vaccination to decrease the risk of COVID-19 is indicated. Counsel the patient on the benefits and risks of vaccination to decrease the risk of COVID-19 and obtain consent. Administer the first dose of the COVID-19 vaccine by intramuscular injection in the upper arm. Monitor the patient for any adverse reaction. Update the patient's immunization record (and registry when applicable) to reflect the vaccine administered.

## Clinical Example (0002A)

A 33-year-old individual seeks immunization against SARS-CoV-2 to decrease the risk of contracting this disease, consistent with evidence-supported guidelines. The individual is offered and accepts an intramuscular injection of SARS-CoV-2 vaccine for this purpose.

## Description of Procedure (0002A)

The physician or other QHP reviews the patient's chart to confirm that vaccination to decrease the risk of COVID-19 is indicated. Counsel the patient on the benefits and risks of vaccination to decrease the risk of COVID-19 and obtain consent. Administer the second dose of the COVID-19 vaccine by intramuscular injection in the upper arm. Monitor the patient for any adverse reaction. Update the patient's immunization record (and registry when applicable) to reflect the vaccine administered.

## Clinical Example (0011A)

A 33-year-old individual seeks immunization against SARS-CoV-2 to decrease the risk of contracting this disease, consistent with evidence-supported guidelines. The individual is offered and accepts an intramuscular injection of SARS-CoV-2 vaccine for this purpose.

## Description of Procedure (0011A)

The physician or other QHP reviews the patient's chart to confirm that vaccination to decrease the risk of COVID-19 is indicated. Counsel the patient on the benefits and risks of vaccination to decrease the risk of COVID-19 and obtain consent. Administer the first dose of the COVID-19 vaccine by intramuscular injection in the upper arm. Monitor the patient for any adverse reaction. Update the patient's immunization record (and registry when applicable) to reflect the vaccine administered.

## Clinical Example (0012A)

A 33-year-old individual seeks immunization against SARS-CoV-2 to decrease the risk of contracting this disease, consistent with evidence-supported guidelines. The individual is offered and accepts an intramuscular injection of SARS-CoV-2 vaccine for this purpose.

## Description of Procedure (0012A)

The physician or other QHP reviews the patient's chart to confirm that vaccination to decrease the risk of COVID-19 is indicated. Counsel the patient on the benefits and risks of vaccination to decrease the risk of COVID-19 and obtain consent. Administer the second dose of the COVID-19 vaccine by intramuscular injection in the upper arm. Monitor the patient for any adverse reaction. Update the patient's immunization record (and registry when applicable) to reflect the vaccine administered.

## Clinical Example (0021A)

A 33-year-old individual seeks immunization against SARS-CoV-2 to decrease the risk of contracting this disease, consistent with evidence-supported guidelines. The individual is offered and accepts an intramuscular injection of SARS-CoV-2 vaccine for this purpose.

## Description of Procedure (0021A)

The physician or other QHP reviews the patient's chart to confirm that vaccination to decrease the risk of COVID-19 is indicated. Counsel the patient on the benefits and risks of vaccination to decrease the risk of COVID-19 and obtain consent. Administer the first dose of the COVID-19 vaccine by intramuscular injection in the upper arm. Monitor the patient for any adverse reaction. Update the patient's immunization record (and registry when applicable) to reflect the vaccine administered.

## Clinical Example (0022A)

A 33-year-old individual seeks immunization against SARS-CoV-2 to decrease the risk of contracting this disease, consistent with evidence-supported guidelines. The individual is offered and accepts an intramuscular injection of SARS-CoV-2 vaccine for this purpose.

## Description of Procedure (0022A)

The physician or other QHP reviews the patient's chart to confirm that vaccination to decrease the risk of COVID-19 is indicated. Counsel the patient on the benefits and risks of vaccination to decrease the risk of COVID-19 and obtain consent. Administer the second dose of the COVID-19 vaccine by intramuscular injection in the upper arm. Monitor the patient for any adverse reaction. Update the patient's immunization record (and registry when applicable) to reflect the vaccine administered.

## Clinical Example (0031A)

A 33-year-old individual seeks immunization against SARS-CoV-2 to decrease the risk of contracting this disease, consistent with evidence-supported guidelines. The individual is offered and accepts an intramuscular injection of SARS-CoV-2 vaccine for this purpose.

## Description of Procedure (0031A)

The physician or other QHP reviews the patient's chart to confirm that vaccination to decrease the risk of COVID-19 is indicated. Counsel the patient on the benefits and risks of vaccination to decrease the risk of COVID-19 and obtain consent. Administer the single-dose COVID-19 vaccine by intramuscular injection in the upper arm. Monitor the patient for any adverse reaction. Update the patient's immunization record (and registry when applicable) to reflect the vaccine administered.

## Clinical Example (0041A)

A 33-year-old individual seeks immunization against SARS-CoV-2 to decrease the risk of contracting this disease, consistent with evidence-supported guidelines. The individual is offered and accepts an intramuscular injection of SARS-CoV-2 vaccine for this purpose.

## Description of Procedure (0041A)

The physician or other QHP reviews the patient's chart to confirm that vaccination to decrease the risk of COVID-19 is indicated. Counsel the patient on the benefits and risks of vaccination to decrease the risk of COVID-19 and obtain consent. Administer the first dose of the COVID-19 vaccine by intramuscular injection in the upper arm. Monitor the patient for any adverse reaction. Update the patient's immunization record (and registry when applicable) to reflect the vaccine administered.

## Clinical Example (0042A)

A 33-year-old individual seeks immunization against SARS-CoV-2 to decrease the risk of contracting this disease, consistent with evidence-supported guidelines. The individual is offered and accepts an intramuscular injection of SARS-CoV-2 vaccine for this purpose.

## Description of Procedure (0042A)

The physician or other QHP reviews the patient's chart to confirm that vaccination to decrease the risk of COVID-19 is indicated. Counsel the patient on the benefits and risks of vaccination to decrease the risk of COVID-19 and obtain consent. Administer the second dose of the COVID-19 vaccine by intramuscular injection in the upper arm. Monitor the patient for any adverse reaction. Update the patient's immunization record (and registry when applicable) to reflect the vaccine administered.

# Vaccines, Toxoids

To assist users to report the most recent new or revised vaccine product codes, the American Medical Association (AMA) currently uses the CPT website (ama-assn.org/cpt-cat-i-vaccine-codes), which features updates of CPT Editorial Panel actions regarding these products. See the Introduction section of the CPT code set for a complete list of the dates of release and implementation.

The CPT Editorial Panel, in recognition of the public health interest in vaccine products, has chosen to publish new vaccine product codes prior to approval by the US Food and Drug Administration (FDA). These codes are indicated with the ⚡ symbol and will be tracked by the AMA to monitor FDA approval status. Once the FDA status changes to approval, the ⚡ symbol will be removed. CPT users should refer to the AMA CPT website (ama-assn.org/cpt-cat-i-vaccine-codes) for the most up-to-date information on codes with the ⚡ symbol.

►Codes 90476-90759, 91300, 91301, 91302, 91303, 91304 identify the vaccine product **only**. To report the administration of a vaccine/toxoid other than SARS-CoV-2 (coronavirus disease [COVID-19]), the vaccine/toxoid product codes (90476-90759) must be used in addition to an immunization administration code(s) (90460, 90461, 90471, 90472, 90473, 90474). To report the administration of a SARS-CoV-2 (coronavirus disease [COVID-19]) vaccine, the vaccine/toxoid product codes (91300, 91301, 91302, 91303, 91304) should be reported with the corresponding immunization administration codes (0001A, 0002A, 0011A, 0012A, 0021A, 0022A, 0031A, 0041A, 0042A). All SARS-CoV-2 (coronavirus disease [COVID-19]) vaccine codes in this section are listed in Appendix Q with their associated vaccine code descriptors, vaccine administration codes, vaccine manufacturer, vaccine name(s), NDC Labeler Product ID, and interval between doses. In order to report these codes, the vaccine must fulfill the code descriptor and must be the vaccine represented by the manufacturer and vaccine name listed in Appendix Q.

Do not report 90476-90759 in conjunction with the SARS-CoV-2 (coronavirus disease [COVID-19]) immunization administration codes 0001A, 0002A, 0011A, 0012A, 0021A, 0022A, 0031A, 0041A, 0042A unless both a SARS-CoV-2 (coronavirus disease [COVID-19]) vaccine/toxoid product and at least one vaccine/toxoid product from 90476-90759 are administered at the same encounter.

Modifier 51 should not be reported with vaccine/toxoid codes 90476-90759, 91300, 91301, 91302, 91303, 91304 when reported in conjunction with administration codes 90460, 90461, 90471, 90472, 90473, 90474, 0001A, 0002A, 0011A, 0012A, 0021A, 0022A, 0031A, 0041A, 0042A.◄

If a significantly separately identifiable Evaluation and Management (E/M) service (eg, office or other outpatient services, preventive medicine services) is performed, the appropriate E/M service code should be reported in addition to the vaccine and toxoid administration codes.

To meet the reporting requirements of immunization registries, vaccine distribution programs, and reporting systems (eg, Vaccine Adverse Event Reporting System) the exact vaccine product administered needs to be reported. Multiple codes for a particular vaccine are provided in the CPT codebook when the schedule (number of doses or timing) differs for two or more products of the same vaccine type (eg, hepatitis A, Hib) or the vaccine product is available in more than one chemical formulation, dosage, or route of administration.

The "when administered to" age descriptions included in CPT vaccine codes are not intended to identify a product's licensed age indication. The term "preservative free" includes use for vaccines that contain no preservative and vaccines that contain trace amounts of preservative agents that are not present in a sufficient concentration for the purpose of preserving the final vaccine formulation. The absence of a designation regarding a preservative does not necessarily indicate the presence or absence of preservative in the vaccine. Refer to the product's prescribing information (PI) for the licensed age indication before administering vaccine to a patient.

Separate codes are available for combination vaccines (eg, Hib-HepB, DTap-IPV/Hib). It is inappropriate to code each component of a combination vaccine separately. If a specific vaccine code is not available, the unlisted procedure code should be reported, until a new code becomes available.

►The vaccine/toxoid abbreviations listed in codes 90476-90759, 91300, 91301, 91302, 91303, 91304 reflect the most recent US vaccine abbreviation references used in the Advisory Committee on Immunization Practices (ACIP) recommendations at the time of CPT code set publication. Interim updates to vaccine code descriptors will be made following abbreviation approval by the ACIP on a timely basis via the AMA CPT website (ama-assn.org/cpt-cat-i-vaccine-codes). The accuracy of the ACIP vaccine abbreviation designations in the CPT code set does not affect the validity of the vaccine code and its reporting function.◄

(For immune globulins, see 90281-90399. For administration of immune globulins, see 96365-96375)

#● **91300** Severe acute respiratory syndrome coronavirus 2 (SARS-CoV-2) (coronavirus disease [COVID-19]) vaccine, mRNA-LNP, spike protein, preservative free, 30 mcg/0.3 mL dosage, diluent reconstituted, for intramuscular use

▶(Report 91300 with administration codes 0001A, 0002A)◀

#● **91301** Severe acute respiratory syndrome coronavirus 2 (SARS-CoV-2) (coronavirus disease [COVID-19]) vaccine, mRNA-LNP, spike protein, preservative free, 100 mcg/0.5 mL dosage, for intramuscular use

▶(Report 91301 with administration codes 0011A, 0012A)◀

#✗● **91302** Severe acute respiratory syndrome coronavirus 2 (SARS-CoV-2) (coronavirus disease [COVID-19]) vaccine, DNA, spike protein, chimpanzee adenovirus Oxford 1 (ChAdOx1) vector, preservative free, 5x1010 viral particles/0.5 mL dosage, for intramuscular use

▶(Report 91302 with administration codes 0021A, 0022A)◀

#● **91303** Severe acute respiratory syndrome coronavirus 2 (SARS-CoV-2) (coronavirus disease [COVID-19]) vaccine, DNA, spike protein, adenovirus type 26 (Ad26) vector, preservative free, 5x1010 viral particles/0.5 mL dosage, for intramuscular use

▶(Report 91303 with administration code 0031A)◀

#✗● **91304** Severe acute respiratory syndrome coronavirus 2 (SARS-CoV-2) (coronavirus disease [COVID-19]) vaccine, recombinant spike protein nanoparticle, saponin-based adjuvant, preservative free, 5 mcg/0.5 mL dosage, for intramuscular use

▶(Report 91304 with administration codes 0041A, 0042A)◀

## Rationale

To accommodate the addition of new codes for reporting COVID-19 vaccine products, codes 91300-91304 and associated parenthetical notes have been added and the existing vaccines/toxoids guidelines have been revised.

Refer to the codebook and the Rationale for codes 0001A-0042A for a full discussion of these changes.

## Clinical Example (91300)

A 33-year-old individual seeks immunization against severe acute respiratory syndrome coronavirus 2 (SARS-CoV-2) virus to decrease the risk of contracting this disease, consistent with evidence-supported guidelines. The individual is offered and accepts an intramuscular injection of the SARS-CoV-2 vaccine for this purpose.

## Description of Procedure (91300)

The physician or other QHP determines that the SARS-CoV-2 vaccine is appropriate for this patient and dispenses the vaccine according to the dose scheduled in the administration code for the SARS-CoV-2 vaccine.

## Clinical Example (91301)

A 33-year-old individual seeks immunization against SARS-CoV-2 virus to decrease the risk of contracting this disease, consistent with evidence-supported guidelines. The individual is offered and accepts an intramuscular injection of the SARS-CoV-2 vaccine for this purpose.

## Description of Procedure (91301)

The physician or other QHP determines that the SARS-CoV-2 vaccine is appropriate for this patient and dispenses the vaccine according to the dose scheduled in the administration code for the SARS-CoV-2 vaccine.

## Clinical Example (91302)

A 33-year-old individual seeks immunization against SARS-CoV-2 virus to decrease the risk of contracting this disease, consistent with evidence-supported guidelines. The individual is offered and accepts an intramuscular injection of the SARS-CoV-2 vaccine for this purpose.

## Description of Procedure (91302)

The physician or other QHP determines that the SARS-CoV-2 vaccine is appropriate for this patient and dispenses the vaccine according to the dose scheduled in the administration code for the SARS-CoV-2 vaccine.

## Clinical Example (91303)

A 33-year-old individual seeks immunization against SARS-CoV-2 virus to decrease the risk of contracting this disease, consistent with evidence-supported guidelines. The individual is offered and accepts an intramuscular injection of the SARS-CoV-2 vaccine for this purpose.

## Description of Procedure (91303)

The physician or other QHP determines that the SARS-CoV-2 vaccine is appropriate for this patient and dispenses the vaccine according to the dose scheduled in the administration code for the SARS-CoV-2 vaccine.

## Clinical Example (91304)

A 33-year-old individual seeks immunization against SARS-CoV-2 virus to decrease the risk of contracting this disease, consistent with evidence-supported guidelines. The individual is offered and accepts an intramuscular injection of the SARS-CoV-2 vaccine for this purpose.

## Description of Procedure (91304)

The physician or other QHP determines that the SARS-CoV-2 vaccine is appropriate for this patient and dispenses the vaccine according to the dose scheduled in the administration code for the SARS-CoV-2 vaccine.

| | |
|---|---|
| **90476** | Adenovirus vaccine, type 4, live, for oral use |
| **90626** | Code is out of numerical sequence. See 90714-90717 |
| **90627** | Code is out of numerical sequence. See 90714-90717 |
| ✔● **90671** | Pneumococcal conjugate vaccine, 15 valent (PCV15), for intramuscular use |

### Rationale

Code 90671 has been established in the Vaccines, Toxoids subsection to report a pneumococcal conjugate vaccine. This new code describes a 15-valent (PCV15) vaccine. Code 90671 includes the ✔ symbol; therefore, interim updates on the FDA status of this code will be reflected on the AMA CPT website (https://www.ama-assn.org/practice-management/cpt/category-i-vaccine-codes) on a semiannual basis (July 1 and January 1).

Administration of the vaccine is reported separately with immunization administration for vaccines/toxoids codes 90460-90472.

### Clinical Example (90671)

A 50-year-old male with a high-risk condition is prescribed the pneumococcal 15-valent (PCV15) vaccine.

### Description of Procedure (90671)

The physician or other QHP administers a single 0.5-mL dose of the PCV15 vaccine through intramuscular injection.

| | |
|---|---|
| #● **90677** | Pneumococcal conjugate vaccine, 20 valent (PCV20), for intramuscular use |

### Rationale

Code 90677 has been established in the Vaccines, Toxoids subsection to report a conjugate pneumococcal vaccine. This code describes a 20-valent (PCV20) vaccine for intramuscular use. Code 90677 includes the ✔ symbol; therefore, interim updates on the FDA status of this code will be reflected on the AMA CPT website (https://www.ama-assn.org/practice-management/cpt/category-i-vaccine-codes) on a semiannual basis (July 1 and January 1).

Administration of the vaccine is reported separately with immunization administration for vaccines/toxoids codes 90460-90472.

### Clinical Example (90677)

A 65-year-old male presents for an annual physical. The physician or other QHP reviews the patient's immunization record and determines he should receive the pneumococcal conjugate vaccine, 20-valent (PCV20) vaccine and orders its administration.

### Description of Procedure (90677)

Administer the PCV20 vaccine by intramuscular injection.

| | |
|---|---|
| **90676** | Rabies vaccine, for intradermal use |
| **90677** | Code is out of numerical sequence. See 90670-90676 |
| #✔● **90626** | Tick-borne encephalitis virus vaccine, inactivated; 0.25 mL dosage, for intramuscular use |
| #✔● **90627** | 0.5 mL dosage, for intramuscular use |

### Rationale

Codes 90626 and 90627 have been established in the Vaccines, Toxoids subsection to report the tick-borne encephalitis virus vaccine. Code 90626 is used for an inactivated 0.25-mL dose and code 90627 is used for a 0.5-mL dose. Codes 90626 and 90627 include the ✔ symbol; therefore, interim updates on the FDA status of these codes will be reflected on the AMA CPT website (https://www.ama-assn.org/practice-management/cpt/category-i-vaccine-codes) on a semiannual basis (July 1 and January 1).

Administration of the vaccine is reported separately with immunization administration for vaccines/toxoids codes 90460-90472.

### Clinical Example (90626)

A 14-year-old male presents for traveler's vaccines before spending the summer camping in Europe. The physician or other QHP reviews the patient's immunization record and determines he should receive the tick-borne encephalitis (TBE) virus vaccine and orders the administration of the vaccine series.

### Description of Procedure (90626)

Administer a 0.25-mL dose of the TBE virus vaccine by intramuscular injection.

## Clinical Example (90627)

A 23-year-old male presents for traveler's vaccines before spending the summer camping in Europe. The physician or other QHP reviews the patient's immunization record and determines he should receive the TBE virus vaccine and orders the administration of the vaccine series.

## Description of Procedure (90627)

Administer a 0.5-mL dose of the TBE virus vaccine by intramuscular injection.

---

**90746**   Hepatitis B vaccine (HepB), adult dosage, 3 dose schedule, for intramuscular use

**# ✔● 90759**   Hepatitis B vaccine (HepB), 3-antigen (S, Pre-S1, Pre-S2), 10 mcg dosage, 3 dose schedule, for intramuscular use

### Rationale

Code 90759 has been established in the Vaccines, Toxoids subsection to report hepatitis B vaccine (HepB). This code describes a 3-antigen (S, Pre-S1, Pre-S2), 3-dose schedule for hepatitis B vaccination and uses a 10-mcg dose. Code 90759 includes the ✔ symbol; therefore, interim updates on the FDA status of this code will be reflected on the AMA CPT website (https://www.ama-assn.org/practice-management/cpt/category-i-vaccine-codes) on a semiannual basis (July 1 and January 1).

Administration of the vaccine is reported separately with immunization administration for vaccines/toxoids codes 90460-90472.

## Clinical Example (90759)

A 35-year-old male presents for a preventive medicine visit. In accordance with national recommendations for immunizations, the clinician reviews the patient's immunization record and determines that the patient should receive the hepatitis B vaccine (HepB), 3-antigen (S, Pre-S1, Pre-S2) 3-dose schedule, for intramuscular use and orders its administration.

## Description of Procedure (90759)

The physician or other QHP administers a single dose of hepatitis B vaccine (HepB), 3-antigen (S, Pre-S1, Pre-S2), 10-mcg dosage, 3-dose schedule, through intramuscular injection.

---

**90747**   Hepatitis B vaccine (HepB), dialysis or immunosuppressed patient dosage, 4 dose schedule, for intramuscular use

**90748**   Hepatitis B and Haemophilus influenzae type b vaccine (Hib-HepB), for intramuscular use

**# ● 90758**   Zaire ebolavirus vaccine, live, for intramuscular use

### Rationale

Code 90758 has been established in the Vaccines, Toxoids subsection to report Zaire ebolavirus vaccine. Code 90758 describes a live vaccine that is administered through an intramuscular injection. Administration of the vaccine is reported separately with one of the immunization administration codes, as appropriate, for vaccines/toxoids represented by codes 90460-90472.

## Clinical Example (90758)

A healthy 45-year-old female physician intends to travel to West Africa as part of a team of health care professionals responding to an outbreak of Ebola virus disease.

## Description of Procedure (90758)

The physician or other QHP administers a single 1-mL dose of Zaire ebolavirus vaccine, live, through intramuscular injection.

---

**90758**   Code is out of numerical sequence. See 90747-90749

**90759**   Code is out of numerical sequence. See 90744-90748

# Psychiatry

## Interactive Complexity

▶Code 90785 is an add-on code for interactive complexity to be reported in conjunction with codes for diagnostic psychiatric evaluation (90791, 90792), psychotherapy (90832, 90833, 90834, 90836, 90837, 90838), and group psychotherapy (90853).

Interactive complexity refers to specific communication factors that complicate the delivery of a psychiatric procedure. Common factors include more difficult communication with discordant or emotional family members and engagement of young and verbally undeveloped or impaired patients. Typical patients are those who have third parties, such as parents, guardians, other family members, agencies, court officers, or schools involved in their psychiatric care.

Psychiatric procedures may be reported "with interactive complexity" when at least one of the following is present:

1. The need to manage maladaptive communication (related to, eg, high anxiety, high reactivity, repeated questions, or disagreement) among participants that complicates delivery of care.

2. Caregiver emotions or behavior that interferes with the caregiver's understanding and ability to assist in the implementation of the treatment plan.

3. Evidence or disclosure of a sentinel event and mandated report to third party (eg, abuse or neglect with report to state agency) with initiation of discussion of the sentinel event and/or report with patient and other visit participants.

4. Use of play equipment or other physical devices to communicate with the patient to overcome barriers to therapeutic or diagnostic interaction between the physician or other qualified health care professional and a patient who has not developed, or has lost, either the expressive language communication skills to explain his/her symptoms and response to treatment, or the receptive communication skills to understand the physician or other qualified health care professional if he/she were to use typical language for communication.

Interactive complexity must be reported in conjunction with an appropriate psychiatric diagnostic evaluation or psychotherapy service, for the purpose of reporting increased complexity of the service due to specific communication factors which can result in barriers to diagnostic or therapeutic interaction with the patient.

When provided in conjunction with the psychotherapy services (90832-90838), the amount of time spent by a physician or other qualified health care professional providing interactive complexity services should be reflected in the timed service code for psychotherapy (90832, 90834, 90837) or the psychotherapy add-on code (90833, 90836, 90838) performed with an evaluation and management service and must relate to the psychotherapy service only. Interactive complexity is not a service associated with evaluation and management services when provided without psychotherapy.◄

★✚ **90785** Interactive complexity (List separately in addition to the code for primary procedure)

►(Use 90785 in conjunction with codes for diagnostic psychiatric evaluation [90791, 90792], psychotherapy [90832, 90833, 90834, 90836, 90837, 90838], and group psychotherapy [90853])◄

►(Use 90785 in conjunction with 90853 for the specified patient when group psychotherapy includes interactive complexity)◄

►(Do not report 90785 in conjunction with 90839, 90840, psychological and neuropsychological testing [96130, 96131, 96132, 96133, 96134, 96136, 96137, 96138, 96139, 96146], or E/M services when no psychotherapy service is also reported)◄

(Do not report 90785 in conjunction with 90839, 90840, 97151, 97152, 97153, 97154, 97155, 97156, 97157, 97158, 0362T, 0373T)

## Rationale

The guidelines in the Interactive Complexity subsection have been revised to indicate that these services should be reported in conjunction with an appropriate psychiatric diagnostic evaluation or psychotherapy service. In accordance with the revision of the guidelines, two parenthetical notes following code 90785 have been revised to reflect these changes. In addition, a new parenthetical note following code 90785 has been established to instruct users to use code 90785 in conjunction with code 90853 for specified patient when group psychotherapy includes interactive complexity.

# Dialysis

(For therapeutic apheresis for white blood cells, red blood cells, platelets and plasma pheresis, see 36511, 36512, 36513, 36514)

(For therapeutic apheresis extracorporeal adsorption procedures, use 36516)

►(For therapeutic ultrafiltration, use 0692T)◄

## Rationale

In support of the establishment of code 0692T for reporting therapeutic ultrafiltration, a cross-reference parenthetical note has been added following the Dialysis subheading in the Medicine section to direct users to report code 0692T for this procedure.

Refer to the codebook and the Rationale for code 0692T for a full discussion of these changes.

(90918, 90922 have been deleted. To report ESRD-related services for patients younger than 2 years of age, see 90951-90953, 90963, 90967)

(90919, 90923 have been deleted. To report ESRD-related services for patients between 2 and 11 years of age, see 90954-90956, 90964, 90968)

(90920, 90924 have been deleted. To report ESRD-related services for patients between 12 and 19 years of age, see 90957-90959, 90965, 90969)

(90921, 90925 have been deleted. To report ESRD-related services for patients 20 years of age and older, see 90960-90962, 90966, 90970)

## End-Stage Renal Disease Services

Codes 90951-90962 are reported **once** per month to distinguish age-specific services related to the patient's ESRD performed in an outpatient setting with three levels of service based on the number of face-to-face visits. ESRD-related services by a physician or other qualified health care professional include establishment of a dialyzing cycle, outpatient evaluation and management of the dialysis visits, telephone calls, and patient management during the dialysis provided during a full month. In the circumstances in which the patient has had a complete assessment visit during the month and services are provided over a period of less than a month, 90951-90962 may be used according to the number of visits performed.

Report inpatient E/M services as appropriate. Dialysis procedures rendered during the hospitalization (July 11-27) should be reported as appropriate (90935-90937, 90945-90947).

▶(Do not report 90951-90970 during the same month in conjunction with 99424, 99425, 99426, 99427, 99437, 99439, 99487, 99489, 99490, 99491)◀

**90951**  End-stage renal disease (ESRD) related services monthly, for patients younger than 2 years of age to include monitoring for the adequacy of nutrition, assessment of growth and development, and counseling of parents; with 4 or more face-to-face visits by a physician or other qualified health care professional per month

### Rationale

To accommodate the addition of the new principal care management codes and other changes made for clarification regarding reporting these services, a parenthetical note within the End-Stage Renal Disease Services subsection of the Medicine section has been revised.

Refer to the codebook and the Rationale for codes 99424-99427 for a full discussion of these changes.

# Gastroenterology

**91110**  Gastrointestinal tract imaging, intraluminal (eg, capsule endoscopy), esophagus through ileum, with interpretation and report

▶(Do not report 91110 in conjunction with 91111, 91113 0651T)◀

▶(Incidental visualization of the colon is not reported separately)◀

(Append modifier 52 if the ileum is not visualized)

**91111**  Gastrointestinal tract imaging, intraluminal (eg, capsule endoscopy), esophagus with interpretation and report

▶(Do not report 91111 in conjunction with 91110, 91113 0651T)◀

▶(Incidental visualization of the esophagus, stomach, duodenum, ileum, and/or colon is not reported separately)◀

(For measurement of gastrointestinal tract transit times or pressure using wireless capsule, use 91112)

#● **91113**  Gastrointestinal tract imaging, intraluminal (eg, capsule endoscopy), colon, with interpretation and report

▶(Do not report 91113 in conjunction with 91110, 91111)◀

▶(Incidental visualization of the esophagus, stomach, duodenum, and/or ileum is not reported separately)◀

**91112**  Gastrointestinal transit and pressure measurement, stomach through colon, wireless capsule, with interpretation and report

(Do not report 91112 in conjunction with 83986, 91020, 91022, 91117)

**91113**  Code is out of numerical sequence. See 91110-91117

### Rationale

Category III code 0355T has been converted to Category I code 91113. In support of this change, parenthetical notes have been added and revised in the Gastroenterology subsection.

Code 91113 has been established to report intraluminal colon imaging, also called colon capsule endoscopy. Colon capsule endoscopy is often performed in instances when a colonoscopy using a scope is performed but cannot be completed due to unforeseen circumstances. To perform capsule endoscopy, the capsule is administered to the patient and the recording device is activated. The images are recorded on a device worn by the patient. At the conclusion of the recording period, the images are downloaded for subsequent review by the physician.

★ = Telemedicine   ✚ = Add-on code   ✗ = FDA approval pending   # = Resequenced code   ⊘ = Modifier 51 exemp

In addition to the establishment of this new code, the exclusionary parenthetical note following code 91110 has been revised to restrict the reporting of code 91113 with code 91110. The instructional parenthetical note following code 91110 has also been revised to include the term "incidental."

The exclusionary parenthetical note following code 91111 has been revised to restrict the reporting of code 91113 with code 91111, and a new instructional parenthetical note has also been added.

Finally, in accordance with the deletion of Category III code 0355T, parenthetical notes have been added in the Category III section to refer users to the new Category I code.

## Clinical Example (91113)

A 60-year-old female is referred for a diagnostic optical colonoscopy. The patient completes an effective bowel-preparation regimen; however, due to angulation and fixation of colonic loops or difficult colonic anatomy, the colonoscopy is unable to be completed. The patient is referred for colon capsule endoscopy to complete visualization of the colon.

## Description of Procedure (91113)

The physician reviews the images with the localization software activated to input the esophagogastric junction, pylorus, and ileocecal valve locations. The physician scans the study and keys annotated anatomic landmarks (eg, esophagogastric junction, first gastric image, first duodenal image, ileocecal valve, first cecal image, hepatic flexure, splenic flexure, and last rectal image) to identify potentially positive findings and determine gastric, small bowel, and colonic transit times. Once the landmarks are determined, view all images with the two different capsule cameras (front and back). This is in effect reviewing two capsule studies: one from the forward-view camera and one from the trailing-view camera. When the physician identifies an abnormality, measure it and create a thumbnail. Note key findings or abnormalities. Carefully analyze and reconcile images or abnormalities that are noted on the two different viewing cameras to determine if they represent two distinct pathologies or the same pathology from two different vantage points. This is critically important to avoid false-positive findings. Determine localization by the passage of time or by capsule-localization software.

## Other Procedures

**91300**   Code is out of numerical sequence. See 90473-90477

**91301**   Code is out of numerical sequence. See 90473-90477

**91302**   Code is out of numerical sequence. See 90473-90477

**91303**   Code is out of numerical sequence. See 90473-90477

**91304**   Code is out of numerical sequence. See 90473-90477

# Ophthalmology

## Special Ophthalmological Services

▲ **92065**   Orthoptic training

### Rationale

In accordance with current medical practice, code 92065 has been revised to delete the phrases "and/or pleoptic" and "with continuing medical direction and evaluation." Based on this change, code 92065 should only be used to report orthoptic training.

Orthoptics is a broad term that defines visually based oculomotor tasks or vision training designed to improve the function of the eye muscles or binocular vision. Vision-training procedures are useful in the treatment of binocular vision disorders, including convergence insufficiency, some forms of strabismus such as esotropia and exotropia, and other eye-movement disorders.

Pleoptics refers to treatments designed to improve impaired vision, especially from amblyopia, by using a light source to dazzle parts of the retina to enable the adjacent areas to begin functioning. Because this technique is no longer used widely, the descriptor has been revised to reflect current medical practice.

# Special Otorhinolaryngologic Services

Diagnostic or treatment procedures that are reported as evaluation and management services (eg, otoscopy, anterior rhinoscopy, tuning fork test, removal of non-impacted cerumen) are not reported separately.

Special otorhinolaryngologic services are those diagnostic and treatment services not included in an evaluation and management service, including office or other outpatient services (99202-99215) or office or other outpatient consultations (99241-99245).

►Codes 92507, 92508, 92520, 92521, 92522, 92523, 92524, and 92526 are used to report evaluation and treatment of speech sound production, receptive language, and expressive language abilities, voice and resonance production, speech fluency, and swallowing. Evaluations may include examination of speech sound production, articulatory movements of oral musculature, oral-pharyngeal swallowing function, qualitative analysis of voice and resonance, and measures of frequency, type, and duration of stuttering. Evaluations may also include the patient's ability to understand the meaning and intent of written and verbal expressions, as well as the appropriate formulation and utterance of expressive thought.◄

## Rationale

The special otorhinolaryngologic services guidelines in the Medicine section have been revised with the removal of the reporting instructions regarding codes 92626 and 92627. The descriptors of codes 92626 and 92627 were revised in the CPT 2020 code set to create a more precise description of their intended use. Because the code descriptors were revised, reference to these codes in the special otorhinolaryngologic services guidelines is no longer applicable. While the guidelines have been updated to remove references to these codes, codes 92626 and 92627 should continue to be reported for evaluation of auditory function for surgically implanted device procedures.

Codes 92626 and 92627 were revised in the CPT 2020 code set to describe evaluation of auditory function for surgically implanted device candidacy or postoperative status of a surgically implanted device. Previously, these two codes described an evaluation of auditory rehabilitation status. The intent of the evaluation is to determine whether a patient is a suitable candidate for a surgically implanted device, such as a cochlear implant.

(For laryngoscopy with stroboscopy, use 31579)

**92502**   Otolaryngologic examination under general anesthesia

**92511**   Nasopharyngoscopy with endoscope (separate procedure)

▶(Do not report 92511 in conjunction with 31575, 42975, 43197, 43198)◄

(For nasopharyngoscopy, surgical, with dilation of eustachian tube, see 69705, 69706)

## Rationale

In support of the establishment of code 42975, the exclusionary parenthetical note following code 92511 has been revised to include code 42975 for reporting drug-induced sleep endoscopy flexible, diagnostic.

Refer to the codebook and the Rationale for code 42975 for a full discussion of these changes.

## Audiologic Function Tests

▶The audiometric tests listed below require the use of calibrated electronic equipment, recording of results, and a report with interpretation. Hearing tests (such as whispered voice, tuning fork) that are otorhinolaryngologic evaluation and management services are not reported separately. All services include testing of both ears. Use modifier 52 if a test is applied to one ear instead of two ears.◄

(For evaluation of speech, language, and/or hearing problems through observation and assessment of performance, see 92521, 92522, 92523, 92524)

**92557**   Comprehensive audiometry threshold evaluation and speech recognition (92553 and 92556 combined)

(For hearing aid evaluation and selection, see 92590-92595)

(For automated audiometry, see 0208T-0212T)

**92558**   Code is out of numerical sequence. See 92583-92588

▶(92559 has been deleted. To report, use 92700)◄

▶(92560, 92561 have been deleted. To report, use 92700)◄

**92562**   Loudness balance test, alternate binaural or monaural

**92563**   Tone decay test

▶(92564 has been deleted. To report, use 92700)◄

## Rationale

Codes 92559-92561 and 92564 were added to the CPT code set more than 30 years ago. Given their longevity and as clinical practice has changed over time, these codes have become outdated and obsolete. For example, the tests listed in codes 92560, 92561, and 92564 are no longer part of the battery of tests that audiologists use and have been replaced by auditory evoked potential (AEP) testing (92650-92653).

As a result, codes 92559-92561 and 92564 have been deleted from the CPT 2022 code set. In support of this change, the audiology guidelines have also been revised. Several deletion parenthetical notes have been added to instruct users to see code 92700, *Unlisted otorhinolaryngological service or procedure.*

**92567**   Tympanometry (impedance testing)

**# 92650**   Auditory evoked potentials; screening of auditory potential with broadband stimuli, automated analysis

**# 92651**   for hearing status determination, broadband stimuli, with interpretation and report

★ = Telemedicine   ✚ = Add-on code   ⵯ = FDA approval pending   # = Resequenced code   ⊘ = Modifier 51 exempt

►(Do not report 92651 in conjunction with 92652, 92653)◄

# **92652**     for threshold estimation at multiple frequencies, with interpretation and report

►(Do not report 92652 in conjunction with 92651, 92653)◄

# **92653**     neurodiagnostic, with interpretation and report

►(Do not report 92653 in conjunction with 92651, 92652)◄

## Rationale

Two exclusionary parenthetical notes have been added following codes 92651 and 92653, and the exclusionary parenthetical note following code 92652 has been revised to instruct users on the correct use of these codes.

Codes 92650-92653 were established in the CPT 2021 code set to report auditory evoked potentials. Since this addition, there have been questions from users regarding whether code 92653 should be reported in conjunction with codes 92651 and 92652 for the evaluation of waveform latency and neural integrity. The AEP response is evaluated using moderate- to high-level stimulus, which is part of the procedure described in codes 92651-92653. Therefore, reporting codes 92651 and 92652 in conjunction with code 92653 would be inappropriate.

# Cardiovascular

## Therapeutic Services and Procedures

### Coronary Therapeutic Services and Procedures

# **92941**     Percutaneous transluminal revascularization of acute total/subtotal occlusion during acute myocardial infarction, coronary artery or coronary artery bypass graft, any combination of intracoronary stent, atherectomy and angioplasty, including aspiration thrombectomy when performed, single vessel

(For additional vessels treated, see 92920-92938, 92943, 92944)

►(For transcatheter intra-arterial hyperoxemic reperfusion/supersaturated oxygen therapy [SSO₂], use 0659T)◄

## Rationale

In support of the addition of code 0659T to report intra-arterial hyperoxemic reperfusion, a parenthetical note has been added following code 92941 to instruct users to report code 0659T for transcatheter intra-arterial hyperoxemic reperfusion or supersaturated oxygen therapy.

Refer to the codebook and the Rationale for code 0659T for a full discussion of these changes.

## Implantable, Insertable, and Wearable Cardiac Device Evaluations

Cardiac device evaluation services are diagnostic medical procedures using in-person and remote technology to assess device therapy and cardiovascular physiologic data. Codes 93260, 93261, 93279-93298 describe this technology and technical/professional and service center practice. Codes 93260, 93261, 93279-93292 are reported per procedure. Codes 93293, 93294, 93295, 93296 are reported no more than **once** every 90 days. Do not report 93293, 93294, 93295, 93296, if the monitoring period is less than 30 days. Codes 93297, 93298 are reported no more than **once** up to every 30 days, per patient. Do not report 93297, 93298, if the monitoring period is less than 10 days. Do not report 93264 if the monitoring period is less than 30 days. Code 93264 is reported no more than once up to every 30 days, per patient.

►For body surface–activation mapping to optimize electrical synchrony of a biventricular pacing or biventricular pacing-defibrillator system at the time of follow-up device interrogation or programming evaluation, also report 0696T in conjunction with the appropriate code (ie, 93279, 93281, 93284, 93286, 93287, 93288, 93289)◄

A service center may report 93296 during a period in which a physician or other qualified health care professional performs an in-person interrogation device evaluation. The same individual may not report an in-person and remote interrogation of the same device during the same period. Report only remote services when an in-person interrogation device evaluation is performed during a period of remote interrogation device evaluation. A period is established by the initiation of the remote monitoring or the 91st day of a pacemaker or implantable defibrillator monitoring or the 31st day of monitoring a subcutaneous cardiac rhythm monitor or implantable cardiovascular physiologic monitor, and extends for the subsequent 90 or 30 days respectively, for which remote monitoring is occurring. Programming device evaluations and in-person interrogation device evaluations may not be reported on the same date by the same individual. Programming device evaluations and remote interrogation device evaluations may both be reported during the remote interrogation device evaluation period.

For monitoring by wearable devices, see 93224-93272.

ECG rhythm derived elements are distinct from physiologic data, even when the same device is capable of producing both. Implantable cardiovascular physiologic monitor services are always separately reported from implantable defibrillator services. When cardiac rhythm data are derived from an implantable defibrillator or pacemaker, do not report subcutaneous cardiac rhythm monitor services with pacemaker or implantable defibrillator services.

**93279**    Programming device evaluation (in person) with iterative adjustment of the implantable device to test the function of the device and select optimal permanent programmed values with analysis, review and report by a physician or other qualified health care professional; single lead pacemaker system or leadless pacemaker system in one cardiac chamber

(Do not report 93279 in conjunction with 93286, 93288)

**93280**    dual lead pacemaker system

(Do not report 93280 in conjunction with 93286, 93288)

**93281**    multiple lead pacemaker system

►(Use 93281 in conjunction with 0696T when body surface–activation mapping to optimize electrical synchrony is also performed)◄

(Do not report 93281 in conjunction with 93286, 93288)

**93282**    single lead transvenous implantable defibrillator system

(Do not report 93282 in conjunction with 93260, 93287, 93289, 93745)

**93283**    dual lead transvenous implantable defibrillator system

(Do not report 93283 in conjunction with 93287, 93289)

**93284**    multiple lead transvenous implantable defibrillator system

►(Use 93284 in conjunction with 0696T when body surface–activation mapping to optimize electrical synchrony is also performed)◄

(Do not report 93284 in conjunction with 93287, 93289)

**# 93260**    implantable subcutaneous lead defibrillator system

(Do not report 93260 in conjunction with 93261, 93282, 93287)

(Do not report 93260 in conjunction with pulse generator and lead insertion or repositioning codes 33240, 33241, 33262, 33270, 33271, 33272, 33273)

**93285**    subcutaneous cardiac rhythm monitor system

►(Do not report 93285 in conjunction with 33285, 93279-93284, 93291, 0650T)◄

►(For programming device evaluation [remote] of subcutaneous cardiac rhythm monitor system, use 0650T)◄

**93286**    Peri-procedural device evaluation (in person) and programming of device system parameters before or after a surgery, procedure, or test with analysis, review and report by a physician or other qualified health care professional; single, dual, or multiple lead pacemaker system, or leadless pacemaker system

(Report 93286 once before and once after surgery, procedure, or test, when device evaluation and programming is performed before and after surgery, procedure, or test)

(Do not report 93286 in conjunction with 93279-93281, 93288, 0408T, 0409T, 0410T, 0411T, 0414T, 0415T)

**93287**    single, dual, or multiple lead implantable defibrillator system

►(Use 93286, 93287 in conjunction with 0696T when body surface–activation mapping to optimize electrical synchrony is also performed)◄

(Report 93287 once before and once after surgery, procedure, or test, when device evaluation and programming is performed before and after surgery, procedure, or test)

(Do not report 93287 in conjunction with 93260, 93261, 93282, 93283, 93284, 93289, 0408T, 0409T, 0410T, 0411T, 0414T, 0415T)

**93288**    Interrogation device evaluation (in person) with analysis, review and report by a physician or other qualified health care professional, includes connection, recording and disconnection per patient encounter; single, dual, or multiple lead pacemaker system, or leadless pacemaker system

(Do not report 93288 in conjunction with 93279-93281, 93286, 93294, 93296)

**93289**    single, dual, or multiple lead transvenous implantable defibrillator system, including analysis of heart rhythm derived data elements

►(Use 93288, 93289 in conjunction with 0696T when body surface–activation mapping to optimize electrical synchrony is also performed)◄

(For monitoring physiologic cardiovascular data elements derived from an implantable defibrillator, use 93290)

(Do not report 93289 in conjunction with 93261, 93282, 93283, 93284, 93287, 93295, 93296)

**# 93261**        implantable subcutaneous lead defibrillator system

(Do not report 93261 in conjunction with 93260, 93287, 93289)

(Do not report 93261 in conjunction with pulse generator and lead insertion or repositioning codes 33240, 33241, 33262, 33270, 33271, 33272, 33273)

**93290**        implantable cardiovascular physiologic monitor system, including analysis of 1 or more recorded physiologic cardiovascular data elements from all internal and external sensors

(For heart rhythm derived data elements, use 93289)

(Do not report 93290 in conjunction with 93297)

**93291**        subcutaneous cardiac rhythm monitor system, including heart rhythm derived data analysis

▶(Do not report 93291 in conjunction with 33285, 93288-93290, 93298, 0650T)◀

## Rationale

In accordance with the establishment of code 0696T, the implantable, insertable, and wearable cardiac device evaluations guidelines have been revised to state that when body surface–activation mapping is performed to optimize electrical synchrony of a biventricular pacing or biventricular pacing-defibrillator system at the time of follow-up device interrogation or programming evaluation, code 0696T is reported with code 93279, 93281, 93284, or 93286-93289, as appropriate. Conditional inclusionary parenthetical notes have been added following codes 93281, 93284, 93287, and 93289, instructing users to report code 0696T when body surface–activation mapping to optimize electrical synchrony is also performed.

Also, in accordance with the addition of Category III code 0650T, exclusionary parenthetical notes following codes 93285 and 93291 have been revised to include 0650T.

Refer to the codebook and the Rationale for codes 0650T and 0696T for a full discussion of these changes.

## Echocardiography

**93315**        Transesophageal echocardiography for congenital cardiac anomalies; including probe placement, image acquisition, interpretation and report

(Do not report 93315 in conjunction with 93355)

**93316**        placement of transesophageal probe only

(Do not report 93316 in conjunction with 93355)

**93317**        image acquisition, interpretation and report only

(Do not report 93317 in conjunction with 93355)

**#+● 93319**        3D echocardiographic imaging and postprocessing during transesophageal echocardiography, or during transthoracic echocardiography for congenital cardiac anomalies, for the assessment of cardiac structure(s) (eg, cardiac chambers and valves, left atrial appendage, interatrial septum, interventricular septum) and function, when performed (List separately in addition to code for echocardiographic imaging)

▶(Use 93319 in conjunction with 93303, 93304, 93312, 93314, 93315, 93317)◀

▶(Do not report 93319 in conjunction with 76376, 76377, 93325, 93355)◀

## Rationale

A new add-on code (93319) has been established to report three-dimensional (3D) imaging for the assessment of cardiac structure, and inclusionary and exclusionary parenthetical notes have been added to provide instruction regarding the appropriate reporting of this procedure.

Code 93319 has been established to capture the additional physician work and practice expense associated with real-time 3D echocardiography.

To support appropriate reporting guidance, an inclusionary parenthetical note has been added following code 93319 that lists the base codes that may be reported with code 93319. An exclusionary parenthetical note has also been added to indicate the services that should not be reported in conjunction with code 93319. In addition, exclusionary parenthetical notes following codes 76376 and 76377 have been revised to include code 93319.

## Clinical Example (93319)

A 70-year-old male, who has a history of mitral valve prolapse and mitral regurgitation, presents with dyspnea on exertion. A complete transthoracic echocardiogram shows moderate to severe mitral regurgitation. A transesophageal echocardiogram (TEE) with three-dimensional (3D) imaging is requested to better assess the mechanism and severity of the mitral regurgitation.

## Description of Procedure (93319)

Prepare the two-dimensional (2D) images for 3D imaging by optimizing the image quality and gain for each of the views. The physician acquires real-time 3D images (narrow sector with display of pyramidal volume, focused wide sector [a zoomed image]) to give a focused, wide-sector view of the cardiac structures and obtain full-volume electrocardiographic-gated multiple-beat 3D images. For the zoomed image, use and adjust the biplane mode to ensure the structure of interest is centered on the orthogonal view. Review and acquire the images, including real-time 3D images with en-face views of the valvular structure. Review, rotate, and crop the focused wide-sector views as needed for the best en-face views of the cardiac structures. Rotate the images for proper orientation and en-face views concurrent with image acquisition from the physician. Reacquire 3D images with color flow Doppler with multi-beat acquisition to obtain 3D color flow Doppler sets to evaluate cardiac valvular function. Analyze the 3D images with specialized software. Crop or transect the full-volume data set acquired to remove tissue planes to better visualize the structures or to visualize cross-sectional views and orthogonal planes. Manipulate the color 3D data sets on the 3D software system to orient the data perpendicularly and parallel to the regurgitant or antegrade flow orifice to assess valvular function, such as the severity of mitral valve regurgitation. Acquire and save the images to the patient's study.

---

**93318**   Echocardiography, transesophageal (TEE) for monitoring purposes, including probe placement, real time 2-dimensional image acquisition and interpretation leading to ongoing (continuous) assessment of (dynamically changing) cardiac pumping function and to therapeutic measures on an immediate time basis

(Do not report 93318 in conjunction with 93355)

**93319**   Code is out of numerical sequence. See 93316-93321

## Cardiac Catheterization

►Cardiac catheterization is a diagnostic medical procedure which includes introduction, positioning and repositioning, when necessary, of catheter(s), within the vascular system, recording of intracardiac and/or intravascular pressure(s), and final evaluation and report of procedure. There are two code families for cardiac catheterization: one for congenital heart disease and one for all other conditions. For cardiac catherization for congenital heart defects (93593, 93594, 93595, 93596, 93597, 93598), see the **Medicine/Cardiovascular/ Cardiac Catheterization for Congenital Heart Defects** subsection. The following guidelines apply to cardiac catheterization performed for indications other than the evaluation of congenital heart defects.

***Right heart catherization for indications other than the evaluation of congenital heart defects (93453, 93456, 93457, 93460, 93461):*** includes catheter placement in one or more right-sided cardiac chamber(s) or structures (ie, the right atrium, right ventricle, pulmonary artery, pulmonary wedge), obtaining blood samples for measurement of blood gases, and cardiac output measurements (Fick or other method), when performed. For placement of a flow directed catheter (eg, Swan-Ganz) performed for hemodynamic monitoring

purposes not in conjunction with other catheterization services, use 93503. Do not report 93503 in conjunction with other diagnostic cardiac catheterization codes. Right heart catheterization does not include right ventricular or right atrial angiography (93566).

For right heart catheterization as part of catheterization to evaluate congenital heart defects, see 93593, 93594, 93596, 93597, 93598. For reporting purposes, when the morphologic left ventricle is in a subpulmonic position (eg, certain cases of transposition of the great arteries) due to congenital heart disease, catheter placement with hemodynamic assessment in this structure during right heart catheterization is considered part of that procedure, and does not constitute left heart catheterization. When the subpulmonic ventricle also connects to the aorta (eg, double outlet right ventricle), catheter placement with hemodynamic assessment of this ventricle during right heart catheterization is considered part of that procedure, while catheter placement with hemodynamic assessment of that same ventricle from the arterial approach is considered left heart catheterization. Report the appropriate code for right and left heart catheterization if catheter placement with hemodynamic assessment of the double outlet right ventricle is performed both during the right heart catheterization and separately from the arterial approach. Right heart catheterization for congenital heart defects does not typically involve thermodilution cardiac output assessments. When thermodilution cardiac output is performed in this setting it may be separately reported using 93598.

***Left heart catheterization for indications other than congenital heart defects (93452, 93453, 93458, 93459, 93460, 93461):*** involves catheter placement in a left-sided (systemic) cardiac chamber(s) (left ventricle or left atrium) and includes left ventricular/left atrial angiography, imaging supervision, and interpretation, when performed. For reporting purposes, when the morphologic right ventricle is in a systemic (subaortic) position due to congenital heart disease (eg, certain cases of transposition of the great arteries), catheter placement with hemodynamic assessment of the subaortic ventricle performed during left heart catheterization is considered part of the procedure and does not constitute right heart catheterization. If additional catheterization of right heart structures (eg, atrium, pulmonary artery) is performed at the same setting, report the appropriate code for right and left heart catheterization. When left heart catheterization is performed using either transapical puncture of the left ventricle or transseptal puncture of an intact septum, report 93462 in conjunction with 93452, 93453, 93458, 93459, 93460, 93461, 93596, 93597. For left heart catheterization services for the evaluation of congenital heart defects, see 93565, 93595, 93596, 93597.

*Catheter placement and injection procedures:* For a listing of the injection procedures included in specific cardiac catheterization procedures, please refer to the table on pages 771-773.

Cardiac catheterization (93451-93461), other than for the evaluation of congenital heart defects, includes: (a) all roadmapping angiography in order to place the catheters; (b) any injections for angiography of the left ventricle, left atrium, native coronary arteries or bypass grafts listed as inherent to the procedure in the cardiac catheterization table located on pages 771-773; and (c) imaging supervision, interpretation, and report. Do not report 93563, 93564, 93565 in conjunction with 93452, 93453, 93454, 93455, 93456, 93457, 93458, 93459, 93460, 93461. The cardiac catheterization codes do not include contrast injection(s) and imaging supervision, interpretation, and report for imaging that is separately identified by other specific procedure code(s).

Catheter placement(s) in coronary artery(ies) involves selective engagement of the origins of the native coronary artery(ies) for the purpose of coronary angiography. Catheter placement(s) in bypass graft(s) (venous, internal mammary, free arterial graft[s]) involves selective engagement of the origins of the graft(s) for the purpose of bypass angiography. Bypass graft angiography is typically performed only in conjunction with coronary angiography of native vessels.

Codes for catheter placement(s) in native coronary arteries (93454-93461), and bypass graft(s) (93455, 93457, 93459, 93461) include intraprocedural injection(s) for coronary/bypass graft angiography, imaging supervision, and interpretation, except when these catheter placements are performed during cardiac catheterization for the evaluation of congenital heart defects. Do not report 93563-93565 in conjunction with 93452-93461.

For right ventricular or right atrial angiography performed in conjunction with right heart catheterization for noncongenital heart disease (93451, 93453, 93456, 93457, 93460, 93461) or for the evaluation of congenital heart defects (93593, 93594, 93596, 93597), use 93566. For reporting purposes, angiography of the morphologic right ventricle or morphologic right atrium is reported with 93566, whether these structures are in the standard prepulmonic position or in a systemic (subaortic) position. Left heart catheterization performed for noncongenital heart disease (93452, 93453, 93458, 93459, 93460, 93461) includes left ventriculography, when performed. For reporting purposes, angiography of the morphologic left ventricle or morphologic left atrium is reported with 93565, whether these structures are in the standard systemic (subaortic) position or in a prepulmonic position. Do not report 93565 in conjunction with 93452, 93453, 93454, 93455, 93456, 93457, 93458, 93459, 93460, 93461. For cardiac catheterization performed for the evaluation of congenital

heart defects, left ventriculography is separately reported with 93565. For both congenital and noncongenital cardiac catheterization, supravalvular aortography is reported with 93567. For both congenital and noncongenital cardiac catheterization, pulmonary angiography is reported with 93568 plus the appropriate right heart catheterization code.

When contrast injection(s) are performed in conjunction with cardiac catheterization for congenital heart disease (93593, 93594, 93595, 93596, 93597), see 93563, 93564, 93565, 93566, 93567, 93568. Injection procedures 93563, 93564, 93565, 93566, 93567, 93568 represent separate identifiable services and may be reported in conjunction with one another when appropriate. Codes 93563, 93564, 93565, 93566, 93567, 93568 include imaging supervision, interpretation, and report.

For angiography of noncoronary arteries and veins, performed as a distinct service, use appropriate codes from the Radiology section and the Vascular Injection Procedures subsection in the Surgery/Cardiovascular System section.

*Adjunctive hemodynamic assessments:* When cardiac catheterization is combined with pharmacologic agent administration with the specific purpose of repeating hemodynamic measurements to evaluate hemodynamic response, use 93463 in conjunction with 93451-93453 and 93456-93461,93593, 93594, 93595, 93596, 93597. Do not report 93463 for intracoronary administration of pharmacologic agents during percutaneous coronary interventional procedures, during intracoronary assessment of coronary pressure, flow or resistance, or during intracoronary imaging procedures. Do not report 93463 in conjunction with 92920-92944, 92975, 92977.

When cardiac catheterization is combined with exercise (eg, walking or arm or leg ergometry protocol) with the specific purpose of repeating hemodynamic measurements to evaluate hemodynamic response, report 93464 in conjunction with 93451-93453, 93456-93461, 93593, 93594, 93595, 93596, 93597.◄

Contrast injection to image the access site(s) for the specific purpose of placing a closure device is inherent to the catheterization procedure and not separately reportable. Closure device placement at the vascular access site is inherent to the catheterization procedure and not separately reportable.

**93451**     Right heart catheterization including measurement(s) of oxygen saturation and cardiac output, when performed

(Do not report 93451 in conjunction with 33289, 93453, 93456, 93457, 93460, 93461, 0613T, 0632T)

▶(Do not report 93451 in conjunction with 33418, 0345T, 0483T, 0484T, 0544T, 0545T, 0643T, for diagnostic right heart catheterization procedures intrinsic to the valve repair, annulus reconstruction procedure, or left ventricular restoration device implantation)◀

**93452** Left heart catheterization including intraprocedural injection(s) for left ventriculography, imaging supervision and interpretation, when performed

(Do not report 93452 in conjunction with 93453, 93458-93461, 0408T, 0409T, 0410T, 0411T, 0414T, 0415T)

▶(Do not report 93452 in conjunction with 33418, 0345T, 0483T, 0484T, 0544T, 0545T, 0643T, for diagnostic left heart catheterization procedures intrinsic to the valve repair, annulus reconstruction procedure, or left ventricular restoration device implantation)◀

**93453** Combined right and left heart catheterization including intraprocedural injection(s) for left ventriculography, imaging supervision and interpretation, when performed

(Do not report 93453 in conjunction with 93451, 93452, 93456-93461, 0408T, 0409T, 0410T, 0411T, 0414T, 0415T)

▶(Do not report 93453 in conjunction with 33418, 0345T, 0483T, 0484T, 0544T, 0545T, 0643T, for diagnostic left and right heart catheterization procedures intrinsic to the valve repair, annulus reconstruction procedure, or left ventricular restoration device implantation)◀

**93454** Catheter placement in coronary artery(s) for coronary angiography, including intraprocedural injection(s) for coronary angiography, imaging supervision and interpretation;

▶(Do not report 93454 in conjunction with 33418, 0345T, 0483T, 0484T, 0544T, 0545T, 0643T, for coronary angiography intrinsic to the valve repair, annulus reconstruction procedure, or left ventricular restoration device implantation)◀

**93455** with catheter placement(s) in bypass graft(s) (internal mammary, free arterial, venous grafts) including intraprocedural injection(s) for bypass graft angiography

▶(Do not report 93455 in conjunction with 33418, 0345T, 0483T, 0484T, 0544T, 0545T, 0643T, for coronary angiography intrinsic to the valve repair, annulus reconstruction procedure, or left ventricular restoration device implantation)◀

**93456** with right heart catheterization

▶(Do not report 93456 in conjunction with 33418, 0345T, 0483T, 0484T, 0544T, 0545T, 0643T, for diagnostic coronary angiography or right heart catheterization procedures intrinsic to the valve repair, annulus reconstruction procedure, or left ventricular restoration device implantation)◀

**93457** with catheter placement(s) in bypass graft(s) (internal mammary, free arterial, venous grafts) including intraprocedural injection(s) for bypass graft angiography and right heart catheterization

▶(Do not report 93457 in conjunction with 33418, 0345T, 0483T, 0484T, 0544T, 0545T, 0643T, for diagnostic coronary angiography or right heart catheterization procedures intrinsic to the valve repair, annulus reconstruction procedure, or left ventricular restoration device implantation)◀

**93458** with left heart catheterization including intraprocedural injection(s) for left ventriculography, when performed

▶(Do not report 93458 in conjunction with 33418, 0345T, 0483T, 0484T, 0544T, 0545T, 0643T, for diagnostic coronary angiography or left heart catheterization procedures intrinsic to the valve repair, annulus reconstruction procedure, or left ventricular restoration device implantation)◀

(Do not report 93458 in conjunction with 0408T, 0409T, 0410T, 0411T, 0414T, 0415T)

**93459** with left heart catheterization including intraprocedural injection(s) for left ventriculography, when performed, catheter placement(s) in bypass graft(s) (internal mammary, free arterial, venous grafts) with bypass graft angiography

▶(Do not report 93459 in conjunction with 33418, 0345T, 0483T, 0484T, 0544T, 0545T, 0643T, for diagnostic coronary angiography or left heart catheterization procedures intrinsic to the valve repair, annulus reconstruction procedure, or left ventricular restoration device implantation)◀

(Do not report 93459 in conjunction with 0408T, 0409T, 0410T, 0411T, 0414T, 0415T)

**93460** with right and left heart catheterization including intraprocedural injection(s) for left ventriculography, when performed

▶(Do not report 93460 in conjunction with 33418, 0345T, 0483T, 0484T, 0544T, 0545T, 0643T, for diagnostic coronary angiography or left and right heart catheterization procedures intrinsic to the valve repair, annulus reconstruction procedure, or left ventricular restoration device implantation)◀

(Do not report 93460 in conjunction with 0408T, 0409T, 0410T, 0411T, 0414T, 0415T)

**93461** with right and left heart catheterization including intraprocedural injection(s) for left ventriculography, when performed, catheter placement(s) in bypass graft(s) (internal mammary, free arterial, venous grafts) with bypass graft angiography

▶(Do not report 93461 in conjunction with 33418, 0345T, 0483T, 0484T, 0544T, 0545T, 0643T, for diagnostic coronary angiography or left and right heart catheterization procedures intrinsic to the valve repair, annulus reconstruction procedure, or left ventricular restoration device implantation)◀

(Do not report 93461 in conjunction with 0408T, 0409T, 0410T, 0411T, 0414T, 0415T)

★ = Telemedicine    ✚ = Add-on code    ✗ = FDA approval pending    # = Resequenced code    ⊘ = Modifier 51 exempt

**+ 93462**    Left heart catheterization by transseptal puncture through intact septum or by transapical puncture (List separately in addition to code for primary procedure)

▶(Use 93462 in conjunction with 33477, 33741, 33745, 93452, 93453, 93458, 93459, 93460, 93461, 93582, 93595, 93596, 93597, 93653, 93654)◀

(Use 93462 in conjunction with 93590, 93591 for transapical puncture performed for left heart catheterization and percutaneous transcatheter closure of paravalvular leak)

▶(Use 93462 in conjunction with 93581 for transseptal or transapical puncture performed for percutaneous transcatheter closure of ventricular septal defect)◀

(Do not report 93462 in conjunction with 93590 for transeptal puncture through intact septum performed for left heart catheterization and percutaneous transcatheter closure of paravalvular leak)

(Do not report 93462 in conjunction with 93656)

▶(Do not report 93462 in conjunction with 33418, 0345T, 0544T, unless transapical puncture is performed)◀

**+ 93463**    Pharmacologic agent administration (eg, inhaled nitric oxide, intravenous infusion of nitroprusside, dobutamine, milrinone, or other agent) including assessing hemodynamic measurements before, during, after and repeat pharmacologic agent administration, when performed (List separately in addition to code for primary procedure)

▶(Use 93463 in conjunction with 33477, 93451-93453, 93456-93461, 93580, 93581, 93582, 93593, 93594, 93595, 93596, 93597)◀

(Report 93463 only once per catheterization procedure)

(Do not report 93463 for pharmacologic agent administration in conjunction with coronary interventional procedure 92920-92944, 92975, 92977)

**+ 93464**    Physiologic exercise study (eg, bicycle or arm ergometry) including assessing hemodynamic measurements before and after (List separately in addition to code for primary procedure)

▶(Use 93464 in conjunction with 33477, 93451-93453, 93456-93461, 93593, 93594, 93595, 93596, 93597)◀

(Report 93464 only once per catheterization procedure)

(For pharmacologic agent administration, use 93463)

**93503**    Insertion and placement of flow directed catheter (eg, Swan-Ganz) for monitoring purposes

(Do not report 93503 in conjunction with 0632T)

(For subsequent monitoring, see 99356-99357)

**93505**    Endomyocardial biopsy

▶(93530 has been deleted. To report, see 93593, 93594)◀

▶(93531, 93532, 93533 have been deleted. To report, see 93462, 93596, 93597)◀

## Rationale

In accordance with the establishment of the Cardiac Catheterization for Congenital Heart Defects subsection with new guidelines and new codes 93593-93598, the Cardiac Catheterization subsection has been substantially revised to reflect these changes. Codes 93530-93533 have been deleted, the cardiac catheterization guidelines have been revised, and several parenthetical notes have been revised or added.

Prior to 2022, codes 93530-93533 described heart catheterization procedures for congenital cardiac anomalies. Effective in 2022, codes 93530-93533 have been deleted and replaced with codes 93593-93597, which more accurately describe heart catheterization for congenital heart defects. A deletion parenthetical note has been added for code 93530, directing users to codes 93593 and 93594, and a deletion parenthetical note has been added for codes 93531-93533, directing users to codes 93462, 93596, and 93597.

The cardiac catheterization guidelines have been revised to clearly distinguish cardiac catheterization performed for indications other than congenital heart defects from cardiac catheterization that is performed for congenital heart defects. Specifically, the definitions for right heart catheterization and adjunctive hemodynamic assessments have been clarified and expanded, and definitions for left heart catheterization and catheterization and injection procedures have been added.

A new instructional parenthetical note has been added, instructing users to report code 93462 with code 93581 for transseptal or transapical puncture performed for percutaneous transcatheter closure of ventricular septal defect. Parenthetical notes following codes 93462-93464 have been revised to reflect the deletion of codes 93531-93533 and the establishment of codes 93593-93597.

Also, in accordance with the establishment of Category III code 0643T, the conditional exclusionary parenthetical notes following codes 93452-93461 have been revised with the addition of code 0643T.

Refer to the codebook and the Rationale for codes 93593-93598 and 0643T for a full discussion of these changes.

▶(93561, 93562 have been deleted. For cardiac output measurement[s], thermodilution, or other indicator dilution method performed during cardiac catheterization for the evaluation of congenital heart defects, use 93598)◀

(For radioisotope method of cardiac output, see 78472, 78473, or 78481)

**+ 93563** Injection procedure during cardiac catheterization including imaging supervision, interpretation, and report; for selective coronary angiography during congenital heart catheterization (List separately in addition to code for primary procedure)

▶(Use 93563 in conjunction with 33741, 33745, 93582, 93593, 93594, 93595, 93596, 93597)◀

**+ 93564** for selective opacification of aortocoronary venous or arterial bypass graft(s) (eg, aortocoronary saphenous vein, free radial artery, or free mammary artery graft) to one or more coronary arteries and in situ arterial conduits (eg, internal mammary), whether native or used for bypass to one or more coronary arteries during congenital heart catheterization, when performed (List separately in addition to code for primary procedure)

▶(Use 93564 in conjunction with 93582, 93593, 93594, 93595, 93596, 93597)◀

(Do not report 93563, 93564 in conjunction with 33418, 0345T, 0483T, 0484T, 0544T, 0545T for coronary angiography intrinsic to the valve repair or annulus reconstruction procedure)

**+ 93565** for selective left ventricular or left atrial angiography (List separately in addition to code for primary procedure)

▶(Use 93565 in conjunction with 33741, 33745, 93582, 93593, 93594, 93595, 93596, 93597)◀

(Do not report 93563-93565 in conjunction with 93452-93461)

**+ 93566** for selective right ventricular or right atrial angiography (List separately in addition to code for primary procedure)

. ▶(Use 93566 in conjunction with 33741, 33745, 93451, 93453, 93456, 93457, 93460, 93461, 93582, 93593, 93594, 93595, 93596, 93597)◀

(Do not report 93566 in conjunction with 33274 for right ventriculography performed during leadless pacemaker insertion)

(Do not report 93566 in conjunction with 0545T for right ventricular or right atrial angiography procedures intrinsic to the annulus reconstruction procedure)

**+ 93567** for supravalvular aortography (List separately in addition to code for primary procedure)

▶(Use 93567 in conjunction with 33741, 33745, 93451-93461, 93593, 93594, 93595, 93596, 93597)◀

(For non-supravalvular thoracic aortography or abdominal aortography performed at the time of cardiac catheterization, use the appropriate radiological supervision and interpretation codes [36221, 75600-75630])

**+ 93568** for pulmonary angiography (List separately in addition to code for primary procedure)

▶(Use 93568 in conjunction with 33741, 33745, 93451, 93453, 93456, 93457, 93460, 93461, 93580, 93581, 93582, 93583, 93593, 93594, 93595, 93596, 93597)◀

(Do not report 93568 in conjunction with 0632T)

**+ 93571** Intravascular Doppler velocity and/or pressure derived coronary flow reserve measurement (coronary vessel or graft) during coronary angiography including pharmacologically induced stress; initial vessel (List separately in addition to code for primary procedure)

▶(Use 93571 in conjunction with 92920, 92924, 92928, 92933, 92937, 92941, 92943, 92975, 93454-93461, 93563, 93564, 93593, 93594, 93595, 93596, 93597)◀

(Do not report 93571 in conjunction with 0523T)

**+ 93572** each additional vessel (List separately in addition to code for primary procedure)

## Rationale

In accordance with the new catheter placement and injection procedures definition added to the cardiac catheterization guidelines, the Injection Procedures subsection and guidelines have been deleted. Codes 93563-93568, 93571, and 93572 are now listed in the Cardiac Catheterization subsection.

In accordance with the establishment of code 93598, codes 93561 and 93562 have been deleted and a cross-reference parenthetical note has been added to reflect these changes.

Refer to the codebook and the Rationale for the new catheter placement and injection procedures definition and code 93598 for a full discussion of these changes.

## Repair of Structural Heart Defect

**93580** Percutaneous transcatheter closure of congenital interatrial communication (ie, Fontan fenestration, atrial septal defect) with implant

▶(Percutaneous transcatheter closure of atrial septal defect includes a right heart catheterization procedure. Code 93580 includes injection of contrast for atrial and ventricular angiograms. Codes 93451-93453,93456, 93457, 93458, 93459, 93460, 93461, 93565, 93566, 93593, 93594, 93595, 93596, 93597, 93598 should not be reported separately in addition to 93580)◀

▶(For other cardiac angiographic procedures performed at the time of transcatheter atrial septal defect closure, see 93563, 93564, 93567, 93568, as appropriate)◀

**93581** Percutaneous transcatheter closure of a congenital ventricular septal defect with implant

▶(Percutaneous transcatheter closure of ventricular septal defect includes a right heart catheterization procedure. Code 93581 includes injection of contrast for atrial and ventricular angiograms. Codes 93451-93453, 93456, 93457, 93458, 93459, 93460, 93461, 93565, 93566, 93593, 93594, 93595, 93596, 93597, 93598 should not be reported separately in addition to 93581)◀

▶(For other cardiac angiographic procedures performed at the time of transcatheter closure of ventricular septal defect, see 93563, 93564, 93567, 93568, as appropriate)◀

(For echocardiographic services performed in addition to 93580, 93581, see 93303-93317, 93662 as appropriate)

**93582** Percutaneous transcatheter closure of patent ductus arteriosus

(93582 includes congenital right and left heart catheterization, catheter placement in the aorta, and aortic arch angiography, when performed)

▶(Do not report 93582 in conjunction with 36013, 36014, 36200, 75600, 75605, 93451,93453, 93456, 93457, 93458, 93459, 93460, 93461, 93567, 93593, 93594, 93595, 93596, 93597, 93598)◀

(For other cardiac angiographic procedures performed at the time of transcatheter PDA closure, see 93563, 93564, 93565, 93566, 93568 as appropriate)

(For repair of patent ductus arteriosus by ligation, see 33820, 33822, 33824)

(For intracardiac echocardiographic services performed at the time of transcatheter PDA closure, use 93662. Other echocardiographic services provided by a separate individual are reported using the appropriate echocardiography service codes, 93315, 93316, 93317)

**93583** Percutaneous transcatheter septal reduction therapy (eg, alcohol septal ablation) including temporary pacemaker insertion when performed

(93583 includes insertion of temporary pacemaker, when performed, and left heart catheterization)

▶(Do not report 93583 in conjunction with 33210, 93452, 93453, 93458, 93459, 93460, 93461, 93565, 93595, 93596, 93597)◀

(93583 includes left anterior descending coronary angiography for the purpose of roadmapping to guide the intervention. Do not report 93454, 93455, 93456, 93457, 93458, 93459, 93460, 93461, 93563 for coronary angiography performed during alcohol septal ablation for the purpose of roadmapping, guidance of the intervention, vessel measurement, and completion angiography)

▶(Diagnostic cardiac catheterization procedures may be separately reportable when no prior catheter-based diagnostic study of the treatment zone is available, the prior diagnostic study is inadequate, or the patient's condition with respect to the clinical indication has changed since the prior study or during the intervention. Use the appropriate codes from 93451, 93454, 93455, 93456, 93457, 93563, 93564, 93566, 93567, 93568, 93593, 93594, 93598)◀

## Rationale

In accordance with the deletion of codes 93531-93533 and the establishment of codes 93593-93598, the instructional parenthetical notes following codes 93580-93583 have been revised to reflect these changes. Cross-reference parenthetical notes have been added following codes 93580 and 93581, directing users to codes 93563, 93564, 93567, and 93568 for other cardiac angiographic procedures performed at the time of transcatheter atrial septal defect closure.

Refer to the codebook and the Rationale for codes 93593-93598 for a full discussion of these changes.

### Transcatheter Closure of Paravalvular Leak

Codes 93590, 93591, 93592 are used to report transcatheter closure of paravalvular leak (PVL). Codes 93590 and 93591 include, when performed, percutaneous access, placing the access sheath(s), advancing the delivery system to the paravalvular leak, positioning the closure device, repositioning the closure device as needed, and deploying the device.

Codes 93590 and 93591 include, when performed, fluoroscopy (76000), angiography, radiological supervision and interpretation services performed to guide the PVL closure (eg, guiding the device placement and documenting completion of the intervention).

▶Code 93590 includes transseptal puncture and left heart catheterization/left ventriculography (93452, 93453, 93458, 93459, 93460, 93461, 93565, 93595, 93596, 93597), when performed. Transapical left heart catheterization (93462) may be reported separately, when performed.

Code 93591 includes, when performed, supravalvular aortography (93567), left heart catheterization/left ventriculography (93452, 93453, 93458, 93459, 93460, 93461, 93565, 93595, 93596, 93597). Transapical left heart catheterization (93462) may be reported separately, when performed.

Diagnostic right heart catheterization codes (93451, 93456, 93457, 93593, 93594, 93598) and diagnostic coronary angiography codes (93454, 93455, 93456, 93457, 93563, 93564) may be reported with 93590, 93591, representing separate and distinct services from PVL closure, if:

1. No prior study is available and a full diagnostic study is performed, or

2. A prior study is available, but as documented in the medical record:

   a. There is inadequate visualization of the anatomy and/or pathology, or

   b. The patient's condition with respect to the clinical indication has changed since the prior study, or

   c. There is a clinical change during the procedure that requires new evaluation.◄

## Rationale

In accordance with the deletion of codes 93530-93533 and the establishment of codes 93593-93598, the transcatheter closure of paravalvular leak guidelines have been revised to reflect these changes.

Refer to the codebook and the Rationale for codes 93593-93598 for a full discussion of these changes.

## ►Cardiac Catheterization for Congenital Heart Defects◄

►Cardiac catheterization for the evaluation of congenital heart defect(s) is reported with 93593, 93594, 93595, 93596, 93597, 93598. Cardiac catheterization services for anomalous coronary arteries arising from the aorta or off of other coronary arteries, patent foramen ovale, mitral valve prolapse, and bicuspid aortic valve, in the absence of other congenital heart defects, are reported with 93451-93464, 93566, 93567, 93568. However, when these conditions exist in conjunction with other congenital heart defects, 93593, 93594, 93595, 93596, 93597 may be reported. Evaluation of anomalous coronary arteries arising from the pulmonary arterial system is reported with the cardiac catheterization for congenital heart defects codes.

***Right heart catheterization for congenital heart defects (93593, 93594, 93596, 93597):*** includes catheter placement in one or more right-sided cardiac chamber(s) or structures (ie, the right atrium, right ventricle, pulmonary artery, pulmonary wedge), obtaining blood samples for measurement of blood gases, and Fick cardiac output measurements, when performed. While the morphologic right atrium and morphologic right ventricle are typically the right heart structures supplying blood flow to the pulmonary artery, in congenital heart disease the subpulmonic ventricle may be a morphologic left ventricle and the subpulmonic atrium may be a morphologic left atrium. For reporting purposes, when the morphologic left ventricle or left atrium is in a subpulmonic position due to congenital heart disease, catheter placement in either of these structures is considered part of right heart catheterization and does not constitute left heart catheterization. Right heart catheterization for congenital cardiac anomalies does not typically involve thermodilution cardiac output assessments. When thermodilution cardiac output is performed in this setting, it may be separately reported using add-on code 93598. Right heart catheterization does not include right ventricular or right atrial angiography. When right ventricular or right atrial angiography is performed, use 93566. For reporting purposes, angiography of the morphologic right ventricle or morphologic right atrium is reported with 93566, whether these structures are in the standard pre-pulmonic position or in a systemic (subaortic) position. For placement of a flow directed catheter (eg, Swan-Ganz) performed for hemodynamic monitoring purposes not in conjunction with other catheterization services, use 93503. Do not report 93503 in conjunction with 93453, 93456, 93457, 93460, 93461, 93593, 93594, 93595, 93596, 93597.

Right heart catheterization for congenital heart defects may be performed in patients with normal or abnormal connections. The terms *normal* and *abnormal* native connections are used to define the variations in the anatomic connections from the great veins to the atria, atria to the ventricles, and ventricles to the great arteries. This designation as normal or abnormal is used to determine the appropriate code to report right heart catheterization services in congenital heart disease.

Normal native connections exist when the pathway of blood flow follows the expected course through the right and left heart chambers and great vessels (ie, superior vena cava/inferior vena cava to right atrium, then right ventricle, then pulmonary arteries for the right heart; left atrium to left ventricle, then aorta for the left heart). Examples of congenital heart defects with normal connections would include acyanotic defects such as isolated atrial septal defect, ventricular septal defect, or patent ductus arteriosus. Services including right heart catheterization for congenital cardiac anomalies with normal connections are reported with 93593, 93596.

Abnormal native connections exist when there are alternative connections for the pathway of blood flow through the heart and great vessels. Abnormal connections are typically present in patients with cyanotic congenital heart defects, any variation of single ventricle anatomy (eg, hypoplastic right or left heart, double outlet right ventricle), unbalanced atrioventricular canal (endocardial cushion) defect, transposition of the great

★ = Telemedicine    ✚ = Add-on code    ✚ = FDA approval pending    # = Resequenced code    ⊘ = Modifier 51 exempt

arteries, valvular atresia, tetralogy of Fallot with or without major aortopulmonary collateral arteries (MAPCAs), total anomalous pulmonary veins, truncus arteriosus, and any lesions with heterotaxia and/or dextrocardia. Examples of right heart catheterization through abnormal connections include accessing the pulmonary arteries via surgical shunts, accessing the pulmonary circulation from the aorta via MAPCAs, or accessing isolated pulmonary arteries through a patent ductus arteriosus. Other examples would include right heart catheterization through cavopulmonary anastomoses, Fontan conduits, atrial switch conduits (Mustard/Senning), or any variations of single ventricle anatomy/physiology. Services including right heart catheterization for congenital heart defects with abnormal connections are reported with 93594, 93597.

***Left heart catheterization for congenital heart defects (93595, 93596, 93597):*** involves catheter placement in a left-sided (systemic) cardiac chamber(s) (ventricle or atrium). The systemic chambers channel oxygenated blood to the aorta. In normal physiology, the systemic chambers include the morphologic left atrium and left ventricle. In congenital heart disease, the systemic chambers may include a morphologic right atrium or morphologic right ventricle which is connected to the aorta due to transposition or other congenital anomaly. These may be termed *subaortic* chambers. For the purposes of reporting, the term left ventricle or left atrium is meant to describe the systemic (subaortic) ventricle or atrium. When left heart catheterization is performed using either transapical puncture of the left ventricle or transseptal puncture of an intact septum, report 93462 in conjunction with 93595, 93596, 93597. Left heart catheterization for congenital heart defects does not include left ventricular/left atrial angiography when performed. Left ventriculography or left atrial angiography performed during cardiac catheterization for congenital heart defects is separately reported with 93565. For reporting purposes, angiography of the morphologic left ventricle or morphologic left atrium is reported with 93565, whether these structures are in the standard systemic (subaortic) position or in a pre-pulmonic position. For left heart catheterization only, in patients with congenital heart defects, with either normal or abnormal connections, use 93595. When combined left and right heart catheterization is performed to evaluate congenital heart defects, use 93596 for normal native connections, or 93597 for abnormal native connections.

***Catheter placement and injection procedures:*** The work of imaging guidance, including fluoroscopy and ultrasound guidance for vascular access and to guide catheter placement for hemodynamic evaluation, is included in the cardiac catheterization for congenital heart defects codes, when performed by the same operator.

For cardiac catheterization for congenital heart defects, injection procedures are separately reportable due to the marked variability in the cardiovascular anatomy encountered.

When contrast injection(s) are performed in conjunction with cardiac catheterization for congenital heart defects, see injection procedure codes 93563, 93564, 93565, 93566, 93567, 93568, or use appropriate codes from the Radiology section and the Vascular Injection Procedures subsection in the Surgery/Cardiovascular System section. Codes 93563, 93564, 93565, 93566, 93567, 93568 include imaging supervision, interpretation, and report.

Injection procedures 93563, 93564, 93565, 93566, 93567, 93568 represent separate, identifiable services and may be reported in conjunction with one another when appropriate. For angiography of noncoronary arteries and veins, performed as a distinct service, use appropriate codes from the Radiology section and the Vascular Injection Procedures subsection in the Surgery/Cardiovascular System section.

Angiography of the native coronary arteries or bypass grafts during cardiac catheterization for congenital heart defects is reported with 93563, 93564. Catheter placement(s) in coronary artery(ies) or bypass grafts involves selective engagement of the origins of the native coronary artery(ies) or bypass grafts for the purpose of coronary angiography.◄

● **93593** Right heart catheterization for congenital heart defect(s) including imaging guidance by the proceduralist to advance the catheter to the target zone; normal native connections

● **93594**     abnormal native connections

● **93595** Left heart catheterization for congenital heart defect(s) including imaging guidance by the proceduralist to advance the catheter to the target zone, normal or abnormal native connections

● **93596** Right and left heart catheterization for congenital heart defect(s) including imaging guidance by the proceduralist to advance the catheter to the target zone(s); normal native connections

● **93597**     abnormal native connections

+● **93598** Cardiac output measurement(s), thermodilution or other indicator dilution method, performed during cardiac catheterization for the evaluation of congenital heart defects (List separately in addition to code for primary procedure)

    ►(Use 93598 in conjunction with 93593, 93594, 93595, 93596, 93597)◄

    ►(Do not report 93598 in conjunction with 93451-93461)◄

    ►(For pharmacologic agent administration during cardiac catheterization for congenital heart defect[s], use 93463)◄

►(For physiological exercise study with cardiac catheterization for congenital heart defect[s], use 93464)◄

►(For indicator dilution studies such as thermodilution for cardiac output measurement during cardiac catheterization for congenital heart defect[s], use 93598)◄

►(For contrast injections during cardiac catheterization for congenital heart defect[s], see 93563, 93564, 93565, 93566, 93567, 93568)◄

►(For angiography or venography not described in the 90000 series code section, see appropriate codes from the Radiology section and the Vascular Injection Procedures subsection in the Surgery/Cardiovascular System section)◄

►(For transseptal or transapical access of the left atrium during cardiac catheterization for congenital heart defect[s], use 93462 in conjunction with 93595, 93596, 93597, as appropriate)◄

## Rationale

A new subsection with guidelines and six new codes (93593-93598) has been added for cardiac catheterization for congenital heart defects. Prior to 2022, codes 93530-93533 described heart catheterization procedures for congenital cardiac anomalies. In accordance with advances in the treatment of congenital heart defects, codes 93530-93531 have been deleted and replaced with a more granular code structure to accurately describe current practice.

Codes 93593-93597 are organized based on treatment of normal native connections vs abnormal native connections. When blood flows along the expected course through the right and left heart chambers and the great vessels, normal native connections exist. In some patients with atypical cardiac anatomy (eg, hypoplastic right or left heart, tetralogy of Fallot), abnormal native connections exist. Refer to the new guidelines for a full discussion of normal and abnormal native connections.

Codes 93593 and 93594 describe right heart catheterization, code 93595 describes left heart catheterization, and codes 93596 and 93597 describe right and left heart catheterization. Imaging guidance by the proceduralist to advance the catheter to the target zone(s) of treatment is included in the service described by codes 93593-93597 and not reported separately. Add-on code 93598 has been established to report cardiac output measurements performed via thermodilution or other indicator dilution method during cardiac catheterization for evaluation of congenital heart defects. An inclusionary parenthetical note has been added following code 93598, instructing users to report code 93598 with codes

93593-93597. An exclusionary parenthetical note has also been added, restricting the reporting of code 93598 with codes 93451-93461.

The guidelines in the new Cardiac Catheterization For Congenital Heart Defects subsection define right heart catheterization, left heart catheterization, and catheter placement and injection procedures for congenital heart defects. The guidelines and new parenthetical notes provide instruction on the appropriate reporting of services performed during cardiac catheterization for congenital heart defects (eg, pharmacologic agent administration, physiologic exercise study, contrast injections, transseptal or transapical access of the left atrium). It is important to review the guidelines and parenthetical instructions carefully when reporting codes 93593-93598.

## Clinical Example (93593)

A 7-kg 9-month-old male, who has a known pulmonary valve stenosis and failure to thrive, is brought to the cardiac catheterization laboratory for evaluation. This cardiac catheterization is requested to measure the right heart hemodynamics and severity of valvular stenosis to determine if intervention is indicated.

## Description of Procedure (93593)

Conduct the vast majority of all procedures under general anesthesia. Palpate and identify the access-site landmarks and administer local anesthesia. Obtain access percutaneously using the Seldinger technique into the internal jugular, subclavian, axillary, or femoral venous systems. When necessary, use ultrasound guidance for vascular access depending on the vessel to be accessed and the age of the patient. Once the vessel is punctured, pass a guidewire into the vessel. Introduce the vascular sheath into the vein, remove the guidewire and dilator, and flush the sheath with sterile heparinized saline. Pass a diagnostic catheter through this sheath under fluoroscopic guidance. Direct the catheter from the venous system into any of the typical right heart structures, including the inferior and superior vena cava, right atrium, right ventricle, right and left pulmonary arteries, and pulmonary capillary wedge position(s).

Conduct baseline measurements and blood sampling in each of these chambers as needed. Calculate cardiac output using the typical Fick method. In patients without intracardiac shunting, cardiac output may be measured by thermodilution (separately reported). As needed, position the patient for angiography in any of the right heart chambers or blood vessels, which includes exchanging the diagnostic catheter used for physiologic data for an angiographic catheter (each are separately reportable). Following measurement of baseline values, pharmacological intervention may be performed (separately reported) and the measurements repeated. Following catheterization, extract the catheter and sheath and achieve compression hemostasis in the catheterization laboratory before taking the patient to the recovery area.

## Clinical Example (93594)

An 8-kg 6-month-old female, who is pulmonary atresia status post prior surgical shunt placement, demonstrates progressive cyanosis, failure to thrive, and worsening cardiac function. She is brought to the cardiac catheterization laboratory for suspected branch pulmonary artery stenosis to determine if further intervention is warranted.

## Description of Procedure (93594)

Conduct the vast majority of all procedures under general anesthesia. Palpate and identify the access-site landmarks and administer local anesthesia. Obtain access percutaneously using the Seldinger technique into the internal jugular, subclavian, axillary, or femoral venous systems. Frequently, multiple attempts must be made because of very small vessels and/or venous thrombosis from previous studies or the presence of central venous access catheters. Additional ultrasound guidance may be necessary and used due to these problems (which is not additionally reportable). In rare cases, the need for hepatic venous access may be necessary due to the lack of any other possible venous access (which is separately reportable). Once the vessel is punctured, pass a guidewire into the vessel. Introduce the vascular sheath into the vein, remove the guidewire and dilator, and flush the sheath with sterile heparinized saline. Pass a diagnostic catheter through this sheath under fluoroscopic guidance. Direct the catheter from the venous system into any of the typical right heart structures, including the inferior and/or superior vena cavae, atria, pulmonary ventricle, right and/or left pulmonary arteries, and pulmonary capillary wedge position(s). Frequently, there are additional venous structures such as a left-sided vena cava, which may have to be catheterized and evaluated selectively. These must be accessed either from an interrupted inferior vena cava, directly from the left internal jugular vein, or through the heart via the coronary sinus.

Conduct baseline measurements and blood sampling in each of these chambers as needed. Calculate cardiac output using the typical Fick method. In patients without intracardiac shunting (eg, post complete repair), cardiac output may be measured by thermodilution (separately reported). As needed, position the patient for angiography in any of the right heart chambers or blood vessels, which includes exchanging the diagnostic catheter used for physiologic data for an angiographic catheter (each is separately reportable). Following measurement of baseline

values, pharmacological intervention (separately reported) may be performed and the measurements repeated. Following catheterization, extract the catheter and achieve compression hemostasis in the catheterization laboratory before taking the patient to the recovery area.

## Clinical Example (93595)

A 2-year-old male with previously repaired coarctation of the aorta undergoes a 2D echocardiogram and Doppler study and a computed tomography (CT) angiogram that demonstrates restenosis of the proximal descending thoracic aorta. This cardiac catheterization is performed to measure the left heart hemodynamics to determine if surgical versus transcatheter intervention is indicated.

## Description of Procedure (93595)

Conduct the vast majority of procedures under general anesthesia. Palpate and identify the access site landmarks and administer local anesthesia. Obtain access percutaneously using the Seldinger technique. When necessary, use ultrasound guidance for vascular access (which is not additionally reportable). Typically, the femoral artery is punctured. Pass a guidewire into the vessel. Introduce the vascular sheath into the artery, remove the guidewire and dilator, and flush the sheath with sterile heparinized saline. If needed, obtain additional arterial access in one of the radial or axillary arteries; occasionally, carotid arterial access is used. Frequently, multiple attempts must be made because of very small vessels and/or arterial thrombosis from previous procedures or postoperative arterial monitoring. Pass a diagnostic end-hole catheter with a guidewire through this sheath under fluoroscopic guidance and direct it from the arterial system into the descending aorta, across the stenosis, around the aortic arch to the ascending aorta, and further across the aortic valve into the left ventricle.

Conduct baseline measurements and blood sampling in each of these chambers as needed. Use the end-hole guide catheter to precisely assess the location of pressure gradients to rule out any additional areas of stenosis. Use the end-hole catheter to again cross the coarctation and secure wire position either in the left ventricle, aortic root, or subclavian artery. Exchange the diagnostic catheter over the wire for an angiographic catheter (separately reported). Perform angiography, typically in the aortic arch, but location can vary due to the presence of multiple or long segment lesions (each separately reported). Perform additional angiography of the coronary arteries, carotid and subclavian arteries, or descending abdominal aorta as necessary (separately reported). In other conditions, angiography of the pulmonary arteries may be performed from the left heart (eg, across a systemic-pulmonary surgical shunt), which is separately reported. Following measurement of

Medicine 90281-99607

baseline values, pharmacological intervention may be performed (separately reported) and repeat the hemodynamic measurements. Following the conduct of the catheterization proper, remove the catheter and achieve compression hemostasis in the catheterization laboratory before taking the patient to the recovery area.

## Clinical Example (93596)

An 18-month-old male, who was noted to have a heart murmur, demonstrated a large ventricular septal defect in a 2D echocardiogram and Doppler study. A cardiac catheterization is performed to measure the magnitude of the left-to-right shunt and to measure the pulmonary artery pressure and resistance to determine if reparative surgery is indicated.

## Description of Procedure (93596)

Conduct the vast majority of all procedures under general anesthesia. Palpate and identify the access site landmarks and administer local anesthesia. Obtain access percutaneously using the Seldinger technique into the internal jugular, subclavian, brachial, and femoral venous systems, as well as femoral arterial access. Ultrasound guidance may be necessary and used for vascular access. Once the vessel is punctured, pass a guidewire into the vessel. Introduce the vascular sheath into the vessel, remove the guidewire and dilator, and flush the sheath with sterile heparinized saline. Pass a diagnostic catheter through this sheath under fluoroscopic guidance. Direct the catheter into any of the right heart structures including the inferior and superior vena cavae, right atrium, right ventricle, right and left pulmonary arteries, and pulmonary capillary wedge positions. If an atrial septal communication is present, it may be crossed for purpose of sampling the left atrium, individual pulmonary veins, and left ventricle. If an atrial communication is not present and the left atrial or pulmonary venous sampling is required, perform a trans-septal perforation (additionally reported). For the retrograde left heart catheterization, pass a diagnostic catheter through the sheath under fluoroscopic guidance, direct it in retrograde fashion into any of the left heart structures or vessels including the systemic arterial (usually left) ventricle, and then pull it back into the ascending aorta and further to the descending aorta. Baseline pressures may be recorded and blood sampling may be conducted in each of these chambers and vessels to be used later for hemodynamic calculations. Once hemodynamic data is collected, remove the diagnostic catheter and insert and use an angiographic catheter for any necessary angiography of these chambers or vessels (each separately reported). Calculate cardiac output using the Fick equation. In patients without intracardiac shunting, cardiac output may be measured by thermodilution (separately reported). Following the completion of the

catheterization proper, remove all catheters and sheaths and achieve compression hemostasis in the catheterization laboratory before taking the patient to the recovery area.

## Clinical Example (93597)

A 3-year-old male, who has tricuspid atresia, secundum atrial septal defect, ventricular septal defect, pulmonary artery stenosis, and a hypoplastic right ventricle, and is status post stage II bidirectional Glenn procedure, is referred for a cardiac catheterization for hemodynamic evaluation to determine if a total right heart bypass (Fontan procedure) is the next appropriate step.

## Description of Procedure (93597)

Conduct the vast majority of all procedures under general anesthesia. Palpate and identify the access site landmarks and administer local anesthesia. Obtain access percutaneously using the Seldinger technique into the internal jugular, subclavian, axillary, or femoral venous systems, as well as arterial access in the femoral, radial, or axillary arteries, and occasionally, carotid arterial access. Frequently, multiple attempts must be made because of very small vessels and/or vascular thrombosis from previous studies or the presence of indwelling catheters. Use additional ultrasound guidance for vascular access when necessary due to these problems. In rare cases, the need for hepatic venous access may be necessary due to lack of any other possible venous access (separately reported). Once the vessel is punctured, pass a guidewire into the vessel. Introduce the vascular sheath into the vessel, remove the guidewire and dilator, and flush the sheath with sterile heparinized saline. Pass a diagnostic catheter through this sheath under fluoroscopic guidance. Perform catheter introductions through these sheaths and manipulate them into the necessary positions. For the right heart catheterization, pass a catheter through the sheath under fluoroscopic guidance and direct it into any necessary venous structures and chambers comprising the right heart, which will vary depending on the congenital heart defect. Frequently, there are additional vessels not encountered in patients with normal connections that must also selectively be catheterized, such as a left-sided vena cava. If an atrial septal communication is present, it may be crossed for purpose of sampling the left-sided atrium, individual pulmonary veins, and left-sided ventricle. If an atrial communication is not present and the left atrial or pulmonary venous sampling is required, perform a trans-septal perforation (additionally reportable).

For the left heart catheterization, pass a diagnostic catheter through the sheath under fluoroscopic guidance, direct it typically in retrograde fashion into the systemic (right or left) ventricle, then pull it back into the ascending aorta and further to the descending aorta.

Frequently, the pulmonary arteries must be accessed from the left heart catheterization due to the presence of an aortopulmonary surgical shunt. Alternatively, both the systemic arterial and pulmonary arterial catheterization must be performed from the same ventricle in patients with transposition of the great arteries and a surgical right ventricle to pulmonary artery (Sano) shunt. In these scenarios, catheter placement across the systemic to pulmonary shunts can be very poorly tolerated, as the pulmonary blood flow is obstructed by the catheter. Great care must be taken, as well as close communication between the cardiologist and anesthesiologist, to ensure stable hemodynamics are maintained.

Frequently, patients require catheterization from both venous (right heart) and arterial (left heart) to identify all possible sources of pulmonary blood supply. In these situations, perform selective catheterizations of numerous individual vessels for sampling and angiography (each being separately reported). Baseline pressures may be recorded and blood sampling may be conducted in each of these chambers and vessels to be used later for hemodynamic calculations. Positioning for angiography may occur in any of the heart chambers or blood vessels, which includes exchanging the diagnostic catheter used for physiologic data for an angiographic catheter (each are separately reportable). Calculate cardiac output, typically using the Fick equation. In patients without intracardiac shunting, cardiac output may be measured by thermodilution (separately reported). Following the completion of the procedure, remove all catheters and sheaths and achieve compression hemostasis in the catheterization laboratory before taking the patient to the recovery area.

## Clinical Example (93598)

A 3-year-old female, who has a history of prematurity, chronic lung disease, and a previously repaired ventricular septal defect, undergoes diagnostic right and left heart catheterization to evaluate her congenital heart disease. Proper calculation of cardiac index by the Fick method is compromised because an accurate oxygen consumption cannot be measured. Therefore, following completion of the diagnostic hemodynamic evaluation, thermodilution studies are performed to confirm cardiac index. Pulmonary vasoreactivity testing is then performed (separately reported).

## Description of Procedure (93598)

Following completion of a congenital right heart catheterization or combined right and left heart catheterization (separately reported), remove the diagnostic catheter previously used and introduce a Swan-Ganz catheter from the venous sheath. Advance the catheter through the right heart and place it into the pulmonary artery for the purpose of assessing cardiac

output by thermodilution. Connect the catheter to the hemodynamic recording system. The operator performs a series of saline injections through the proximal port. Record the results. Perform and evaluate multiple injections (typically between three and six). If there is consistency in the initial three or four, average the injections. If not, perform additional injections until the operator is satisfied that enough measurements have been obtained to represent the true cardiac output. If there are clinical changes in the patient's condition or changes in the level of anesthesia, administer pressers and a repeat thermodilution assessment may be performed (which is not additionally reportable). Following completion of the cardiac catheterization, evaluate the cardiac output data, convert the results to a cardiac index, and enter the data as part of the official catheterization report.

# Intracardiac Electrophysiological Procedures/Studies

**+ 93613** Intracardiac electrophysiologic 3-dimensional mapping (List separately in addition to code for primary procedure)

▶(Use 93613 in conjunction with 93620)◀

(Do not report 93613 in conjunction with 93609, 93654)

## Rationale

In support of the revision of codes 93653, 93654, and 93656 to report cardiac ablation services bundling, the parenthetical note following add-on code 93613 has been revised with the deletion of codes 93653 and 93656.

Refer to the codebook and the Rationale for codes 93653, 93654, and 93656 for a full discussion of these changes.

**93620** Comprehensive electrophysiologic evaluation including insertion and repositioning of multiple electrode catheters with induction or attempted induction of arrhythmia; with right atrial pacing and recording, right ventricular pacing and recording, His bundle recording

(Do not report 93620 in conjunction with 93600, 93602, 93603, 93610, 93612, 93618, 93619, 93653, 93654, 93655, 93656, 93657)

**+ 93621** with left atrial pacing and recording from coronary sinus or left atrium (List separately in addition to code for primary procedure)

▶(Use 93621 in conjunction with 93620)◀

(Do not report 93621 in conjunction with 93656)

## Rationale

In support of the revision of codes 93653, 93654, and 93656 to report cardiac ablation services bundling, the parenthetical note following add-on code 93621 has been revised with the deletion of codes 93653 and 93654.

Refer to the codebook and the Rationale for codes 93653, 93654, and 93656 for a full discussion of these changes.

▲ **93653**   Comprehensive electrophysiologic evaluation with insertion and repositioning of multiple electrode catheters, induction or attempted induction of an arrhythmia with right atrial pacing and recording and catheter ablation of arrhythmogenic focus, including intracardiac electrophysiologic 3-dimensional mapping, right ventricular pacing and recording, left atrial pacing and recording from coronary sinus or left atrium, and His bundle recording, when performed; with treatment of supraventricular tachycardia by ablation of fast or slow atrioventricular pathway, accessory atrioventricular connection, cavo-tricuspid isthmus or other single atrial focus or source of atrial re-entry

▶(Do not report 93653 in conjunction with 93600, 93602, 93603, 93610, 93612, 93613, 93618, 93619, 93620, 93621, 93654, 93656)◀

▲ **93654**   with treatment of ventricular tachycardia or focus of ventricular ectopy including left ventricular pacing and recording, when performed

▶(Do not report 93654 in conjunction with 93279-93284, 93286-93289, 93600-93603, 93609, 93610, 93612, 93613, 93618-93620, 93622, 93653, 93656)◀

+ **93655**   Intracardiac catheter ablation of a discrete mechanism of arrhythmia which is distinct from the primary ablated mechanism, including repeat diagnostic maneuvers, to treat a spontaneous or induced arrhythmia (List separately in addition to code for primary procedure)

(Use 93655 in conjunction with 93653, 93654, 93656)

▲ **93656**   Comprehensive electrophysiologic evaluation including transseptal catheterizations, insertion and repositioning of multiple electrode catheters with intracardiac catheter ablation of atrial fibrillation by pulmonary vein isolation, including intracardiac electrophysiologic 3-dimensional mapping, intracardiac echocardiography including imaging supervision and interpretation, induction or attempted induction of an arrhythmia including left or right atrial pacing/recording, right ventricular pacing/recording, and His bundle recording, when performed

▶(Do not report 93656 in conjunction with 93279, 93280, 93281, 93282, 93283, 93284, 93286, 93287, 93288, 93289, 93462, 93600, 93602, 93603, 93610, 93612, 93613, 93618, 93619, 93620, 93621, 93653, 93654, 93662)◀

## Rationale

Codes 93653, 93654, and 93656 have been revised to report cardiac ablation services bundling.

These codes were identified for revision by the AMA/Specialty Society Relative Value Scale (RVS) Update Committee (RUC) Relativity Assessment Workgroup (RAW) after a survey identified code 93656, which describes comprehensive electrophysiologic evaluation including transseptal catheterizations, insertion, and repositioning of multiple electrode catheters (atrial fibrillation ablation), for its rapid increase in growth. As a result, it was determined that some of the work described by code 93656 should be bundled into existing codes, as they were being billed together more than 75% of the time.

Following a review of the volume data, it was determined that code 93653, which describes comprehensive electrophysiologic evaluation with insertion and repositioning of multiple electrode catheters (supraventricular [SVT] ablation), would also need these services bundled within it. In support of the revision of codes 93653, 93654, and 93656 to report cardiac ablation services bundling, the parenthetical notes following these codes have been revised to reflect those changes.

In addition to the revision of codes 93653, 93654, and 93656, a table with the elements of cardiac ablation codes and the procedure and services included with ablations has been added to provide guidance on how to correctly report these revised codes.

### Clinical Example (93653)

A 64-year-old female has recurrent palpitations. An event monitor has documented supraventricular tachycardia (SVT). A comprehensive electrophysiologic evaluation with catheter ablation is ordered.

### Description of Procedure (93653)

Confirm that direct current cardioversion/defibrillation and electrophysiology (EP) testing/ablation equipment is present and in proper working order. Test fluoroscopic equipment that will be used to visualize catheter movement and location. Administer local analgesia with anesthesia that is appropriate for the patient, including moderate sedation. Obtain venous access. Arterial access to monitor blood pressure and to facilitate retrograde aortic access to the left ventricle may be obtained. Advance the multielectrode catheters from the access sheaths into the respective cardiac chambers where they will be used to pace and record. Perform pacing and sensing in the right atrium, left atrium, and right ventricle. Obtain a recording of the bundle of His and measure the refractory periods. Attempt arrhythmia induction via maneuvers such as burst pacing and

★ = Telemedicine   ✛ = Add-on code   ✗ = FDA approval pending   # = Resequenced code   ⊘ = Modifier 51 exempt

premature pacing using programmed electrical stimulation at multiple drive-cycle lengths from multiple atrial and ventricular sites. Once the SVT is induced, perform pacing maneuvers to elucidate the mechanism of the tachycardia. Perform a combination of diagnostic maneuvers and generate a high-definition anatomical map of the chamber(s) of interest. Perform voltage and electrical activation in the arrhythmia and/or in sinus rhythm to identify normal activation, the location of the scar, and the mechanism of the arrhythmia, and then perform catheter ablation. Maneuver the ablation catheter from the sites of vascular access to the appropriate cardiac location to facilitate delivery of ablative energy. Deliver multiple lesions to ensure eradication of the arrhythmia focus and provide consolidation lesions in the surrounding tissue. During the course of the EP procedure, an induced arrhythmia requires the use an advanced 3D computer mapping system to assist in identifying the arrhythmia circuit and localizing the origin (for focal arrhythmias) or the critical isthmus (for reentrant arrhythmias). Calibrate the 3D mapping system and obtain recordings during sinus rhythm (to identify normal activation and location of the scar) and during each distinct arrhythmia. The physician analyzes the computer-generated map to ensure the electrograms are annotated correctly and the display parameters are correct for the specific arrhythmia being mapped. Based on the data from the 3D mapping system, endocardial electrograms, the surface ECG, and the response of the SVT to pacing maneuvers, advance the ablation catheter to the point of earliest activation as localized by the mapping system to identify a mid-diastolic potential, Kent potential, and/or similar paced maps. When a reentrant circuit is identified, perform and evaluate entrainment mapping studies to confirm the catheter location is within the reentrant circuit, and then perform radiofrequency (or cryo) ablation. If initial mapping in one chamber does not lead to complete identification of the essential arrhythmia circuit (either based on analysis of the map or based on an incomplete ablation result), move the mapping catheter(s) into another cardiac chamber and generate an additional 3D map to aid in diagnosis; repeat the procedure until the arrhythmia mechanism is fully characterized and ablation is deemed completely successful. Prepare a final report that includes the mapping procedure and findings.

To record left atrial activity, the femoral venous access site is already prepared for a related procedure. Achieve central venous access and place a sheath in the femoral vein using standard percutaneous techniques, changing to subclavian or jugular access if that fails. Introduce the catheter into the sheath and advance into the right atrium where the ostium of the coronary sinus is engaged. Advance the catheter into the coronary sinus. Use the multielectrode catheter to record electrical activity from the left atrium and, at times, pace the left atrium to attempt arrhythmia induction. Reposition the catheter as necessary throughout the course of the cardiac EP procedure to optimize recordings and pacing thresholds. At the conclusion of the procedure, remove the catheter. Include a description of this additional work and catheter use and associated findings in the procedure report. Throughout the ablation, monitor the patient for hemodynamic compromise due to cardiac perforation or tachyarrhythmias, embolic phenomena, or damage to cardiac or vascular structures. Following the ablation portion of the procedure, perform repeat electrophysiologic testing to assess the outcome of ablation using decremental, burst, and premature pacing maneuvers. Repeat these procedures at the conclusion of a 30-minute waiting period following the final ablation lesion. If the tachycardia demonstrates recovery or incomplete suppression, perform repeat mapping and ablation as described above, and repeat these steps until the tachycardia is rendered durably suppressed. Remove the sheaths, achieve appropriate hemostasis, and perform a follow-up assessment of the patient for any complications.

## Clinical Example (93654)

A 73-year-old male, who has a history of New York Heart Association (NYHA) Class III heart failure due to ischemic dilated cardiomyopathy (ejection fraction [EF] 25%) and prior myocardial infarction (MI), presents with recurrent implantable cardioverter-defibrillator (ICD) therapies for drug-refractory ventricular tachycardia (VT).

## Description of Procedure (93654)

Confirm that direct current cardioversion/defibrillation and EP testing/ablation equipment is present and in proper working order. Test the fluoroscopic equipment that will be used to visualize catheter movement and location. Test and confirm that the 3D mapping equipment is functioning normally. Administer local analgesia. For patients with ICDs, reprogram and/or transiently deactivate their devices at the start of the case to minimize adverse consequences resulting from electromagnetic interference from radiofrequency current application. Obtain venous access. Obtain arterial access to monitor blood pressure (BP) and to facilitate retrograde aortic access to the left ventricle. Advance the multielectrode catheters from the access sheaths and into the respective cardiac chambers where they will be used to pace and record. Place an intracardiac echocardiography (ICE) probe via a femoral venous access approach. Perform ICE in conjunction with the 3D mapping system to create a 3D shell of the right or left ventricle that includes the aortic root, aortic valve leaflets, coronary sinus, and mitral valve annulus. Also record the papillary muscles in the 3D anatomical ultrasound map. Perform pacing and sensing in the right atrium and right ventricle. Obtain a recording of the bundle of His and measure the refractory periods. Attempt to induce VT via burst pacing, decremental pacing, and premature pacing using programmed electrical stimulation at multiple drive-cycle lengths from multiple ventricular sites.

To record left atrial activity, the femoral venous access site is already prepared for a related procedure. Achieve central venous access and place a sheath in the femoral vein using standard percutaneous techniques, changing to subclavian or jugular access if that fails. Introduce the catheter into the sheath and advance it into the right atrium where the ostium of the coronary sinus is engaged. Advance the catheter into the coronary sinus. Use the multielectrode catheter to record electrical activity from the left atrium and, at times, pace the left atrium to attempt arrhythmia induction. Reposition the catheter as necessary throughout the course of the cardiac EP procedure to optimize recordings and pacing thresholds. At the conclusion of the procedure, remove the catheter. Include a description of this additional work, catheter use, and associated findings in the procedure report. Once an arrhythmia is induced, perform pacing maneuvers to elucidate the mechanism of the VT. When an arrhythmia is induced during the course of the EP procedure, use the 3D computer-mapping system to assist in identifying the arrhythmia circuit and localizing the origin (for focal arrhythmias) or the critical isthmus (for reentrant arrhythmias). Calibrate the 3D mapping system and obtain recordings during sinus rhythm (to identify normal activation and location of the scar) and during each distinct arrhythmia. The physician analyzes the computer-generated map to ensure the electrograms are annotated correctly and the display parameters are correct for the specific arrhythmia being mapped. Based on the data from the 3D mapping system, endocardial electrograms, the surface ECG, and the response of the SVT to pacing maneuvers, advance the ablation catheter to the point of earliest activation as localized by the mapping system to identify a mid-diastolic potential, Kent potential, and/or similar paced maps. When a reentrant circuit is identified, perform and evaluate entrainment mapping studies to confirm the catheter location is within the reentrant circuit, and then perform radiofrequency (or cryo) ablation. If initial mapping in one chamber does not lead to complete identification of the essential arrhythmia circuit (either based on analysis of the map or based on incomplete ablation result), move the mapping catheter(s) into another cardiac chamber and generate an additional 3D map to aid in diagnosis; repeat the procedure until the arrhythmia mechanism is fully characterized and ablation is deemed completely successful. (Occasional mapping of the epicardial surface of the heart is necessary.) Prepare a final report that includes the mapping procedure and findings.

Next, map the electrical activation sequence with the 3D electroanatomical mapping system and superimpose the activation timing on the 3D echocardiogram previously obtained. Administer anticoagulation once the catheters have been placed on the left side of the heart. Once the VT circuit is localized, move a catheter to the appropriate location or region of abnormal myocardium to deliver ablative energy. Deliver multiple lesions to ensure eradication of the arrhythmia focus and to provide consolidation lesions in the surrounding tissue. Throughout the ablation, monitor the patient for hemodynamic compromise due to cardiac perforation or tachyarrhythmias, embolic phenomena, or damage to cardiac or vascular structures. Following the ablation portion of the procedure, perform repeat electrophysiologic testing to assess the outcome of ablation using decremental, burst, and premature pacing maneuvers. Repeat these procedures at the conclusion of a 30-minute waiting period following the final ablation lesion. If the tachycardia demonstrates recovery or incomplete suppression, perform repeat mapping and ablation as described above, and repeat these steps until the tachycardia is rendered durably suppressed. Once EP testing and ablation are completed, reverse anticoagulation. Remove the sheaths, achieve appropriate hemostasis, and perform a follow-up assessment of the patient for any complications. For patients with ICDs, reprogram their devices to an active configuration, reprogramming rates as necessary to treat any remaining arrhythmias.

## Clinical Example (93656)

A 62-year-old male, who has a history of hypertension and recurrent atrial fibrillation, remains symptomatic despite rate and rhythm control with antiarrhythmic drugs. A comprehensive EP evaluation with transseptal catheterization and catheter ablation by pulmonary vein isolation for atrial fibrillation is ordered.

## Description of Procedure (93656)

Confirm that direct current cardioversion/defibrillation and EP testing/ablation equipment is present and in proper working order. Test the fluoroscopic equipment that will be used to visualize catheter movement and location. Administer local analgesia. Obtain venous access. Arterial access to monitor BP and to facilitate retrograde aortic access to the left ventricle may be obtained. By means of the venous access sites, position the multielectrode catheters into specific cardiac chambers. Advance an ICE probe into the heart and perform imaging of the heart and pericardium to visualize the right atrium, tricuspid valve, right ventricle, left atrium, aortic valve, left ventricle, pulmonary veins (left upper, left lower, right upper, right lower), pericardium, superior vena cava, and coronary sinus. Use ICE as necessary to guide catheter manipulation, guide

▶Elements of Cardiac Ablation Codes◀

| Procedure/Services Included with Ablations | ▶SVT Ablation (93653) | | | VT Ablation (93654) | | | AF Ablation (93656) | | |
|---|---|---|---|---|---|---|---|---|---|
| | Inherent | Bundled | Not bundled; sometimes performed | Inherent | Bundled | Not bundled; sometimes performed | Inherent | Bundled | Not bundled; sometimes performed |
| Insert/reposition multiple catheters | X | | | X | | | X | | |
| Transseptal catheterization(s) (93462) | | | X | | | X | X | | |
| Induction or attempted induction of arrhythmia with right atrial pacing and recording | X | | | X | | | | | X |
| Intracardiac ablation of arrhythmia | X | | | X | | | X | | |
| SVT ablation | X | | | | | | | | |
| VT ablation | | | | X | | | | | |
| AF ablation | | | | | | | X | | |
| Intracardiac 3D mapping (93613) | | X | | | X | | | X | |
| Right ventricular pacing and recording | | X | | | X | | | X | |
| Left atrial pacing and recording from coronary sinus or left atrium (93621) | | X | | | X | | | X | |
| His bundle recording | | X | | | X | | | X | |
| Left ventricular pacing and recording | | | | | X | | | | |
| Intracardiac echocardiography (93662) | | | X | | | X | | X◀ | |

transseptal puncture, provide visualization of catheter contact during mapping and ablation, and observe for complications throughout the procedure. Place the ICE catheter into the left atrium or right ventricle for additional imaging planes. Perform one or two transseptal catheterizations to achieve access and facilitate placement of both a circular mapping catheter and an ablation catheter in the left atrium. Administer additional anticoagulation and monitor the level of anticoagulation throughout the procedure, administering additional anticoagulation as needed. Measure conduction intervals and refractory periods and attempt to induce arrhythmia. Obtain a recording of the bundle of His and perform ventricular pacing and

sensing. Pass a mapping catheter into the left atrium and assess and record pulmonary vein conduction. Perform selective venography of the pulmonary veins to define anatomy, as necessary. Generate a high-definition 3D anatomical map of the chamber(s) of interest. Perform voltage and relative electrical activation in the arrhythmia and/or sinus as necessary to identify normal activation, the location of the scar, and the mechanism of arrhythmia. In addition, import, segment, and/or register the MRI/CT scan to the 3D map as necessary. Perform high-output pacing to prevent and/or monitor for phrenic nerve damage during ablation. Perform catheter ablation to achieve pulmonary vein isolation. Create point lesions or balloon-administered lesions that

▲=Revised code   ●=New code   ▶ ◀=Contains new or revised text   ✕=Duplicate PLA test   ↕=Category I PLA      American Medical Association   **171**

Medicine 90281-99607

encircle the pulmonary vein region guided by anatomical mapping and electrical signals provided by a circular mapping catheter. Pulmonary vein isolation, as measured by the circular mapping catheter as well as loss of tissue voltage and tissue pacing capture, is the measured endpoint.

When an induced arrhythmia requires the use of advanced 3D computer-assisted mapping system to localize the arrhythmia origin during the course of an EP procedure, place the mapping system in the cardiac chamber of interest using standard percutaneous techniques. Calibrate the system and obtain recordings during sinus rhythm to identify normal activation and location of the scar during each distinct tachycardia. Display the computer-generated map, make modifications in the computer parameters and display, and identify the tachycardia origin. Move the ablation catheter to the point of early activation that was localized by the mapping system and identify a mid-diastolic potential, Kent potential, and/or similar paced maps. When a reentrant circuit is identified, perform and evaluate entrainment mapping studies to confirm the catheter location is within the reentrant circuit. Create additional mappings to confirm arrhythmia origin and to study additional arrhythmias at the conclusion of the procedure. Prepare a final report that includes the mapping procedure and findings.

Throughout the ablation, monitor the patient for hemodynamic compromise due to cardiac perforation or tachyarrhythmias, embolic phenomena, thrombus formation, or damage to cardiac or vascular structures. Pay particular attention to lesion delivery within the pulmonary vein or close to the esophagus. Following the ablation portion of the procedure, perform additional electrophysiologic testing to assess the outcome of ablation. Repeat these procedures at the conclusion of a 30-minute waiting period following the final ablation lesion. If the pulmonary veins demonstrate recovery of conduction, perform repeat mapping and ablation as described above, and repeat these steps until the pulmonary veins are rendered durably isolated. Once EP testing and ablation are completed, reverse anticoagulation. Remove the sheaths, achieve appropriate hemostasis, and perform a follow-up assessment of the patient for any complications.

**93660**     Evaluation of cardiovascular function with tilt table evaluation, with continuous ECG monitoring and intermittent blood pressure monitoring, with or without pharmacological intervention

▶(For testing of autonomic nervous system function, see 95921, 95924)◀

## Rationale

To support the deletion of code 95943, the cross-reference parenthetical note following code 93660 has been updated to reflect the deletion of this code from the CPT code set.

Refer to the codebook and the Rationale for code 95943 for a full discussion of these changes.

**+ 93662**     Intracardiac echocardiography during therapeutic/diagnostic intervention, including imaging supervision and interpretation (List separately in addition to code for primary procedure)

▶(Use 93662 in conjunction with 33274, 33275, 33340, 33361, 33362, 33363, 33364, 33365, 33366, 33418, 33477, 33741, 33745, 92986, 92987, 92990, 92997, 93451, 93452, 93453, 93454, 93455, 93456, 93457, 93458, 93459, 93460, 93461, 93505, 93580, 93581, 93582, 93583, 93590, 93591, 93593, 93594, 93595, 93596, 93597, 93620, 93653, 93654, 93656, 0345T, 0483T, 0484T, 0543T, 0544T, 0545T, as appropriate)◀

(Do not report 93662 in conjunction with 92961, 0569T, 0570T, 0613T)

## Rationale

The inclusionary parenthetical note following add-on code 93662 has been revised with the removal of codes 93462, 93621, and 93622 and the addition of several codes.

Code 93662 was established in the CPT 2001 code set. Since 2001, many cardiac catheterization procedures and electrophysiologic procedures during which intracardiac echocardiography would be performed have been added to the code set. These codes have been added to the inclusionary parenthetical note consistent with current clinical practice. In accordance with the establishment of codes 93593-93597, the parenthetical note has also been revised to reflect these changes.

Refer to the codebook and the Rationale for codes 93593-93597 for a full discussion of these changes.

# Pulmonary

## ►Pulmonary Diagnostic Testing, Rehabilitation, and Therapies◄

**94621**    Cardiopulmonary exercise testing, including measurements of minute ventilation, $CO_2$ production, $O_2$ uptake, and electrocardiographic recordings

(Do not report 94617, 94619, 94621 in conjunction with 93000, 93005, 93010, 93040, 93041, 93042 for ECG monitoring performed during the same session)

(Do not report 94617, 94619, 94621 in conjunction with 93015, 93016, 93017, 93018)

(Do not report 94621 in conjunction with 94680, 94681, 94690)

(Do not report 94617, 94618, 94619, 94621 in conjunction with 94760, 94761)

● **94625**    Physician or other qualified health care professional services for outpatient pulmonary rehabilitation; without continuous oximetry monitoring (per session)

● **94626**      with continuous oximetry monitoring (per session)

►(Do not report 94625, 94626 in conjunction with 94760, 94761)◄

**94640**    Pressurized or nonpressurized inhalation treatment for acute airway obstruction for therapeutic purposes and/or for diagnostic purposes such as sputum induction with an aerosol generator, nebulizer, metered dose inhaler or intermittent positive pressure breathing (IPPB) device

### Rationale

Codes 94625 and 94626 have been added to report outpatient pulmonary rehabilitation without (94625) and with (94626) continuous oximetry monitoring for exercise. An exclusionary parenthetical note has also been added to restrict reporting these services in conjunction with other pulse oximetry services. In addition, the subheading has been revised with the addition of the term "Rehabilitation" to "Pulmonary Diagnostic Testing, Rehabilitation, and Therapies" in order to accommodate the new service.

Codes 94625 and 94626 are used to report the physician or other QHP services associated with providing outpatient pulmonary rehabilitation. Because continuous oximetry monitoring is commonly (but not always) provided with this service, the code descriptor reflects the provision of these services with (94626) or without (94625) the oximetry monitoring, as well as the intent for reporting (ie, for each session). In addition, because language has been included regarding provision of oximetry monitoring, the

exclusionary parenthetical note also restricts reporting of either service in conjunction with noninvasive ear or pulse oximetry services.

### Clinical Example (94625)

A 67-year-old male, who has severe chronic obstructive pulmonary disease (COPD), is enrolled in a pulmonary rehabilitation program without oximetry monitoring 45 days after hospitalization for an exacerbation.

### Description of Procedure (94625)

Perform a review of systems and review and confirm key information from the patient's medical records with the patient. The physician reviews the patient's current vital signs including oxygen saturation (SpO2) at rest and during exercise and compares them with previous readings. The physician decides whether the patient is fit to participate in the pulmonary rehabilitation program, and whether the patient will require monitoring during the exercise and strengthening portion of the program. The physician is required to be immediately available during the exercise session, and the physician will perform face-to-face evaluation of the patient for any acute issues that arise, including oxygen desaturations beyond baseline, tachypnea or respiratory distress, tachycardia, hypertension or hypotension, or symptoms of acute illness, such as developing acute exacerbation of COPD.

### Clinical Example (94626)

A 67-year-old male, who has severe COPD, is enrolled in a pulmonary rehabilitation program with oximetry monitoring 45 days after hospitalization for an exacerbation.

### Description of Procedure (94626)

Perform a review of systems and confirm key information from the patient's medical records with the patient. The physician reviews the current vital signs including SpO2 at rest and during exercise and compares them with previous readings. The physician decides whether or not the patient is fit to participate in the pulmonary rehabilitation program, and whether the patient will require supplemental oxygen (and the amount of oxygen) and monitoring during the exercise and strengthening portion of the program. The physician is required to be immediately available during the exercise session, and the physician will perform face-to-face evaluation of the patient for any acute issues that arise, including oxygen desaturations beyond baseline or despite supplemental oxygen, tachypnea or respiratory distress, tachycardia, hypertension or hypotension, or symptoms of acute illness, such as developing acute exacerbation of COPD.

# Neurology and Neuromuscular Procedures

## Autonomic Function Tests

**95921**  Testing of autonomic nervous system function; cardiovagal innervation (parasympathetic function), including 2 or more of the following: heart rate response to deep breathing with recorded R-R interval, Valsalva ratio, and 30:15 ratio

**95924**  combined parasympathetic and sympathetic adrenergic function testing with at least 5 minutes of passive tilt

(Do not report 95924 in conjunction with 95921 or 95922)

▶(95943 has been deleted. To report testing other than autonomic nervous system function testing, use 95999)◀

### Rationale

Code 95943 and all related references have been deleted from the CPT 2022 code set.

Code 95943, *Simultaneous, independent, quantitative measures of both parasympathetic function and sympathetic function, based on time-frequency analysis of heart rate variability concurrent with time-frequency analysis of continuous respiratory activity, with mean heart rate and blood pressure measures, during rest, paced (deep) breathing, Valsalva maneuvers, and head-up postural change,* was established in the CPT 2013 code set to differentiate the service from code 93660, *Evaluation of cardiovascular function with tilt table evaluation, with continuous ECG monitoring and intermittent blood pressure monitoring, with or without pharmacological intervention.* However, subsequent utilization analyses reveal that the service described in code 95943 is not widely performed. Therefore, code 95943 and all related references to code 95943 have been deleted from the CPT 2022 code set. A deletion parenthetical note has been added to reflect this change.

When reporting testing other than autonomic nervous system function testing, a parenthetical note has been added to direct users to report code 95999, *Unlisted neurological or neuromuscular diagnostic procedure.*

In accordance with the deletion of code 95943, the cross-reference parenthetical note following code 93660 has been revised to delete the reference to code 95943.

## Neurostimulators, Analysis-Programming

Code 95980 describes intraoperative electronic analysis of an implanted gastric neurostimulator pulse generator system, with programming; code 95981 describes subsequent analysis of the device; code 95982 describes subsequent analysis and reprogramming. For electronic analysis and reprogramming of gastric neurostimulator, lesser curvature, see 95980-95982.

Codes 95971, 95972, 95976, 95977, 95983, 95984 are reported when programming a neurostimulator is performed by a physician or other qualified health care professional. Programming may be performed in the operating room, postoperative care unit, inpatient, and/or outpatient setting. Programming a neurostimulator in the operating room is not inherent in the service represented by the implantation code and may be reported by either the implanting surgeon or other qualified health care professional, when performed.

▶Test stimulations are typically performed during an implantation procedure (43647, 43648, 43881, 43882, 61850, 61860, 61863, 61864, 61867, 61868, 61880, 61885, 61886, 61888, 63650, 63655, 63661, 63662, 63663, 63664, 63685, 63688, 64553, 64555, 64561, 64566, 64568, 64569, 64570, 64575, 64580, 64581, 64582, 64583, 64584, 64585, 64590, 64595) to confirm correct target site placement of the electrode array(s) and/or to confirm the functional status of the system. Test stimulation is not considered electronic analysis or programming of the neurostimulator system (test stimulation is included in the service described by the implantation code) and should not be reported with 95970, 95971, 95972, 95980, 95981, 95982, 95983, 95984. Electronic analysis of a device (95970) is not reported separately at the time of implantation.◀

▶(For insertion of neurostimulator pulse generator, see 61885, 61886, 63685, 64568, 64582, 64590)◀

▶(For revision or removal of neurostimulator pulse generator or receiver, see 61888, 63688, 64569, 64570, 64583, 64584, 64595)◀

▶(For implantation of neurostimulator electrodes, see 43647, 43881, 61850-61868, 63650, 63655, 64553-64581. For revision or removal of neurostimulator electrodes, see 43648, 43882, 61880, 63661, 63662, 63663, 63664, 64569, 64570, 64583, 64584, 64585)◀

(For analysis and programming of implanted integrated neurostimulation system, posterior tibial nerve, see 0589T, 0590T)

**95970**  Electronic analysis of implanted neurostimulator pulse generator/transmitter (eg, contact group[s], interleaving, amplitude, pulse width, frequency [Hz], on/off cycling, burst, magnet mode, dose lockout, patient selectable parameters, responsive neurostimulation, detection algorithms, closed loop parameters, and passive parameters) by physician or other qualified health care professional; with brain, cranial nerve, spinal cord, peripheral nerve, or sacral nerve, neurostimulator pulse generator/transmitter, without programming

▶(Do not report 95970 in conjunction with 43647, 43648, 43881, 43882, 61850, 61860, 61863, 61864, 61867, 61868, 61880, 61885, 61886, 61888, 63650, 63655, 63661, 63662, 63663, 63664, 63685, 63688, 64553, 64555, 64561, 64566, 64568, 64569, 64570, 64575, 64580, 64581, 64582, 64583, 64584, 64585, 64590, 64595, during the same operative session)◀

## Rationale

In accordance with the deletion of Category III codes 0466T-0468T and addition of Category I codes 64582-64584, guidelines within the Neurostimulators, Analysis-Programming subsection have been revised with the addition of codes 64582-64584. In addition, parenthetical notes following these guidelines and code 95970 have been revised with the addition of codes 64582, 64583, and/or 64584, as appropriate.

Refer to the codebook and the Rationale for codes 64582-64584 for a full discussion of these changes.

# Hydration, Therapeutic, Prophylactic, Diagnostic Injections and Infusions, and Chemotherapy and Other Highly Complex Drug or Highly Complex Biologic Agent Administration

## Therapeutic, Prophylactic, and Diagnostic Injections and Infusions (Excludes Chemotherapy and Other Highly Complex Drug or Highly Complex Biologic Agent Administration)

A therapeutic, prophylactic, or diagnostic IV infusion or injection (other than hydration) is for the administration of substances/drugs. When fluids are used to administer the drug(s), the administration of the fluid is considered incidental hydration and is not separately reportable. These services typically require direct supervision for any or all purposes of patient assessment, provision of

consent, safety oversight, and intra-service supervision of staff. Typically, such infusions require special consideration to prepare, dose or dispose of, require practice training and competency for staff who administer the infusions, and require periodic patient assessment with vital sign monitoring during the infusion. These codes are not intended to be reported by the physician or other qualified health care professional in the facility setting.

See codes 96401-96549 for the administration of chemotherapy or other highly complex drug or highly complex biologic agent services. These highly complex services require advanced practice training and competency for staff who provide these services; special considerations for preparation, dosage or disposal; and commonly, these services entail significant patient risk and frequent monitoring. Examples are frequent changes in the infusion rate, prolonged presence of nurse administering the solution for patient monitoring and infusion adjustments, and frequent conferring with the physician or other qualified health care professional about these issues.

(Do not report 96365-96379 with codes for which IV push or infusion is an inherent part of the procedure [eg, administration of contrast material for a diagnostic imaging study])

▶(For mechanical scalp cooling, see 0662T, 0663T)◀

## Rationale

In support of the establishment of codes 0662T and 0663T to report mechanical scalp cooling, a parenthetical note has been added following the guidelines in the Therapeutic, Prophylactic, and Diagnostic Injections and Infusions (Excludes Chemotherapy and Other Highly Complex Drug or Highly Complex Biologic Agent Administration) subsection to instruct users on the correct use of these codes.

Refer to the codebook and the Rationale for codes 0662T and 0663T for a full discussion of these changes.

96372    Therapeutic, prophylactic, or diagnostic injection (specify substance or drug); subcutaneous or intramuscular

▶(For administration of vaccines/toxoids, see 90460, 90461, 90471, 90472, 0001A, 0002A, 0011A, 0012A, 0021A, 0022A, 0031A, 0041A, 0042A)◀

Medicine 90281-99607

## Rationale

To accommodate the addition of new codes for reporting COVID-19 vaccine products, the parenthetical note following code 96372 has been revised.

Refer to the codebook and the Rationale for codes 0001A-0042A for a full discussion of these changes.

(Report 96372 for non-antineoplastic hormonal therapy injections)

(Report 96401 for anti-neoplastic nonhormonal injection therapy)

(Report 96402 for anti-neoplastic hormonal injection therapy)

▶(For intradermal cancer immunotherapy injection, see 0708T, 0709T)◀

## Rationale

In support of the addition of codes to identify intradermal cancer immunotherapy (0708T, 0709T), a parenthetical note following code 96372 has been added.

Refer to the codebook and the Rationale for codes 0708T and 0709T for a full discussion of these changes.

(Do not report 96372 for injections given without direct physician or other qualified health care professional supervision. To report, use 99211. Hospitals may report 96372 when the physician or other qualified health care professional is not present)

(96372 does not include injections for allergen immunotherapy. For allergen immunotherapy injections, see 95115-95117)

## Chemotherapy and Other Highly Complex Drug or Highly Complex Biologic Agent Administration

### Injection and Intravenous Infusion Chemotherapy and Other Highly Complex Drug or Highly Complex Biologic Agent Administration

**96401** Chemotherapy administration, subcutaneous or intramuscular; non-hormonal anti-neoplastic

▶(For intradermal cancer immunotherapy injection, see 0708T, 0709T)◀

**96402** hormonal anti-neoplastic

## Rationale

In support of the addition of codes to identify intradermal cancer immunotherapy (0708T, 0709T), a parenthetical note following code 96401 has been added.

Refer to the codebook and the Rationale for codes 0708T and 0709T for a full discussion of these changes.

# Non-Face-to-Face Nonphysician Services

## Telephone Services

**98966** Telephone assessment and management service provided by a qualified nonphysician health care professional to an established patient, parent, or guardian not originating from a related assessment and management service provided within the previous 7 days nor leading to an assessment and management service or procedure within the next 24 hours or soonest available appointment; 5-10 minutes of medical discussion

**98967** 11-20 minutes of medical discussion

**98968** 21-30 minutes of medical discussion

▶(Do not report 98966-98968 during the same month with 99426, 99427, 99439, 99487, 99489, 99490, 99491)◀

(Do not report 98966, 98967, 98968 in conjunction with 93792, 93793)

## Rationale

To accommodate the addition of the new principal care management codes and other changes made to clarify the reporting of these services, a parenthetical note within the Telephone Services subsection of the Non-Face-to-Face Nonphysician Services subsection has been revised with the addition of codes 99426 and 99427.

Refer to the codebook and the Rationale for codes 99424-99427 for a full discussion of these changes.

★ = Telemedicine    + = Add-on code    ✗ = FDA approval pending    # = Resequenced code    ⊘ = Modifier 51 exempt

# Qualified Nonphysician Health Care Professional Online Digital Assessment and Management Service

**98970**     Qualified nonphysician health care professional online digital assessment and management, for an established patient, for up to 7 days, cumulative time during the 7 days; 5-10 minutes

**98971**     11-20 minutes

**98972**     21 or more minutes

(Report 98970, 98971, 98972 once per 7-day period)

(Do not report online digital E/M services for cumulative visit time less than 5 minutes)

(Do not count 98970, 98971, 98972 time otherwise reported with other services)

(Do not report 98970, 98971, 98972 for home and outpatient INR monitoring when reporting 93792, 93793)

►(Do not report 98970, 98971, 98972 when using 99091, 99339, 99340, 99374, 99375, 99377, 99378, 99379, 99380, 99426, 99427, 99437, 99439, 99487, 99489, 99490, 99491, for the same communication[s])◄

## Rationale

To accommodate the addition of the new principal care management codes and other changes made to clarify the reporting of these services, a parenthetical note within the Qualified Nonphysician Health Care Professional Online Digital Assessment and Management Service subsection has been revised with the addition of codes 99426, 99427, and 99437.

Refer to the codebook and the Rationale for codes 99424-99427 for a full discussion of these changes.

## ►Remote Therapeutic Monitoring Services◄

►Remote therapeutic monitoring services (eg, musculoskeletal system status, respiratory system status, therapy adherence, therapy response) represent the review and monitoring of data related to signs, symptoms, and functions of a therapeutic response. These data may represent objective device-generated integrated data or subjective inputs reported by a patient. These data are reflective of therapeutic responses that provide a functionally integrative representation of patient status.

Codes 98975, 98976, 98977 are used to report remote therapeutic monitoring services during a 30-day period. To report 98975, 98976, 98977, the service(s) must be ordered by a physician or other qualified health care professional. Code 98975 may be used to report the set-up and patient education on the use of any device(s) utilized for therapeutic data collection. Codes 98976, 98977 may be used to report supply of the device for scheduled (eg, daily) recording(s) and/or programmed alert(s) transmissions. To report 98975, 98976, 98977, the device used must be a medical device as defined by the FDA. Codes 98975, 98976, 98977 are not reported if monitoring is less than 16 days. Do not report 98975, 98976, 98977 with other physiologic monitoring services (eg, 95250 for continuous glucose monitoring requiring a minimum of 72 hours of monitoring or 99453, 99454 for remote monitoring of physiologic parameter[s]).

Code 98975 is reported for each episode of care. For reporting remote therapeutic monitoring parameters, an episode of care is defined as beginning when the remote therapeutic monitoring service is initiated and ends with attainment of targeted treatment goals.◄

● **98975**     Remote therapeutic monitoring (eg, respiratory system status, musculoskeletal system status, therapy adherence, therapy response); initial set-up and patient education on use of equipment

►(Do not report 98975 more than once per episode of care)◄

►(Do not report 98975 for monitoring of less than 16 days)◄

● **98976**     device(s) supply with scheduled (eg, daily) recording(s) and/or programmed alert(s) transmission to monitor respiratory system, each 30 days

● **98977**     device(s) supply with scheduled (eg, daily) recording(s) and/or programmed alert(s) transmission to monitor musculoskeletal system, each 30 days

►(Do not report 98975, 98976, 98977 in conjunction with codes for more specific physiologic parameters [93296, 94760, 99453, 99454])◄

►(Do not report 98976, 98977 for monitoring of less than 16 days)◄

►(For therapeutic monitoring treatment management services, use 98980)◄

►(For remote physiologic monitoring, see 99453, 99454)◄

►(For physiologic monitoring treatment management services, use 99457)◄

►(For self-measured blood pressure monitoring, see 99473, 99474)◄

## ►Remote Therapeutic Monitoring Treatment Management Services◄

►Remote therapeutic monitoring treatment management services are provided when a physician or other qualified health care professional uses the results of remote therapeutic monitoring to manage a patient under a specific treatment plan. To report remote therapeutic monitoring, the service must be ordered by a physician or other qualified health care professional. To report 98980, 98981, any device used must be a medical device as defined by the FDA. Do not use 98980, 98981 for time that can be reported using codes for more specific monitoring services. Codes 98980, 98981 may be reported during the same service period as chronic care management services (99439, 99487, 99489, 99490, 99491), transitional care management services (99495, 99496), principal care management services (99424, 99425, 99426, 99427), and behavioral health integration services (99484, 99492, 99493, 99494). However, time spent performing these services should remain separate and no time should be counted toward the required time for both services in a single month. Codes 98980, 98981 require at least one interactive communication with the patient or caregiver. The interactive communication contributes to the total time, but it does not need to represent the entire cumulative reported time of the treatment management service. For the first completed 20 minutes of physician or other qualified health care professional time in a calendar month report 98980, and report 98981 for each additional completed 20 minutes. Do not report 98980, 98981 for services of less than 20 minutes. Report 98980 once regardless of the number of therapeutic monitoring modalities performed in a given calendar month.

Do not count any time on a day when the physician or other qualified health care professional reports an E/M service (office or other outpatient services [99202, 99203, 99204, 99205, 99211, 99212, 99213, 99214, 99215], domiciliary, rest home services [99324, 99325, 99326, 99327, 99328, 99334, 99335, 99336, 99337], home services [99341, 99342, 99343, 99344, 99345, 99347, 99348, 99349, 99350], inpatient services [99221, 99222, 99223, 99231, 99232, 99233, 99251, 99252, 99253, 99254, 99255]).

Do not count any time related to other reported services (eg, psychotherapy services [90832, 90833, 90834, 90836, 90837, 90838], interrogation device evaluation services [93290], anticoagulant management services [93793], respiratory monitoring services [94774, 94775, 94776, 94777], health behavior assessment and intervention services [96156, 96158, 96159, 96160, 96161, 96164, 96165, 96167, 96168, 96170, 96171], therapeutic interventions that focus on cognitive function services [97129, 97130], adaptive behavior treatment services [97153, 97154, 97155, 97156, 97157, 97158], therapeutic procedures [97110, 97112, 97116, 97530, 97535], tests and measurements [97750, 97755], physical therapy evaluation services [97161, 97162, 97163, 97164], occupational therapy evaluations [97165, 97166, 97167, 97168], orthotic management and training and

prosthetic training services [97760, 97661, 97763], medical nutrition therapy services [97802, 97803, 97804], medication therapy management services [99605, 99606, 99607], critical care services [99291, 99292], principal care management services [99424, 99425, 99426, 99427]) in the cumulative time of the remote therapeutic monitoring treatment management service during the calendar month of reporting.◄

● 98980    Remote therapeutic monitoring treatment management services, physician or other qualified health care professional time in a calendar month requiring at least one interactive communication with the patient or caregiver during the calendar month; first 20 minutes

▶(Report 98980 once each 30 days, regardless of the number of therapeutic parameters monitored)◄

▶(Do not report 98980 for services of less than 20 minutes)◄

▶(Do not report 98980 in conjunction with 93264, 99091 99457, 99458)◄

▶(Do not report 98980 in the same calendar month as 99473, 99474)◄

+● 98981      each additional 20 minutes (List separately in addition to code for primary procedure)

▶(Use 98981 in conjunction with 98980)◄

▶(Do not report 98981 for services of less than an additional increment of 20 minutes)◄

## Rationale

Five new Category I codes (98975-98981) have been established and two new subsections with guidelines and parenthetical notes have been added to the Medicine section of the CPT code set.

Codes 98975-98981 are intended to report remote monitoring of non-physiologic parameters. These new codes have been created to be analogous to remote physiologic monitoring codes 99453, 99454, 99457, and 99458. However, the main difference between these code families is the data parameters that are being reviewed. The existing remote physiologic codes are intended to monitor physiologic parameters (eg, weight, blood pressure, pulse oximetry, respiratory flow rate, etc). The new remote therapeutic monitoring codes (98975-98981) are intended to monitor services (eg, musculoskeletal system status, respiratory system status, therapy adherence, therapy response) representing the review and monitoring of data related to signs, symptoms, and functions of a therapeutic response.

The new Remote Therapeutic Monitoring Services subsection includes codes 98975-98977. Code 98975 is intended to report the initial set-up and patient education on use of the equipment. Codes 98976 and 98977 are intended to report a 30-day device supply with scheduled recordings or programmed alert transmission to monitor the respiratory system (98976) or musculoskeletal system (98977). The new guidelines in this subsection provide clarity on the reporting of these codes.

The future intention is that the CPT code set may be expanded to account for other body systems beyond just respiratory and musculoskeletal. Because these device supply codes (98976, 98977) are reported to describe the cost of the device supplied to the patient, this family of codes was designed to accommodate additional technology and devices that may have variable costs depending on the therapeutic approach taken by the physician and/or other QHP.

The new Remote Therapeutic Monitoring Treatment Management Services subsection includes two new codes (98980, 98981), which are intended to be reported per month for the time spent on remote therapeutic monitoring treatment management services by the physician or other QHP for the first 20 minutes (98980) and each additional 20 minutes thereafter (98981).

## Clinical Example (98975)

A 65-year-old male presents to the physician's or other QHP's office with exacerbation of a chronic condition. Following the visit, the physician initiates a remote therapeutic monitoring program to enable data collection and monitoring to support the therapeutic management of his condition.

## Description of Procedure (98975)

Clinical staff walks the patient through the set-up of the therapeutic monitoring technology. Educate the patient regarding how to use the technology and related daily tasks. For respiratory therapy monitoring, introduce the patient to the device and the mobile app. For musculoskeletal therapy monitoring, educate the patient on setting up the device, reviewing the 3D motion-capture technology, and reviewing the specific exercises as prescribed by the physician or other QHP. Give the patient the opportunity to ask questions.

## Clinical Example (98976)

An 8-year-old female presents to the physician's or other QHP's office with a cough and wheezing. She is diagnosed with a respiratory condition exacerbated by environmental factors. Following the visit, the physician or other QHP initiates a remote therapeutic monitoring program to enable data collection and monitoring to support the therapeutic management of her respiratory condition.

## Description of Procedure (98976)

N/A

## Clinical Example (98977)

A 66-year-old female, who has limited mobility caused by osteoarthritis of her knees, is enrolled in a remote therapeutic monitoring program to enable data collection and monitoring to support the therapeutic management of her musculoskeletal condition.

## Description of Procedure (98977)

N/A

## Clinical Example (98980)

An 8-year-old presents to the physician's or other QHP's office with exacerbation of asthma. The physician or other QHP initiates a remote therapeutic monitoring program to enable data collection and monitoring to support the therapeutic management of the patient's condition.

## Description of Procedure (98980)

The physician or other QHP analyzes and interprets the data. Based on the interpreted data, the physician or other QHP uses medical and clinical decision making to assess the patient's condition, communicate with the patient, and oversee, coordinate, and/or modify the patient's care through shared decision making to achieve established outcomes and goals of care.

## Clinical Example (98981)

An 8-year-old presents to the physician's or other QHP's office with exacerbation of asthma. The physician or other QHP initiates a remote therapeutic monitoring program to enable data collection and monitoring to support the therapeutic management of the patient's condition. [**Note:** This is an add-on service. Only consider the additional work related to the additional physician or other QHP staff time beyond the 20 minutes reported with code 98980.]

## Description of Procedure (98981)

The physician or other QHP analyzes and interprets the data. Based on the interpreted data, the physician or other QHP uses medical and clinical decision making to assess the patient's condition, communicate with the patient, and oversee, coordinate, and/or modify the patient's care through shared decision making to achieve established outcomes and goals of care. Additional time is needed due to the specific needs of the patient's medical condition(s).

# Special Services, Procedures and Reports

## Miscellaneous Services

**99070**   Supplies and materials (except spectacles), provided by the physician or other qualified health care professional over and above those usually included with the office visit or other services rendered (list drugs, trays, supplies, or materials provided)

(For supply of spectacles, use the appropriate supply codes)

▶(For additional supplies, materials, and clinical staff time required during a Public Health Emergency, as defined by law, due to respiratory-transmitted infectious disease, use 99072)◀

**99071**   Educational supplies, such as books, tapes, and pamphlets, for the patient's education at cost to physician or other qualified health care professional

▶Code 99072 is used to report the additional supplies, materials, and clinical staff time over and above the practice expense(s) included in an office visit or other non-facility service(s) when the office visit or other non-facility service(s) is rendered during a Public Health Emergency (PHE), as defined by law, due to respiratory-transmitted infectious disease. These required additional supplies, materials, and clinical staff time are intended to mitigate the transmission of the respiratory disease for which the PHE was declared. These include, but are not limited to, additional supplies, such as face masks and cleaning supplies, as well as clinical staff time for activities such as pre-visit instructions and office arrival symptom checks that support the safe provision of evaluation, treatment, or procedural service(s) during the respiratory infection–focused PHE. When reporting 99072, report only once per in-person patient encounter per day regardless of the number of services rendered at that encounter. Code 99072 may be reported during a PHE when the additional clinical staff duties as described are performed by the physician or other qualified health care professional in lieu of clinical staff.◀

● **99072**   Additional supplies, materials, and clinical staff time over and above those usually included in an office visit or other non-facility service(s), when performed during a Public Health Emergency, as defined by law, due to respiratory-transmitted infectious disease

## Rationale

Code 99072 has been established to report the additional supplies and clinical staff time required to perform evaluation, treatment, or procedural services to mitigate transmission of communicable disease during a Public Health Emergency (PHE). As physician practices across the United States continue to see patients during the COVID-19 PHE, physicians expressed concern about the added practice expense (PE) for personal protective equipment (PPE) required to safely provide in-person medical services to patients.

The additional supplies and clinical staff time described in code 99072 are needed for the safety of all physicians and other QHPs, as well as clinical and administrative staff and patients. Therefore, this new code is intended to be reported in conjunction with the CPT code(s) to report the primary service. It is important to note that code 99072 is not intended to be reported only during the COVID-19 pandemic, but may be reported during any PHE, as defined by law, due to respiratory-transmitted infectious disease.

## Clinical Example (99072)

A 65-year-old female presents to the physician's office, requiring care for an illness, acute injury, or ongoing care for a chronic condition. The encounter occurs during a Public Health Emergency (PHE), as defined by law, due to respiratory-transmitted infectious disease.

## Description of Procedure (99072)

N/A

# Category III Codes

## Summary of Additions, Deletions, and Revisions

The summary of changes shows the actual changes that have been made to the code descriptors.

New codes appear with a bullet (●) and are indicated as "Code added." Revised codes are preceded with a triangle (▲). Within revised codes, or if a code symbol has been deleted, the deleted language and code symbol appear with a ~~strikethrough~~, while new text appears underlined.

The ✓ symbol is used to identify codes for vaccines that are pending FDA approval. The # symbol is used to identify codes that have been resequenced. CPT add-on codes are annotated by the ✚ symbol. The ⊘ symbol is used to identify codes that are exempt from the use of modifier 51. The ★ symbol is used to identify codes that may be used for reporting telemedicine services. The ✖ symbol is used to identify a proprietary laboratory analyses (PLA) test that has an identical descriptor as another PLA test. A PLA code that satisfies Category I code criteria and has been accepted by the CPT Editorial Panel is annotated with the ↕ symbol.

| Code | Description |
|------|-------------|
| ▲0101T | Extracorporeal shock wave involving musculoskeletal system, not otherwise specified~~, high energy~~ |
| ▲0102T | Extracorporeal shock wave~~, high energy,~~ performed by a physician, requiring anesthesia other than local,_ and_ involving <u>the </u>lateral humeral epicondyle |
| #▲0512T | Extracorporeal shock wave for integumentary wound healing, ~~high energy,~~ including topical application and dressing care; initial wound |
| #✚▲0513T | each additional wound (List separately in addition to code for primary procedure) |
| ~~0191T~~ | ~~Insertion of anterior segment aqueous drainage device, without extraocular reservoir, internal approach, into the trabecular meshwork; initial insertion~~ |
| ~~0376T~~ | ~~each additional device insertion (List separately in addition to code for primary procedure)~~ |
| #●0671T | Code added |
| ~~0290T~~ | ~~Corneal incisions in the recipient cornea created using a laser, in preparation for penetrating or lamellar keratoplasty (List separately in addition to code for primary procedure)~~ |
| ~~0355T~~ | ~~Gastrointestinal tract imaging, intraluminal (eg, capsule endoscopy), colon, with interpretation and report~~ |
| ~~0356T~~ | ~~Insertion of drug-eluting implant (including punctal dilation and implant removal when performed) into lacrimal canaliculus, each~~ |
| ~~0423T~~ | ~~Secretory type II phospholipase A2 (sPLA2-IIA)~~ |
| ~~0451T~~ | ~~Insertion or replacement of a permanently implantable aortic counterpulsation ventricular assist system, endovascular approach, and programming of sensing and therapeutic parameters; complete system (counterpulsation device, vascular graft, implantable vascular hemostatic seal, mechano-electrical skin interface and subcutaneous electrodes)~~ |
| ~~0452T~~ | ~~aortic counterpulsation device and vascular hemostatic seal~~ |
| ~~0453T~~ | ~~mechano-electrical skin interface~~ |
| ~~0454T~~ | ~~subcutaneous electrode~~ |

Category III  0042T-0713T

| Code | Description |
|---|---|
| 0455T | ~~Removal of permanently implantable aortic counterpulsation ventricular assist system; complete system (aortic counterpulsation device, vascular hemostatic seal, mechano-electrical skin interface and electrodes)~~ |
| 0456T | ~~aortic counterpulsation device and vascular hemostatic seal~~ |
| 0457T | ~~mechano-electrical skin interface~~ |
| 0458T | ~~subcutaneous electrode~~ |
| 0459T | ~~Relocation of skin pocket with replacement of implanted aortic counterpulsation ventricular assist device, mechano-electrical skin interface and electrodes~~ |
| 0460T | ~~Repositioning of previously implanted aortic counterpulsation ventricular assist device; subcutaneous electrode~~ |
| 0461T | ~~aortic counterpulsation device~~ |
| 0462T | ~~Programming device evaluation (in person) with iterative adjustment of the implantable mechano-electrical skin interface and/or external driver to test the function of the device and select optimal permanent programmed values with analysis, including review and report, implantable aortic counterpulsation ventricular assist system, per day~~ |
| 0463T | ~~Interrogation device evaluation (in person) with analysis, review and report, includes connection, recording and disconnection per patient encounter, implantable aortic counterpulsation ventricular assist system, per day~~ |
| 0466T | ~~Insertion of chest wall respiratory sensor electrode or electrode array, including connection to pulse generator (List separately in addition to code for primary procedure)~~ |
| 0467T | ~~Revision or replacement of chest wall respiratory sensor electrode or electrode array, including connection to existing pulse generator~~ |
| 0468T | ~~Removal of chest wall respiratory sensor electrode or electrode array~~ |
| ▲0493T | <u>Contact N</u>near-infrared spectroscopy studies of lower extremity wounds (eg, for oxyhemoglobin measurement) |
| #●0640T | Code added |
| #●0641T | Code added |
| #●0642T | Code added |
| #●0643T | Code added |
| 0548T | ~~Transperineal periurethral balloon continence device; bilateral placement, including cystoscopy and fluoroscopy~~ |
| 0549T | ~~unilateral placement, including cystoscopy and fluoroscopy~~ |
| 0550T | ~~removal, each balloon~~ |
| 0551T | ~~adjustment of balloon(s) fluid volume~~ |
| #●0646T | Code added |
| ●0644T | Code added |
| ●0645T | Code added |
| ●0647T | Code added |
| ▲0648T | Quantitative magnetic resonance for analysis of tissue composition (eg, fat, iron, water content), including multiparametric data acquisition, data preparation and transmission, interpretation and report, obtained without diagnostic MRI examination of the same anatomy (eg, organ, gland, tissue, target structure) during the same session<u>; single organ</u> |
| #●0697T | Code added |

★ = Telemedicine   ✚ = Add-on code   ✗ = FDA approval pending   # = Resequenced code   ⊘ = Modifier 51 exempt

| Code | Description |
|------|-------------|
| **+▲0649T** | Quantitative magnetic resonance for analysis of tissue composition (eg, fat, iron, water content), including multiparametric data acquisition, data preparation and transmission, interpretation and report, obtained with diagnostic MRI examination of the same anatomy (eg, organ, gland, tissue, target structure); single organ (List separately in addition to code for primary procedure) |
| **#+●0698T** | Code added |
| **●0650T** | Code added |
| **●0651T** | Code added |
| **●0652T** | Code added |
| **●0653T** | Code added |
| **●0654T** | Code added |
| **●0655T** | Code added |
| **●0656T** | Code added |
| **●0657T** | Code added |
| **●0658T** | Code added |
| **●0659T** | Code added |
| **●0660T** | Code added |
| **●0661T** | Code added |
| **●0662T** | Code added |
| **+●0663T** | Code added |
| **●0664T** | Code added |
| **●0665T** | Code added |
| **●0666T** | Code added |
| **●0667T** | Code added |
| **●0668T** | Code added |
| **●0669T** | Code added |
| **●0670T** | Code added |
| **●0672T** | Code added |
| **●0673T** | Code added |
| **●0674T** | Code added |
| **●0675T** | Code added |
| **+●0676T** | Code added |
| **●0677T** | Code added |
| **+●0678T** | Code added |
| **●0679T** | Code added |

Category III 0042T-0713T

| Code | Description |
|---|---|
| ●0680T | Code added |
| ●0681T | Code added |
| ●0682T | Code added |
| ●0683T | Code added |
| ●0684T | Code added |
| ●0685T | Code added |
| ●0686T | Code added |
| ●0687T | Code added |
| ●0688T | Code added |
| ●0689T | Code added |
| ✚●0690T | Code added |
| ●0691T | Code added |
| ●0692T | Code added |
| ●0693T | Code added |
| ●0694T | Code added |
| ●0695T | Code added |
| ●0696T | Code added |
| ●0699T | Code added |
| ●0700T | Code added |
| ✚●0701T | Code added |
| ●0702T | Code added |
| ●0703T | Code added |
| ●0704T | Code added |
| ●0705T | Code added |
| ●0706T | Code added |
| ●0707T | Code added |
| ●0708T | Code added |
| ✚●0709T | Code added |
| ●0710T | Code added |
| ●0711T | Code added |
| ●0712T | Code added |
| ●0713T | Code added |

★ = Telemedicine   ✚ = Add-on code   ✗ = FDA approval pending   # = Resequenced code   ⊘ = Modifier 51 exempt

# Category III Codes

The following section contains a set of temporary codes for emerging technology, services, procedures, and service paradigms. Category III codes allow data collection for these services/procedures. Use of unlisted codes does not offer the opportunity for the collection of specific data. If a Category III code is available, this code must be reported instead of a Category I unlisted code. This is an activity that is critically important in the evaluation of health care delivery and the formation of public and private policy. The use of the codes in this section allows physicians and other qualified health care professionals, insurers, health services researchers, and health policy experts to identify emerging technology, services, procedures, and service paradigms for clinical efficacy, utilization and outcomes.

(For destruction of localized lesion of choroid by transpupillary thermotherapy, use 67299)

(For destruction of macular drusen, photocoagulation, use 67299)

(For application of extracorporeal shock wave involving musculoskeletal system not otherwise specified, use 0101T)

(For application of extracorporeal shock wave involving lateral humeral epicondyle, use 0102T)

(For non-surgical septal reduction therapy, use 93799)

(For pulsed magnetic neuromodulation incontinence treatment, use 53899)

**0100T**  Placement of a subconjunctival retinal prosthesis receiver and pulse generator, and implantation of intraocular retinal electrode array, with vitrectomy

(For initial programming of implantable intraocular retinal electrode array device, use 0472T)

▲ **0101T**  Extracorporeal shock wave involving musculoskeletal system, not otherwise specified

(For extracorporeal shock wave therapy involving integumentary system not otherwise specified, see 0512T, 0513T)

(Do not report 0101T in conjunction 0512T, 0513T, when treating same area)

▲ **0102T**  Extracorporeal shock wave performed by a physician, requiring anesthesia other than local, and involving the lateral humeral epicondyle

#▲ **0512T**  Extracorporeal shock wave for integumentary wound healing, including topical application and dressing care; initial wound

#+▲ **0513T**      each additional wound (List separately in addition to code for primary procedure)

(Use 0513T in conjunction with 0512T)

## Rationale

Code descriptors and parenthetical notes throughout the CPT code set have been revised to reflect current practice of not differentiating between "high" or "low" energy used to perform extracorporeal shock wave procedures. Specifically, codes 0101T, 0102T, 0512T, and 0513T have been revised with deletion of the phrase "high energy." In addition, the descriptor language in code 0102T has been editorially revised.

## Clinical Example (0101T)

A 55-year-old female presents with an injury to the left shoulder that has failed to respond to appropriate conservative therapy. Extracorporeal shock wave therapy (ESWT) is ordered to treat pain and improve function.

## Description of Procedure (0101T)

Place the patient supine on the stretcher and place the affected arm in the lateral position. Point the applicator head of the device downward toward the floor and raise the table to bring the elbow into the F2 area, which is the treatment area of the shock wave. Palpate and designate the area of tenderness with a marking pen. Point the head of the device toward the treatment region. Apply coupling gel to the treatment area. Couple the shock head to the patient's shoulder and position it by the physician. It is important that there is good contact between the patient's anatomy and the shock head to ensure the treatment area remains within F2 throughout the procedure. The physician instructs the technician to set the device to shock wave delivery at a clinically appropriate rate. Treat the entire shoulder region to the proper depth based on the individual patient's anatomy and pathophysiology.

## Clinical Example (0102T)

A 55-year-old patient presents with an injury to the right elbow involving the lateral humeral epicondyle that has failed to respond to appropriate conservative therapy. ESWT is ordered to improve pain and function. The therapy will involve treating the lateral humeral epicondyle, and due to the depth of the tissue to be treated, the patient will receive conscious sedation.

## Description of Procedure (0102T)

Place the patient supine on the stretcher and place the affected arm in the lateral position. Point the applicator head of the device downward toward the floor and raise the table to bring the elbow into the F2 area, which is the treatment area of the shock wave. Induce the patient with either conscious sedation or general anesthesia. Apply coupling gel to the treatment area. Couple the shock head to the patient's elbow and position it by the physician. It is important that there is good contact between the patient's elbow and the shock head to ensure the treatment area remains within F2 throughout the procedure. The physician instructs the technician to set the shock wave delivery rate to 4 Hz. The procedure starts at 0.08 mJ/mm² (millijoule/millimeter) and the energy is increased in increments until reaching a maximum energy flux density of 0.10 mJ/mm² (energy level is adjusted according to the patient's pain level and response). Energy level is not to exceed 0.18 mJ/mm².

Ensure the elbow remains in constant contact with the shock head. The physician moves the affected area within the shock wave path (F2) and pronates and supinates the patient's hand during the procedure to ensure the entire tendon is treated to the proper depth based on the individual patient's anatomy and pathophysiology.

## Clinical Example (0512T)

A 58-year-old female, who has type II diabetes mellitus, presents with a stage II ulcer of greater than 30-day duration on the plantar aspect of the right foot. The ulcer measures 3 × 4 cm (12 cm²). ESWT is ordered to promote wound healing.

## Description of Procedure (0512T)

Examine the patient and cleanse the wound in standard fashion. Perform standard-of-care treatment, including possible debridement as determined by the treating clinician. Take wound measurements and determine shock-count delivery based on wound volume and comorbidities. Prepare the device for treatment. Deliver clinically appropriate shock wave therapy to the wound and to at least 1 cm of the peri-wound. Clean the wound post-application. Perform a final examination of the wound and apply wet-to-moist dressings. A complete course of treatment includes as many as eight applications, typically performed in a 10-week period.

## Clinical Example (0513T)

A 68-year-old male, who has type II diabetes mellitus, presents with a stage II ulcer of 1-year duration on the left foot. The ulcer measures 8 x 14 cm (112 cm²). Medical history includes peripheral vascular disease, peripheral neuropathy, osteomyelitis, and hypothyroidism. The ulcer has shown resistance to multiple treatments, including surgical debridement, advanced dressings, and advanced wound therapies.

## Description of Procedure (0513T)

Examine the patient and cleanse the wound in standard fashion. Perform standard-of-care treatment, including possible debridement as determined by the treating clinician. Take wound measurements and determine

shock-count delivery based on wound volume and comorbidities. Prepare the device for treatment. Deliver ESWT to the wound and to at least 1 cm of the peri-wound. Clean the wound post-application. Perform a final examination of the wound and apply wet-to-moist dressings. A complete course of treatment includes as many as eight applications, typically performed in a 10-week period.

---

(For holotranscobalamin, quantitative, use 84999)

(For inert gas rebreathing for cardiac output measurement during rest, use 93799)

(For inert gas rebreathing for cardiac output measurement during exercise, use 93799)

+ **0174T**  Computer-aided detection (CAD) (computer algorithm analysis of digital image data for lesion detection) with further physician review for interpretation and report, with or without digitization of film radiographic images, chest radiograph(s), performed concurrent with primary interpretation (List separately in addition to code for primary procedure)

**0175T**  Computer-aided detection (CAD) (computer algorithm analysis of digital image data for lesion detection) with further physician review for interpretation and report, with or without digitization of film radiographic images, chest radiograph(s), performed remote from primary interpretation

▶(0191T has been deleted)◀

▶(For anterior segment drainage device implantation without concomitant cataract removal, use 0671T)◀

▶(0376T has been deleted)◀

▶(For insertion of anterior segment aqueous drainage device without extraocular reservoir, internal approach, see 66989, 66991, 0671T)◀

\#● **0671T**  Insertion of anterior segment aqueous drainage device into the trabecular meshwork, without external reservoir, and without concomitant cataract removal, one or more

▶(Do not report 0671T in conjunction with 66989, 66991)◀

▶(For complex extracapsular cataract removal with intraocular lens implant without concomitant aqueous drainage device, use 66982)◀

▶(For extracapsular cataract removal with intraocular lens implant without concomitant aqueous drainage device, use 66984)◀

▶(For insertion of anterior segment drainage device into the subconjunctival space, use 0449T)◀

---

★ = Telemedicine   + = Add-on code   ✎ = FDA approval pending   # = Resequenced code   ⊘ = Modifier 51 exempt

## Rationale

In support of the addition of codes 66989 and 66991, codes 0191T and 0376T have been deleted and code 0671T has been established to report insertion of an anterior segment aqueous drainage device into the trabecular meshwork without external reservoir and without concomitant cataract removal.

Parenthetical notes have been added to direct users to the new code and provide direction regarding the appropriate codes to use when cataract removal is involved. Parenthetical notes have also been added to restrict reporting aqueous drainage device procedures with codes 66989 and 66991. In addition, parenthetical notes have been deleted in accordance with the deletion of codes 0191T and 0376T.

Refer to the codebook and the Rationale for codes 66989 and 66991 for a full discussion of these changes.

## Clinical Example (0671T)

A-57-year-old female, who has a 5-year history of open-angle glaucoma that is poorly controlled on topical intraocular pressure (IOP)–lowering medications, has one or more aqueous drainage devices implanted using an internal approach to achieve the desired IOP reduction.

## Description of Procedure (0671T)

Create a small, temporal clear corneal incision. Use a viscoelastic solution to deepen the anterior chamber. Inspect the angle with a goniolens. The surgeon locates the trabecular meshwork, a narrow (150 microns) circumferential band of tissue that drains aqueous humor from the anterior chamber. Use a viscoelastic solution to clear any blood from the implantation site. Introduce the inserter into the anterior chamber and, under gonioscopy, advance the inserter to the trabecular meshwork. Place the first stent. Implant each additional stent 2 to 3 clock hours away from the previously placed stent into the trabecular meshwork and then withdraw the inserter from the eye. Flush the anterior chamber of any refluxed blood, irrigate the chamber with a balanced salt solution (BSS) to remove all viscoelastic solution, and then infiltrate the chamber with a BSS as needed to achieve physiologic pressure.

(To report insertion of drainage device by external approach, use 66183)

**0278T** Transcutaneous electrical modulation pain reprocessing (eg, scrambler therapy), each treatment session (includes placement of electrodes)

▶(0290T has been deleted)◀

▶(For corneal incisions in the recipient cornea created using a laser in preparation for penetrating or lamellar keratoplasty, use 66999)◀

## Rationale

In accordance with the CPT guidelines for archiving Category III codes, code 0290T has been deleted. Report code 66999, *Unlisted procedure, anterior segment of eye*, if corneal incisions in the recipient cornea are created using laser in preparation for penetrating or lamellar keratoplasty. A cross-reference parenthetical note has been added to reflect these changes.

(For greater than 48 hours of monitoring of external electrocardiographic recording, see 93241, 93242, 93243, 93244, 93245, 93246, 93247, 93248)

(For focused microwave thermotherapy of the breast, use 19499)

**0342T** Therapeutic apheresis with selective HDL delipidation and plasma reinfusion

▶Fluoroscopy (76000) and radiologic supervision and interpretation are inherent to the transcatheter mitral valve repair (TMVR) procedure and are not separately reportable. Diagnostic cardiac catheterization (93451, 93452, 93453, 93454, 93455, 93456, 93457, 93458, 93459, 93460, 93461, 93593, 93594, 93595, 93596, 93597, 93598) should **not** be reported with transcatheter mitral valve repair (0345T) for:

■ Contrast injections, angiography, roadmapping, and/or fluoroscopic guidance for the transcatheter mitral valve repair TMVR),

■ Left ventricular angiography to assess mitral regurgitation for guidance of TMVR, or

■ Right and left heart catheterization for hemodynamic measurements before, during, and after TMVR for guidance of TMVR.

Diagnostic right and left heart catheterization (93451, 93452, 93453, 93456, 93457, 93458, 93459, 93460, 93461, 93593, 93594, 93595, 93596, 93597, 93598) and diagnostic coronary angiography (93454, 93455, 93456, 93457, 93458, 93459, 93460, 93461, 93563, 93564) not inherent to the TMVR may be reported with 0345T, appended with modifier 59, if:

1. No prior study is available and a full diagnostic study is performed, or

2. A prior study is available, but as documented in the medical record:

   a. There is inadequate visualization of the anatomy and/or pathology, or

b. The patient's condition with respect to the clinical indication has changed since the prior study, or

c. There is a clinical change during the procedure that requires new evaluation. ◀

Percutaneous coronary interventional procedures may be reported separately, when performed.

Other cardiac catheterization services may be reported separately, when performed for diagnostic purposes not intrinsic to the TMVR.

When transcatheter ventricular support is required, the appropriate code may be reported with the appropriate ventricular assist device (VAD) procedure (33990, 33991, 33992, 33993, 33995, 33997) or balloon pump insertion (33967, 33970, 33973).

**0345T** Transcatheter mitral valve repair percutaneous approach via the coronary sinus

## Rationale

In accordance with the deletion of codes 93530-93533 and the establishment of codes 93593-93598, the guidelines for Category III code 0345T (transcatheter mitral valve repair) have been revised to reflect these changes.

Refer to the codebook and the Rationale for codes 93593-93598 for a full discussion of these changes.

▶(0355T has been deleted)◀

▶(For gastrointestinal tract imaging, intraluminal [eg, capsule endoscopy] of the colon, use 91113)◀

## Rationale

In accordance with the conversion of Category III code 0355T to Category I code 91113, a deletion parenthetical note and a cross-reference parenthetical note have been added to the Category III section.

Refer to the codebook and the Rationale for code 91113 for a full discussion of these changes.

▶(0356T has been deleted)◀

▶(For insertion of drug-eluting implant including punctal dilation, when performed, into the lacrimal canaliculus, use 68841)◀

## Rationale

In accordance with the conversion of Category III code 0356T to Category I code 68841, a deletion parenthetical note and a cross-reference parenthetical note referencing code 68841 for insertion of drug-eluting implant, including punctal dilation, when performed, have been added to the Category III section.

Refer to the codebook and the Rationale for code 68841 for a full discussion of these changes.

(For placement of drug-eluting insert under the eyelid[s], see 0444T, 0445T)

**0376T** Code is out of numerical sequence. See 0184T-0200T

**0422T** Tactile breast imaging by computer-aided tactile sensors, unilateral or bilateral

▶(0423T has been deleted)◀

▶(For secretory type II phospholipase A2 [sPLA2-IIA], use 84999)◀

## Rationale

In accordance with the CPT guidelines for archiving Category III codes, code 0423T has been deleted. Report code 84999, *Unlisted chemistry procedure,* if secretory type II phospholipase A2 [sPLA2-IIA] is performed. A cross-reference parenthetical note has been added to reflect these changes.

**0445T** Subsequent placement of a drug-eluting ocular insert under one or more eyelids, including re-training, and removal of existing insert, unilateral or bilateral

▶(For insertion and removal of drug-eluting implant into lacrimal canaliculus, use 68841)◀

## Rationale

In accordance with the deletion of Category III code 0356T and the establishment of code 68841, the cross-reference parenthetical note following code 0445T has been revised to reflect these changes.

Refer to the codebook and the Rationale for code 68841 for a full discussion of these changes.

**0449T** Insertion of aqueous drainage device, without extraocular reservoir, internal approach, into the subconjunctival space; initial device

★ = Telemedicine   ✛ = Add-on code   ✗ = FDA approval pending   # = Resequenced code   ⊘ = Modifier 51 exempt

**+ 0450T**    each additional device (List separately in addition to code for primary procedure)

(Use 0450T in conjunction with 0449T)

(For removal of aqueous drainage device without extraocular reservoir, placed into the subconjunctival space via internal approach, use 92499)

▶(For insertion of intraocular anterior segment drainage device into the trabecular meshwork without concomitant cataract removal with intraocular lens implant, use 0671T)◀

## Rationale

In support of the addition of codes 66989, 66991, and 0671T, parenthetical notes have been added to direct users to the new codes.

Refer to the codebook and the Rationale for codes 66989 and 66991 for a full discussion of these changes.

▶(0451T, 0452T, 0453T, 0454T have been deleted)◀

▶(For insertion or replacement of a permanently implantable aortic counterpulsation ventricular assist system, endovascular approach, and programming of sensing and therapeutic parameters, use 33999)◀

▶(0455T, 0456T, 0457T, 0458T have been deleted)◀

▶(For removal of permanently implantable aortic counterpulsation ventricular assist system, use 33999)◀

▶(0459T has been deleted)◀

▶(For relocation of skin pocket with replacement of implanted aortic counterpulsation ventricular assist device, mechano-electrical skin interface and electrodes, use 33999)◀

▶(0460T, 0461T have been deleted)◀

▶(For repositioning of previously implanted aortic counterpulsation ventricular assist device, use 33999)◀

▶(0462T has been deleted)◀

▶(For programming device evaluation [in person] with iterative adjustment of the implantable mechano-electrical skin interface and/or external driver, use 33999)◀

▶(0463T has been deleted)◀

▶(For interrogation device evaluation [in person] with analysis, review, and report, use 33999)◀

## Rationale

In accordance with the CPT guidelines for archiving Category III codes, codes 0451T-0463T and the introductory guidelines that describe the family of services related to the placement and maintenance of permanent aortic counterpulsation ventricular assistance devices have been deleted. Six deletion parenthetical notes have been added and six cross-reference parenthetical notes have been added to direct users to report code 33999, *Unlisted procedure, cardiac surgery,* for this procedure.

In accordance with the deletion of Category III codes 0451T-0463T, parenthetical notes in the Cardiac Assist subsection referencing these codes have also been deleted.

▶(0466T, 0467T, 0468T have been deleted)◀

▶(For insertion, revision or replacement, or removal of chest wall respiratory sensor electrode or electrode array, see 64582, 64583, 64584)◀

## Rationale

In accordance with the addition of codes 64582-64584, codes 0466T-0468T and related parenthetical notes have been deleted, and parenthetical notes have been added to direct users to the new codes. A cross-reference parenthetical note has been added to reflect these changes.

Refer to the codebook and the Rationale for codes 64582-64584 for a full discussion of these changes.

**0481T**    Injection(s), autologous white blood cell concentrate (autologous protein solution), any site, including image guidance, harvesting and preparation, when performed

Codes 0483T, 0484T include vascular access, catheterization, balloon valvuloplasty, deploying the valve, repositioning the valve as needed, temporary pacemaker insertion for rapid pacing, and access site closure, when performed.

Angiography, radiological supervision and interpretation, intraprocedural roadmapping (eg, contrast injections, fluoroscopy) to guide the TMVI, left ventriculography (eg, to assess mitral regurgitation for guidance of TMVI), and completion angiography are included in codes 0483T, 0484T.

▶Diagnostic right and left heart catheterization codes (93451, 93452, 93453, 93456, 93457, 93458, 93459, 93460, 93461, 93593, 93594, 93595, 93596, 93597, 93598) should **not** be used with 0483T, 0484T to report:

1. Contrast injections, angiography, roadmapping, and/ or fluoroscopic guidance for the transcatheter mitral valve implantation (TMVI),

2. Left ventricular angiography to assess or confirm valve positioning and function,

3. Right and left heart catheterization for hemodynamic measurements before, during, and after TMVI for guidance of TMVI.

Diagnostic right and left heart catheterization codes (93451, 93452, 93453, 93456, 93457, 93458, 93459, 93460, 93461, 93593, 93594, 93595, 93596, 93597, 93598) and diagnostic coronary angiography codes (93454, 93455, 93456, 93457, 93458, 93459, 93460, 93461, 93563, 93564) performed at the time of TMVI may be separately reportable, if:

1. No prior study is available and a full diagnostic study is performed, or

2. A prior study is available, but as documented in the medical record:

   a. There is inadequate visualization of the anatomy and/or pathology, or

   b. The patient's condition with respect to the clinical indication has changed since the prior study, or

   c. There is a clinical change during the procedure that requires new evaluation.◄

For same session/same day diagnostic cardiac catheterization services, report the appropriate diagnostic cardiac catheterization code(s) appended with modifier 59, indicating separate and distinct procedural service from TMVI.

When cardiopulmonary bypass is performed in conjunction with TMVI, 0483T, 0484T may be reported with the appropriate add-on code for percutaneous peripheral bypass (33367), open peripheral bypass (33368), or central bypass (33369).

For percutaneous transcatheter tricuspid valve annulus reconstruction, with implantation of adjustable annulus reconstruction device, use 0545T.

**0483T** Transcatheter mitral valve implantation/replacement (TMVI) with prosthetic valve; percutaneous approach, including transseptal puncture, when performed

## Rationale

In accordance with the deletion of codes 93530-93533 and the establishment of codes 93593-93598, the guidelines for Category III code 0483T (transcatheter mitral valve implantation/replacement) have been revised to reflect these changes.

Refer to the codebook and the Rationale for codes 93593-93598 for a full discussion of these changes.

►Near-infrared spectroscopy is used to measure cutaneous vascular perfusion. Code 0493T describes near-infrared spectroscopy of lower extremity wounds that requires direct contact of the spectrometer sensors with the patient's skin. Codes 0640T, 0641T, 0642T describe noncontact near-infrared spectroscopy of skin flaps or wounds for measurement of cutaneous vascular perfusion that does not require direct contact of the spectrometer sensors with the patient's skin.◄

▲ **0493T** Contact near-infrared spectroscopy studies of lower extremity wounds (eg, for oxyhemoglobin measurement)

►(For noncontact near-infrared spectroscopy studies, see 0640T, 0641T, 0642T)◄

#● **0640T** Noncontact near-infrared spectroscopy studies of flap or wound (eg, for measurement of deoxyhemoglobin, oxyhemoglobin, and ratio of tissue oxygenation [StO$_2$]); image acquisition, interpretation and report, each flap or wound

#● **0641T** image acquisition only, each flap or wound

►(Do not report 0641T in conjunction with 0640T, 0642T)◄

#● **0642T** interpretation and report only, each flap or wound

►(Do not report 0642T in conjunction with 0640T, 0641T)◄

►(For contact near-infrared spectroscopy studies, use 0493T)◄

## Rationale

Three new Category III codes (0640T-0642T) with new introductory guidelines have been established to report noncontact near-infrared spectroscopy studies. Code 0493T has been revised to support the addition of these new codes. In addition, several parenthetical notes have been added to provide guidance on the appropriate reporting of these new codes.

As stated in the new introductory guidelines, near-infrared spectroscopy is used to measure cutaneous vascular perfusion.

Code 0493T has been revised to specify the term "Contact" in the code descriptor in order to distinguish between services for noncontact near-infrared spectroscopy studies and contact near-infrared spectroscopy studies. Code 0640T describes the complete study for noncontact near-infrared spectroscopy for a flap or a wound. The examples provided in parentheses within the code descriptor list the types of measurements being performed, including measurement of deoxyhemoglobin, oxyhemoglobin, and ratio of tissue oxygenation (StO$_2$).

★ = Telemedicine   ✚ = Add-on code   ⃫ = FDA approval pending   # = Resequenced code   ⊘ = Modifier 51 exempt

Code 0641T is reported for the image acquisition only of each flap or wound. Code 0642T is reported for the interpretation and report only of each flap or wound.

To assist in the appropriate reporting of this new series of codes, two exclusionary parenthetical notes have been added following codes 0641T and 0642T. The first parenthetical note restricts reporting code 0641T with codes 0640T and 0642T. The second parenethetical note restricts reporting code 0642T with codes 0640T and 0641T. In addition, two cross-reference parenthetical notes have been added to direct users to the appropriate codes to report noncontact and contact near-infrared spectroscopy studies.

## Clinical Example (0640T)

A 65-year-old obese female, who has a history of heart disease, type II diabetes mellitus, and peripheral neuropathy, presents with a left foot ulcer. The oxygenation of the peri-ulcer skin is assessed with noncontact near-infrared spectroscopy.

A 50-year-old female, who is undergoing a bilateral nipple-sparing mastectomy with immediate reconstruction, undergoes evaluation of the oxygenation of the breast flaps using noncontact near-infrared spectroscopy.

## Description of Procedure (0640T)

Power on and calibrate the noncontact near-infrared spectrometer. The physician or other qualified health care professional (QHP) logs in and enters the patient information. Prepare the flap or wound, ensuring it is fully exposed, clean, and dry. Position the spectrometer over the area of interest and acquire images of the flap or peri-wound skin. The physician or other QHP reviews and manipulates the images. Note the biomarker values and assess them for flap or peri-wound skin viability. Incorporate the interpretation of the spectroscopy images in a report and download the report to the patient's record.

## Clinical Example (0641T)

A 65-year-old obese female, who has a history of heart disease, type II diabetes mellitus, and peripheral neuropathy, presents with a left foot ulcer. The oxygenation of the peri-ulcer skin is assessed with noncontact near-infrared spectroscopy.

A 50-year-old female, who is undergoing a bilateral nipple-sparing mastectomy with immediate reconstruction, undergoes evaluation of the oxygenation of the breast flaps using noncontact near-infrared spectroscopy.

## Description of Procedure (0641T)

Power on and calibrate the noncontact near-infrared spectrometer. The physician or other QHP logs in and enters the patient information. Prepare the flap or wound, ensuring it is fully exposed, clean, and dry. Position the spectrometer over the area of interest and acquire images of the flap or peri-wound skin. The physician or other QHP reviews and manipulates the images. Note the biomarker values. Download the images and biomarker data to the patient's record.

## Clinical Example (0642T)

A 65-year-old obese female, who has a history of heart disease, type II diabetes mellitus, and peripheral neuropathy, presents with a left foot ulcer. The oxygenation of the peri-ulcer skin is assessed with noncontact near-infrared spectroscopy.

A 50-year-old female, who is undergoing a bilateral nipple-sparing mastectomy with immediate reconstruction, undergoes evaluation of the oxygenation of the breast flaps using noncontact near-infrared spectroscopy.

## Description of Procedure (0642T)

Interpret and incorporate the spectroscopy images and biomarker values in a report. Download the report to the patient's record and forward it to the ordering physician or other QHP.

| Code | Description |
|------|-------------|
| 0501T | Noninvasive estimated coronary fractional flow reserve (FFR) derived from coronary computed tomography angiography data using computation fluid dynamics physiologic simulation software analysis of functional data to assess the severity of coronary artery disease; data preparation and transmission, analysis of fluid dynamics and simulated maximal coronary hyperemia, generation of estimated FFR model, with anatomical data review in comparison with estimated FFR model to reconcile discordant data, interpretation and report |
| 0502T | data preparation and transmission |
| 0503T | analysis of fluid dynamics and simulated maximal coronary hyperemia, and generation of estimated FFR model |
| 0504T | anatomical data review in comparison with estimated FFR model to reconcile discordant data, interpretation and report |

(Report 0501T, 0502T, 0503T, 0504T one time per coronary CT angiogram)

(Do not report 0501T in conjunction with 0502T, 0503T, 0504T, 0523T)

(For automated quantification and characterization of coronary plaque using coronary computed tomographic angiography data, see 0623T, 0624T, 0625T, 0626T)

▶Automated quantification and characterization of coronary atherosclerotic plaque is a service in which coronary computed tomographic angiography (CTA) data are analyzed using computerized algorithms to assess the extent and severity of coronary artery disease. The computer-generated findings are provided in an interactive format to the physician or other qualified health care professional who performs the final review and report. The coronary CTA is performed and interpreted as a separate service and is not included in the service of automated analysis of coronary CTA.◀

| | | |
|---|---|---|
| # **0623T** | | Automated quantification and characterization of coronary atherosclerotic plaque to assess severity of coronary disease, using data from coronary computed tomographic angiography; data preparation and transmission, computerized analysis of data, with review of computerized analysis output to reconcile discordant data, interpretation and report |
| # **0624T** | | data preparation and transmission |
| # **0625T** | | computerized analysis of data from coronary computed tomographic angiography |
| # **0626T** | | review of computerized analysis output to reconcile discordant data, interpretation and report |

(Use 0623T, 0624T, 0625T, 0626T one time per coronary computed tomographic angiogram)

(Do not report 0623T in conjunction with 0624T, 0625T, 0626T)

(Do not report 0623T, 0624T, 0625T, 0626T in conjunction with 76376, 76377)

(For noninvasive estimated coronary fractional flow reserve [FFR] derived from coronary computed tomography angiography data, see 0501T, 0502T, 0503T, 0504T)

## Rationale

New introductory guidelines have been established in the Category III section before codes 0623T, 0624T, 0625T, and 0626T.

The guidelines describe the process of performing automated quantification and characterization of coronary atherosclerotic plaque from coronary computed tomographic angiography (CTA) data that are analyzed using computerized algorithms to assess the extent and severity of coronary artery disease.

# Wireless Cardiac Stimulation System for Left Ventricular Pacing

A wireless cardiac stimulator system provides biventricular pacing by sensing right ventricular pacing output from a previously implanted conventional device (pacemaker or defibrillator, with univentricular or biventricular leads), and then transmitting an ultrasound pulse to a wireless electrode implanted on the endocardium of the left ventricle, which then emits a left ventricular pacing pulse.

The complete system consists of two components: a wireless endocardial left ventricle electrode and a pulse generator. The pulse generator has two components: a transmitter and a battery. The electrode is implanted transarterially into the left ventricular wall and powered wirelessly using ultrasound delivered by a subcutaneously implanted transmitter. Two subcutaneous pockets are created on the chest wall, one for the battery and one for the transmitter, and these two components are connected by a subcutaneously tunneled cable.

Patients with a wireless cardiac stimulator require programming/interrogation of their existing conventional device, as well as the wireless device. The wireless cardiac stimulator is programmed and interrogated with its own separate programmer and settings.

Code 0515T describes insertion of a complete wireless cardiac stimulator system (electrode and pulse generator, which includes transmitter and battery), including interrogation, programming, pocket creation, revision and repositioning, and all echocardiography and other imaging to guide the procedure, when performed. Use 0516T only when insertion of the electrode is a stand-alone procedure. For insertion of only a new generator or generator component (battery and/or transmitter), use 0517T.

For removal of only the generator or a generator component (battery and/or transmitter) without replacement, use 0518T. For removal and replacement of a generator or a generator component (battery and/or transmitter), use 0519T. For battery and/or generator removal and reinsertion performed together with a new electrode insertion, use 0520T.

All catheterization and imaging guidance (including transthoracic or transesophageal echocardiography) required to complete a wireless cardiac stimulator procedure is included in 0515T, 0516T, 0517T, 0518T, 0519T, 0520T. Do not report 76000, 76998, 93303-93355 in conjunction with 0515T, 0516T, 0517T, 0518T, 0519T, 0520T.

▶Do not report left heart catheterization codes (93452, 93453, 93458, 93459, 93460, 93461, 93595, 93596, 93597) for delivery of a wireless cardiac stimulator electrode into the left ventricle.◀

★ = Telemedicine  ✚ = Add-on code  ✱ = FDA approval pending  # = Resequenced code  ⊘ = Modifier 51 exempt

**0515T** Insertion of wireless cardiac stimulator for left ventricular pacing, including device interrogation and programming, and imaging supervision and interpretation, when performed; complete system (includes electrode and generator [transmitter and battery])

## Rationale

In accordance with the deletion of codes 93531-93533 and the establishment of codes 93595-93597, the guidelines for Category III code 0515T (wireless cardiac stimulator insertion) have been revised to reflect these changes.

Refer to the codebook and the Rationale for codes 93595-93597 for a full discussion of these changes.

---

**0543T** Transapical mitral valve repair, including transthoracic echocardiography, when performed, with placement of artificial chordae tendineae

(For transesophageal echocardiography image guidance, use 93355)

Codes 0544T and 0545T include vascular access, catheterization, deploying and adjusting the reconstruction device(s), temporary pacemaker insertion for rapid pacing if required, and access site closure, when performed.

Angiography, radiological supervision and interpretation, intraprocedural roadmapping (eg, contrast injections, fluoroscopy) to guide the device implantation, ventriculography (eg, to assess target valve regurgitation for guidance of device implantation and adjustment), and completion angiography are included in 0544T and 0545T.

►Diagnostic right and left heart catheterization codes (93451, 93452, 93453, 93454, 93455, 93456, 93457, 93458, 93459, 93460, 93461, 93565, 93566, 93593, 93594, 93595, 93596, 93597, 93598) may not be used in conjunction with 0544T, 0545T to report:

1. Contrast injections, angiography, roadmapping, and/or fluoroscopic guidance for the implantation and adjustment of the transcatheter mitral or tricuspid valve annulus reconstruction device, or

2. Right or left ventricular angiography to assess or confirm transcatheter mitral or tricuspid valve annulus reconstruction device positioning and function, or

3. Right and left heart catheterization for hemodynamic measurements before, during, and after transcatheter mitral or tricuspid valve annulus reconstruction for guidance.

Diagnostic right and left heart catheterization codes (93451, 93452, 93453, 93456, 93457, 93458, 93459, 93460, 93461, 93593, 93594, 93595, 93596, 93597, 93598) and diagnostic coronary angiography codes (93454, 93455, 93456, 93457, 93458, 93459, 93460, 93461, 93563, 93564) performed at the time of transcatheter mitral or tricuspid valve annulus reconstruction may be separately reportable, if:

1. No prior study is available and a full diagnostic study is performed, or

2. A prior study is available, but as documented in the medical record:

   a. There is inadequate visualization of the anatomy and/or pathology, or

   b. The patient's condition with respect to the clinical indication has changed since the prior study, or

   c. There is a clinical change during the procedure that requires new evaluation.◄

Other cardiac catheterization services may be reported separately, when performed for diagnostic purposes not intrinsic to the transcatheter mitral valve annulus reconstruction.

For same session/same day diagnostic cardiac catheterization services, report the appropriate diagnostic cardiac catheterization code(s) appended with modifier 59 indicating separate and distinct procedural service from transcatheter mitral or tricuspid valve annulus reconstruction.

Percutaneous coronary interventional procedures may be reported separately, when performed.

When cardiopulmonary bypass is performed in conjunction with transcatheter mitral valve or tricuspid valve annulus reconstruction, 0544T, 0545T should be reported with the appropriate add-on code for percutaneous peripheral bypass (33367), open peripheral bypass (33368), or central bypass (33369).

When transcatheter ventricular support is required, the appropriate code may be reported with the appropriate ventricular assist device (VAD) procedure (33990, 33991, 33992, 33993) or balloon pump insertion (33967, 33970, 33973).

For percutaneous transcatheter mitral valve repair, use 0345T. For percutaneous transcatheter mitral valve implantation/replacement (TMVI) with prosthetic valve, use 0483T.

**0545T** Transcatheter tricuspid valve annulus reconstruction with implantation of adjustable annulus reconstruction device, percutaneous approach

(Do not report 0544T, 0545T in conjunction with 76000)

►(Do not report 0544T, 0545T in conjunction with 93451, 93452, 93453, 93456, 93457, 93458, 93459, 93460, 93461, 93565, 93566, 93593, 93594, 93595, 93596, 93597, 93598 for diagnostic left and right heart catheterization procedures intrinsic to the annular repair procedure)◄

(Do not report 0544T, 0545T in conjunction with 93454, 93455, 93456, 93457, 93458, 93459, 93460, 93461, 93563, 93564 for coronary angiography procedures intrinsic to the annular repair procedure)

►(For transcatheter left ventricular restoration device implantation from an arterial approach not necessitating transseptal puncture, use 0643T)◄

## Rationale

In accordance with the deletion of codes 93530-93533 and the establishment of codes 93593-93598, the guidelines and the conditional exclusionary parenthetical note for Category III codes 0544T and 0545T (transcatheter valve annulus reconstruction) have been revised to reflect these changes. In accordance with the establishment of Category III code 0643T, a cross-reference parenthetical note has been added following code 0545T directing users to report code 0643T for transcatheter left ventricular restoration device implantation.

Refer to the codebook and the Rationale for codes 93593-93598 and 0643T for a full discussion of these changes.

►Code 0643T includes the primary arterial vascular access and contralateral arterial access and percutaneous access site closure, when performed. Guide catheter(s) and snare wire(s) may be required to advance the device to the treatment zone and are included in 0643T when performed. Left heart catheterization, intracardiac device customization, deploying, cinching, and adjusting the left ventricular restoration device are inherent to the procedure. Right heart catheterization may be performed for guidance of hemodynamics during device placement and is included in the procedure when performed for this purpose. Related angiography, radiological supervision and interpretation, intraprocedural roadmapping (eg, contrast injections, fluoroscopy) to guide the device implantation, ventriculography (eg, to assess ventricular shape, guidance of device implantation and adjustment), and completion angiography are included in 0643T.

Diagnostic right and left heart catheterization codes (93451, 93452, 93453, 93456, 93457, 93458, 93459, 93460, 93461, 93593, 93594, 93595, 93596, 93597), diagnostic coronary angiography codes (93454, 93455, 93456, 93457, 93458, 93459, 93460, 93461, 93563, 93564), and left ventriculography code (93565) may not be used in conjunction with 0643T to report:

1. Contrast injections, angiography, roadmapping, and/or fluoroscopic guidance for the implantation, intracardiac customization, deploying, cinching, and adjustment of the left ventricular restoration device, or

2. Left ventricular angiography to assess or confirm transcatheter left ventricular restoration device positioning and function, or

3. Right and left heart catheterization for hemodynamic measurements before, during, and after transcatheter left ventricular restoration device implantation for guidance.

Diagnostic right and left heart catheterization codes (93451, 93452, 93453, 93456, 93457, 93458, 93459, 93460, 93461, 93593, 93594, 93595, 93596, 93597) and diagnostic coronary angiography codes (93454, 93455, 93456, 93457, 93458, 93459, 93460, 93461, 93563, 93564) performed at the time of transcatheter left ventricular restoration device implantation may be separately reportable, if:

1. No prior study is available and a full diagnostic study is performed, or

2. A prior study is available, but as documented in the medical record:

    a. There is inadequate visualization of the anatomy and/or pathology, or

    b. The patient's condition with respect to the clinical indication has changed since the prior study, or

    c. There is clinical change during the procedure that requires new evaluation.

Other cardiac catheterization services may be reported separately, when performed for diagnostic purposes not intrinsic to transcatheter left ventricular restoration device implantation.

For same session/same day diagnostic cardiac catheterization services not intrinsic to the transcatheter left ventricular restoration device implantation procedure, report the appropriate diagnostic cardiac catheterization code(s) appended with modifier 59, indicating separate and distinct procedural service from transcatheter left ventricular restoration device implantation.

Percutaneous coronary interventional procedures may be reported separately, when performed.

When cardiopulmonary bypass is performed in conjunction with transcatheter left ventricular restoration device implantation, 0643T should be reported with the appropriate add-on code for percutaneous peripheral bypass (33367), open peripheral bypass (33368), or central bypass (33369).

When transcatheter ventricular support is required, the appropriate code may be reported with the appropriate ventricular assist device (VAD) procedure (33990, 33991, 33992, 33993) or balloon pump insertion (33967, 33970, 33973).

For transcatheter mitral valve annulus reconstruction with implantation of adjustable annulus reconstruction device from a venous approach, necessitating transseptal puncture, use 0544T.◄

**# ● 0643T**   Transcatheter left ventricular restoration device implantation including right and left heart catheterization and left ventriculography when performed, arterial approach

▶(Do not report 0643T in conjunction with 76000)◀

▶(Do not report 0643T in conjunction with 93451, 93452, 93453, 93456, 93457, 93458, 93459, 93460, 93461, 93565, 93593, 93594, 93595, 93596, 93597, for diagnostic right and left heart catheterization procedures or ventriculography intrinsic to the left ventricular restoration device implantation procedure)◀

▶(Do not report 0643T in conjunction with 93454, 93455, 93456, 93457, 93458, 93459, 93460, 93461, 93563, 93564, for coronary angiography procedures intrinsic to the left ventricular restoration device implantation procedure)◀

## Rationale

Code 0643T has been established to report transcatheter left ventricular restoration device implantation using an arterial approach. New guidelines and parenthetical notes have been added to provide instructions on the appropriate reporting of code 0643T.

This procedure is intended to treat heart conditions such as left ventricular failure and congestive heart failure. As indicated in the code descriptor, code 0643T includes right and left heart catheterization and left ventriculography, when performed. The new guidelines clarify the work that is included in the procedure, as well as procedures that may be reported separately when performed at the time of the procedure.

Three conditional exclusionary parenthetical notes have also been added following code 0643T to provide further clarification on the codes that may not be reported with code 0643T.

## Clinical Example (0643T)

A 67-year-old female presents with progressive shortness of breath and established symptomatic heart failure with reduced ejection fraction (HFrEF), despite guideline-directed medical therapy. She has been hospitalized due to heart failure during the previous 12 months and had a B-type natriuretic peptide (BNP) of 2500 pg/mL within the past 90 days.

## Description of Procedure (0643T)

Initiate general anesthesia. Obtain vascular access. Advance a guidewire and then a subsequent guide catheter (GC) into the femoral artery. Track the guidewire and GC up the aorta, retrograde across the aortic valve into the left ventricle (LV), settling the guide tip in the anterior subannular space between the left ventricular outflow tract (LVOT) and anterolateral papillary muscle. (In a small percentage [approximately 10%] of cases, contralateral vascular access may also be performed with the subsequent advancement of a guidewire and then a snare wire to assist in device maneuvers.)

Track a specialized navigation catheter and its guidewire through the GC. Traverse the specialized navigation catheter and guidewire around the perimeter of the left ventricle (LV) free wall and intraventricular septum, and then back out the aortic valve. Once properly positioned below the mitral apparatus, exchange the guidewire for a larger diameter guidewire. Exchange the specialized navigation catheter for a specialized windowed catheter over the larger guidewire. Position the curve-shaped specialized windowed catheter along the LV free wall from the guide tip at the LVOT around to the junction of the free wall and septum.

The specialized windowed catheter acts as a template for subsequent anchor placement through pre-cut windows on its outer radius and is in contact with the endocardium along the entire LV basal free wall. The inner tunnel within the specialized windowed catheter has a single window, which can then be incrementally withdrawn to align with each of the outer specialized windowed catheter windows to facilitate anchor exit and delivery at appropriately spaced intervals.

Individually place approximately 13 anchors. Use the specialized windowed catheter to determine the number of anchors to use during the procedure based on each patient's specific anatomy. (The number of anchors that can be placed ranges from approximately 10 to 16 anchors.) Route the cable that comes pre-attached to the first anchor deployed through the eyelets of each subsequent anchor (and sliders) prior to their delivery. Deliver each anchor via a separate specialized delivery catheter. Track the delivery catheter up the specialized windowed catheter to exit through the aligned window and then advance the tip into the left ventricular myocardium to a pre-determined depth for each anchor placed. Deploy the anchor, housed within the tip of the delivery catheter, releasing it from the delivery catheter while allowing its self-expanding nitinol arms to anchor into the myocardium.

Deliver the anchors sequentially from the junction of the LV free wall and septum around to the guide tip adjacent the LVOT, subtending an arc of approximately 220 degrees at the base of the ventricle and along the entire ventricular free wall. Prior to each delivery catheter being tracked, place a slider over the cable such that sliders can be located between each pair of anchors to distribute the applied load among anchors when the implant is cinched.

Once the final anchor has been deployed, remove the specialized windowed catheter and guidewire from the guide and apply tension to the cinch cable using a specialized cinch and lock catheter. Once the implant has been cinched and the LV free wall radius reduced, use the same catheter to actuate a nitinol lock, which maintains the tension within the implant. Use a separate cut catheter to cut the excess cable length prior to removal of the GC.

Remove the remaining catheters and sheaths from the femoral vasculature with antagonism of the heparin anticoagulation with protamine, and close the arteriotomy with standard technique.

**0547T**  Bone-material quality testing by microindentation(s) of the tibia(s), with results reported as a score

▶(0548T, 0549T, 0550T, 0551T have been deleted)◀

▶(To report unilateral or bilateral insertion, removal, or fluid adjustment of a periurethral adjustable balloon continence device, see 53451, 53452, 53453, 53454)◀

## Rationale

In accordance with the conversion of Category III codes 0548T-0551T to Category I codes 53451-53454, codes 0548T-0551T have been deleted. A deletion parenthetical note has been added to reflect these changes. In addition, a cross-reference parenthetical note has been added directing users to report new codes 53451-53454.

Refer to the codebook and the Rationale for codes 53451-53454 for a full discussion of these changes.

**0554T**  Bone strength and fracture risk using finite element analysis of functional data and bone-mineral density utilizing data from a computed tomography scan; retrieval and transmission of the scan data, assessment of bone strength and fracture risk and bone-mineral density, interpretation and report

(Do not report 0554T in conjunction with 0555T, 0556T, 0557T)

**0555T**  retrieval and transmission of the scan data

**0556T**  assessment of bone strength and fracture risk and bone-mineral density

**0557T**  interpretation and report

▶(Do not report 0554T, 0555T, 0556T, 0557T in conjunction with 0691T)◀

## Rationale

In accordance with the addition of Category III code 0691T, the exclusionary parenthetical note following code 0557T has been added to restrict reporting codes 0554T-0557T with code 0691T.

Refer to the codebook and the Rationale for code 0691T for a full discussion of these changes.

**0558T**  Computed tomography scan taken for the purpose of biomechanical computed tomography analysis

▶(Do not report 0558T in conjunction with 71250, 71260, 71270, 71275, 72125, 72126, 72127, 72128, 72129, 72130, 72131, 72132, 72133, 72191, 72192, 72193, 72194, 74150, 74160, 74170, 74174, 74175, 74176, 74177, 74178, 74261, 74262, 74263, 75571, 75572, 75573, 75574, 75635, 78816, 0691T)◀

## Rationale

In accordance with the addition of Category III code 0691T, the exclusionary parenthetical note following code 0558T has been revised with the addition of code 0691T.

Refer to the codebook and the Rationale for code 0691T for a full discussion of these changes.

## Tricuspid Valve Repair

Codes 0569T, 0570T include the work of percutaneous vascular access, placing the access sheath, cardiac catheterization, advancing the repair device system into position, repositioning the prosthesis as needed, deploying the prosthesis, and vascular closure. Code 0569T may only be reported once per session. Add-on code 0570T is reported in conjunction with 0569T for each additional prosthesis placed.

For open tricuspid valve procedures, see 33460, 33463, 33464, 33465, 33468.

Angiography, radiological supervision and interpretation performed to guide transcatheter tricuspid valve repair (TTVr) (eg, guiding device placement and documenting completion of the intervention) are included in these codes.

Intracardiac echocardiography (93662), when performed, is included in 0569T, 0570T. Transesophageal echocardiography (93355) performed by a separate operator for guidance of the procedure may be separately reported.

►Fluoroscopy (76000) and diagnostic right and left heart catheterization codes (93451, 93452, 93453, 93456, 93457, 93458, 93459, 93460, 93461, 93566, 93593, 93594, 93595, 93596, 93597, 93598) may **not** be used with 0569T, 0570T to report the following techniques for guidance of TTVr:

1. Contrast injections, angiography, roadmapping, and/or fluoroscopic guidance for the TTVr,

2. Right ventricular angiography to assess tricuspid regurgitation for guidance of TTVr, or

3. Right and left heart catheterization for hemodynamic measurements before, during, and after TTVr for guidance of TTVr.

Diagnostic right and left heart catheterization codes (93451, 93452, 93453, 93456, 93457, 93458, 93459, 93460, 93461, 93566,93593, 93594, 93595, 93596, 93597, 93598) and diagnostic coronary angiography codes (93454, 93455, 93456, 93457, 93458, 93459, 93460, 93461, 93563, 93564) may be reported with 0569T, 0570T, representing separate and distinct services from TTVr, if:

1. No prior study is available and a full diagnostic study is performed, or

2. A prior study is available but as documented in the medical record:

   a. There is inadequate evaluation of the anatomy and/or pathology, or

   b. The patient's condition with respect to the clinical indication has changed since the prior study, or

   c. There is a clinical change during the procedure that requires new diagnostic evaluation.◄

Other cardiac catheterization services may be reported separately when performed for diagnostic purposes not intrinsic to TTVr.

For same session/same day diagnostic cardiac catheterization services, report the appropriate diagnostic cardiac catheterization code(s) with modifier 59 indicating separate and distinct procedural service from TTVr.

Diagnostic coronary angiography performed at a separate session from an interventional procedure may be separately reportable.

Percutaneous coronary interventional procedures may be reported separately, when performed.

When transcatheter ventricular support is required in conjunction with TTVr, the procedure may be reported with the appropriate ventricular assist device (VAD) procedure code (33990, 33991, 33992, 33993) or balloon pump insertion code (33967, 33970, 33973).

When cardiopulmonary bypass is performed in conjunction with TTVr, 0569T, 0570T may be reported with the appropriate add-on code for percutaneous peripheral bypass (33367), open peripheral bypass (33368), or central bypass (33369).

**0569T** Transcatheter tricuspid valve repair, percutaneous approach; initial prosthesis

**+ 0570T** each additional prosthesis during same session (List separately in addition to code for primary procedure)

## Rationale

In accordance with the deletion of codes 93530-93533 and the establishment of codes 93593-93598, the guidelines for Category III code 0569T (transcatheter tricuspid valve repair) have been revised to reflect these changes.

Refer to the codebook and the Rationale for codes 93593-93598 for a full discussion of these changes.

## ►Tricuspid Valve Implantation/Replacement◄

►Code 0646T includes vascular access, catheterization, repositioning the valve delivery device as needed, deploying the valve, temporary pacemaker insertion for rapid pacing (33210), and access site closure by any method, when performed.

Angiography (eg, peripheral), radiological supervision and interpretation, intraprocedural roadmapping (eg, contrast injections, fluoroscopy, intracardiac echocardiography) to guide the transcatheter tricuspid valve implantation (TTVI)/replacement, right atrial and/or right ventricular angiography (eg, to assess tricuspid regurgitation for guidance of TTVI), and completion angiography are included in 0646T.

Transesophageal echocardiography (93355) performed by a separate operator for guidance of the procedure may be separately reported. Intracardiac echocardiography (93662) is not separately reportable when performed.

Diagnostic right heart catheterization codes (93451, 93453, 93456, 93457, 93460, 93461, 93593, 93594, 93596, 93597) and right atrial/right ventricular angiography code (93566) should not be used with 0646T to report:

1. Contrast injections, angiography, roadmapping, and/or fluoroscopic guidance for the TTVI,

2. Right atrial and/or ventricular angiography to assess or confirm valve positioning and function,

3. Right heart catheterization for hemodynamic measurements before, during, and after TTVI for guidance of TTVI.

Diagnostic right heart catheterization codes (93451, 93453, 93456, 93457, 93460, 93461, 93593, 93594, 93596, 93597) and right atrial/right ventricular angiography code (93566) performed at the time of TTVI may be separately reportable, if:

1. No prior study is available and a full diagnostic study is performed, or

2. A prior study is available, but as documented in the medical record:

   a. There is inadequate visualization of the anatomy and/or pathology,or

   b. The patient's condition with respect to the clinical indication has changed since the prior study, or

   c. There is a clinical change during the procedure that requires new evaluation.

For same session/same day diagnostic cardiac catheterization services, report the appropriate diagnostic cardiac catheterization code(s) appended with modifier 59, indicating separate and distinct procedural service from TTVI.

When transcatheter ventricular support is required in conjunction with TTVI, the procedure may be reported with the appropriate ventricular assist device (VAD) procedure code (33990, 33991, 33992, 33993) or balloon pump insertion code (33967, 33970, 33973).◄

#● **0646T**    Transcatheter tricuspid valve implantation (TTVI)/replacement with prosthetic valve, percutaneous approach, including right heart catheterization, temporary pacemaker insertion, and selective right ventricular or right atrial angiography, when performed

▶(Do not report 0646T in conjunction with 33210, 33211 for temporary pacemaker insertion)◄

▶(Do not report 0646T in conjunction with 93451, 93453, 93456, 93457, 93460, 93461, 93503, 93566, 93593, 93594, 93596, 93597, for diagnostic right heart catheterization procedures intrinsic to the valve repair procedure)◄

▶(Do not report 0646T in conjunction with 93662 for imaging guidance with intracardiac echocardiography)◄

▶(For transcatheter tricuspid valve annulus reconstruction, use 0545T)◄

▶(For transcatheter tricuspid valve repair, see 0569T, 0570T)◄

## Rationale

A new subsection that includes a new code (0646T) and guidelines for tricuspid valve implantation (TTVI)/replacement has been added to the Category III section. Category III code 0646T describes TTVI/replacement with a prosthetic valve.

Three existing Category III codes (0545T, 0569T, 0570T) describe transcatheter tricuspid valve procedures. Code 0545T describes transcatheter reconstruction of the tricuspid valve annulus in which a number of anchors is implanted along the tricuspid valve annulus prior to implantation of an adjustable annulus reconstruction device. Codes 0569T and 0570T describe transcatheter repair of the existing tricuspid valve using prosthetic clip(s), for example. New code 0646T describes a new transcatheter procedure in which a valve prosthesis is implanted, or an existing prosthesis is replaced, within the tricuspid valve.

As indicated in the code descriptor, code 0646T includes right heart catheterization, temporary pacemaker insertion, and selective right ventricular or right atrial angiography, when performed. The new guidelines clarify the work included in the TTVI/replacement procedure, as well as procedures that may be reported separately when performed at the time of the procedure.

Several exclusionary and cross-reference parenthetical notes have been added following code 0646T to provide further instruction on the appropriate reporting of the procedure.

## Clinical Example (0646T)

A 69-year-old female presents with severe symptomatic tricuspid regurgitation and worsening right-sided heart failure. Prior diagnostic transesophageal echocardiography (TEE) demonstrated tricuspid regurgitation with right ventricular dysfunction. Upon evaluation, it is determined that she is at high risk for open valve surgery. She is recommended for transcatheter tricuspid valve implantation.

## Description of Procedure (0646T)

Initiate general anesthesia and place the hemodynamic monitoring lines. Place the TEE probe for guidance (reported separately when performed by a different physician). Obtain femoral vein access. Under fluoroscopic guidance, insert a guidewire into the femoral vein and advance it to the superior vena cava. After serial dilation and upsizing the femoral vein, advance a sheath into the right atrium of the heart and remove the dilator and guidewire.

Using a combination of fluoroscopic and echocardiographic guidance, advance the valve delivery catheter via the vena cava to the right atrium. Confirm entry and positioning in the right atrium by fluoroscopy and TEE. Determine the appropriate position for deployment of the valve within the tricuspid plane by right ventriculography and TEE. Using the appropriate echocardiographic modalities (TEE, intracardiac echocardiography [ICE]) visualization and fluoroscopic guidance, cross the tricuspid valve and position the delivery catheter within the tricuspid valve. Under rapid pacing by a temporary transvenous pacemaker electrode, partially expand the transcatheter tricuspid valve prosthesis to judge the appropriate depth of deployment.

Optimize the position of the prosthetic valve in relation to the patient's anatomy while remaining above the native annulus to enable blood flow prior to full deployment. Under rapid pacing by a temporary transvenous pacemaker electrode, advance the device to the annulus and, using fluoroscopy to monitor expansion of the prosthesis and appropriate echocardiographic modalities (eg, TEE, ICE) to assure proper positioning, fully expand and release the transcatheter tricuspid valve prosthesis.

After deployment of the new valve prosthesis, withdraw the delivery catheter across the valve and from the right atrium. Retract and remove the catheter through the sheath. Confirm proper positioning and functioning of the valve, including any perivalvular leakage, by TEE. Measure and evaluate the degree of regurgitation and resultant gradients. Remove the sheath and close venous access.

**0613T**    Percutaneous transcatheter implantation of interatrial septal shunt device, including right and left heart catheterization, intracardiac echocardiography, and imaging guidance by the proceduralist, when performed

▶(Do not report 0613T in conjunction with 76937, 93313, 93314, 93318, 93355, 93451, 93452, 93453, 93456, 93457, 93458, 93459, 93460, 93461, 93462, 93593, 93594, 93595, 93596, 93597, 93598, 93662)◀

## Rationale

In accordance with the deletion of codes 93530-93533 and the establishment of codes 93593-93598, the exclusionary parenthetical note following Category III code 0613T has been revised to reflect these changes.

Refer to the codebook and the Rationale for codes 93593-93598 for a full discussion of these changes.

**0620T**    Code is out of numerical sequence. See 0503T-0507T

**0626T**    Code is out of numerical sequence. See 0503T-0507T

**0632T**    Percutaneous transcatheter ultrasound ablation of nerves innervating the pulmonary arteries, including right heart catheterization, pulmonary artery angiography, and all imaging guidance

▶(Do not report 0632T in conjunction with 36013, 36014, 36015, 75741, 75743, 75746, 93451, 93453, 93456, 93460, 93503, 93505, 93568, 93593, 93594, 93596, 93597)◀

## Rationale

In accordance with the establishment of codes 93593-93597, the exclusionary parenthetical note following code 0632T has been revised to reflect these changes.

Refer to the codebook and the Rationale for codes 93593-93597 for a full discussion of these changes.

**0640T**    Code is out of numerical sequence. See 0492T-0495T

**0641T**    Code is out of numerical sequence. See 0492T-0495T

**0642T**    Code is out of numerical sequence. See 0492T-0495T

▶Code 0644T is for transcatheter percutaneous removal or debulking of intracardiac vegetations (eg, endocarditis) or mass(es) (eg, thrombus) using a suction device. Code 0644T includes the work of percutaneous access, all associated sheath device introduction, manipulation and positioning of guidewires and selective and non-selective catheterizations (eg, 36140, 36200, 36215, 36216, 36217, 36218, 36245, 36246, 36247, 36248), blood vessel dilation, embolic protection if used, percutaneous venous thrombectomy (eg, 37187, 37188), and closure of the blood vessel by pressure or application of an access vessel arterial closure device.

If an axillary, femoral, or iliac conduit is required to facilitate access of the catheter, 34714, 34716, or 34833 may be reported in addition to 0644T.

Extensive repair or replacement of a blood vessel (eg, 35206, 35226, 35231, 35236, 35256, 35266, 35286, 35302, 35371) may be reported separately.

Fluoroscopic and ultrasound guidance used in conjunction with percutaneous intracardiac mass removal is not separately reported. Transesophageal echocardiography guidance may be reported separately when provided by a separate provider.

The insertion and removal of arterial and/or venous cannula(e) (eg, 33951, 33952, 33953, 33954, 33955, 33956, 33965, 33966, 33969, 33984, 33985, 33986) and initiation (eg, 33946, 33947) of the extracorporeal circuit (veno-arterial or veno-venous) for intraoperative reinfusion of aspirated blood is included in the procedure. If prolonged extracorporeal membrane oxygenation (ECMO) or extracorporeal life support (ECLS) is required at the conclusion of the procedure, then the appropriate ECMO cannula(e) insertion code (eg, 33951, 33952, 33953, 33954, 33955, 33956), removal code (33965, 33966, 33969, 33984, 33985, 33986), and initiation code (eg, 33946, 33947) may be reported in addition to 0644T.

Other interventional procedures performed at the time of percutaneous intracardiac mass removal may be reported separately (eg, removal of infected pacemaker leads, removal of tunneled catheters, placement of dialysis catheters, valve repair, or replacement).

When transcatheter ventricular support is required in conjunction with percutaneous intracardiac mass removal, 0644T may be reported with the appropriate ventricular assist device (VAD) procedure code (33975, 33976, 33990, 33991, 33992, 33993, 33995, 33997, 33999) or balloon pump insertion code (33967, 33970, 33973).

When cardiopulmonary bypass is performed in conjunction with percutaneous intracardiac mass removal, 0644T may be reported with the appropriate add-on code for percutaneous peripheral bypass (33367), open peripheral bypass (33368), or central bypass (33369).◄

**0643T**     Code is out of numerical sequence. See 0544T-0547T

● **0644T**     Transcatheter removal or debulking of intracardiac mass (eg, vegetations, thrombus) via suction (eg, vacuum, aspiration) device, percutaneous approach, with intraoperative reinfusion of aspirated blood, including imaging guidance, when performed

▶(Do not report 0644T in conjunction with 37187, 37188)◄

## Rationale

Code 0644T has been established to report transcatheter removal or debulking of intracardiac mass via suction device through a percutaneous approach. In addition, guidelines have been included and parenthetical notes have been revised and added to provide instructions on the appropriate reporting of this service.

Code 0644T is used to identify percutaneous transcatheter removal or debulking of intracardiac masses using a suction device and includes intraoperative reinfusion of aspirated blood and imaging used for guidance during the procedure. The specificity of the language provides some insight regarding services that are inherently included as part of the procedure and that should not be separately reported.

Common to many cardiovascular services, guidelines that proceed the code listing also provide instruction regarding services that are inherently included. Services such as percutaneous access, sheath device introduction, guidewire manipulation and positioning, selective catheterizations, and guidance via fluoroscopy and/or ultrasound are specifically noted within the guidelines to alert users regarding services that may not be separately reported.

The guidelines also provide instruction regarding the services that are not inherently included. For these services, instruction is provided to direct users to the codes that may be reported separately in addition to the percutaneous intracardiac procedure. These include services such as extensive repair or replacement of a blood vessel, other interventional procedures performed at the time of percutaneous intracardiac mass removal (eg, removal of infected pacemaker leads and removal of tunneled catheters), and transcatheter ventricular support that may be required in conjunction with the percutaneous intracardiac mass removal.

Guidelines also provide instruction regarding special circumstances that may exist, allowing separate reporting of services that are ordinarily included and that allow use of certain add-on procedure codes in conjunction with the percutaneous intracardiac mass removal codes. A guideline instructs that transesophageal echocardiography guidance may be separately reported when provided by a separate provider allowing separate reporting of ultrasound imaging guidance services, which would ordinarily be included as part of the percutaneous intracardiac mass removal procedure, when completed by a provider who does not perform the mass removal procedure. Also provided is instruction that specifies that cardiopulmonary bypass services performed in conjunction with percutaneous intracardiac mass removal procedures may be reported with add-on codes for the percutaneous (33367), open peripheral (33368), or central (33369) bypass procedures.

To accommodate the addition of code 0644T and confirm the appropriate reporting of code 0644T with add-on codes 33367-33369, the add-on instructional parenthetical notes following these codes have been updated with the addition of code 0644T.

## Clinical Example (0644T)

A 27-year-old female presents with active intravenous (IV) drug use, fever, and bacteremia. An echocardiogram shows a 1.5-cm mobile mass on her tricuspid valve with embolic evidence to her lungs, which requires oxygen. After an appropriate trial of antibiotics, the cardiac lesion has not cleared. A consultation is made for the removal of the intracardiac mass. Due to her active drug use and pulmonary condition, she is not an ideal candidate for traditional open-heart surgery.

## Description of Procedure (0644T)

Take the patient to a suite with the capability to perform fluoroscopy and TEE. Administer general anesthesia. A qualified transesophageal echocardiographer is required for this procedure. Prepare and drape the patient from the patient's ears to her knees. Use ultrasound guidance for bilateral femoral vein access. Place a 6- to 7-French (Fr) catheter into each vessel over a wire, and exchange the wire for a stiffer, longer wire. Use fluoroscopy and

★ = Telemedicine    ✚ = Add-on code    ◢ = FDA approval pending    # = Resequenced code    ⊘ = Modifier 51 exempt

TEE to guide the longer wire into the heart. Administer heparin and measure activated clotting time (ACT) with a goal of achieving an ACT of greater than 250 seconds. In one femoral vein, use a modified Seldinger technique to dilate the return cannula to the size necessary (14- to 20-Fr) based on the patient's body-surface area. In the contralateral femoral vein, use a modified Seldinger technique to insert a 26-Fr dry-seal catheter, which will accommodate the 24-Fr aspiration thrombectomy cannula. Prepare and insert the vacuum cannula into the dry-seal catheter, and using fluoroscopy or TEE, guide the cannula into the cavoatrial junction. Initiate flows on the extracorporeal circuit between 2.5 to 4 liters per minute (lpm). Both a perfusionist and physician knowledgeable in cardiopulmonary bypass physiology are required for this procedure. Once flows are established and hemodynamics are stable, direct the device toward the material in the heart and continue aspiration until satisfactory results are obtained. Decrease flows until the circuit is off. Remove the cannulae and achieve hemostasis in the access vessels by placing deep sutures through the skin and applying manual compression. Capture the removed material within the device filter and send it for pathological and microbiological analysis upon completion of the case.

▶Code 0645T describes transcatheter implantation of a coronary sinus reduction device and includes vascular access, ultrasound guidance, vascular closure, right heart catheterization, coronary sinus catheterization, venography, coronary sinus angiography, right atrial or right ventricular angiography, any interventions in the coronary sinus, and any other imaging required for guidance of the coronary sinus reduction device placement.

Intracardiac echocardiography (93662), when performed, is included in 0645T. Transesophageal echocardiography (93355) performed by a separate operator for guidance of the procedure may be separately reported.

Diagnostic right heart catheterization codes (93451, 93453, 93456, 93457, 93460, 93461, 93566, 93593, 93594, 93596, 93597, 93598) should **not** be used in conjunction with 0645T to report contrast injections, angiography, roadmapping, fluoroscopic guidance for the coronary sinus reduction device implantation, right atrial, right ventricular, or coronary sinus angiography to assess or confirm device positioning and function, or right heart catheterization for hemodynamic measurements before, during, and after coronary sinus reduction device implantation for guidance of the procedure.

Diagnostic right and left heart catheterization codes (93451, 93452, 93453, 93456, 93457, 93458, 93459, 93460, 93461, 93566, 93593, 93594, 93595, 93596, 93597, 93598) and diagnostic coronary angiography

codes (93454, 93455, 93456, 93457, 93458, 93459, 93460, 93461, 93563, 93564) performed at the time of coronary sinus reduction device implantation may be separately reportable, if:

1. No prior study is available and a full diagnostic study is performed, or

2. A prior study is available, but as documented in the medical record:

    a. There is inadequate visualization of the anatomy and/or pathology, or

    b. The patient's condition with respect to the clinical indication has changed since the prior study, or

    c. There is a clinical change during the procedure that requires new evaluation.

For same session/same day diagnostic cardiac catheterization services, report the appropriate diagnostic cardiac catheterization code(s) appended with modifier 59, indicating separate and distinct procedural service from transcatheter coronary sinus reduction implantation.◀

● **0645T**     Transcatheter implantation of coronary sinus reduction device including vascular access and closure, right heart catheterization, venous angiography, coronary sinus angiography, imaging guidance, and supervision and interpretation, when performed

         ▶(Do not report 0645T in conjunction with 36010, 36011, 36012, 36013, 37246, 37247, 37252, 37253, 75827, 75860, 76000, 76499, 76937, 77001, 93451, 93453, 93456, 93457, 93460, 93461, 93566, 93593, 93594, 93596, 93597, 93598, 93662)◀

## Rationale

Code 0645T has been established to report the transcatheter implantation of a coronary sinus reduction device. Code 0645T describes a new procedure not previously described in the CPT code set; therefore, new guidelines have been added to describe the work included in the procedure and to provide guidance on the appropriate reporting of this new code.

As indicated in the code descriptor, code 0645T includes vascular access and closure, right heart catheterization, venous angiography, coronary sinus angiography, and imaging guidance, supervision and interpretation, when performed. The new guidelines clarify the work that is included in the coronary sinus device implantation procedure, as well as procedures that may be reported separately when performed at the time of the procedure. An exclusionary parenthetical note has been added to indicate the codes that may not be reported with code 0645T.

## Clinical Example (0645T)

A 65-year-old male, who has dyslipidemia and hypertension, presents with recurrent angina despite optimal medical therapy. He has a history of obstructive coronary artery disease with multiple percutaneous coronary intervention (PCIs) and a coronary artery bypass graft (CABG). Ischemia is noted on an exercise treadmill test. The patient is not a candidate for further cardiac revascularization. A coronary sinus (CS) reduction device is implanted to treat symptoms of refractory angina.

## Description of Procedure (0645T)

Under local anesthesia and ultrasound guidance, obtain access in the right internal jugular vein and insert a 9-Fr introducer sheath. Insert a 6-Fr diagnostic catheter that was flushed with sterile heparinized normal saline into the right atrium (RA). Measure and record RA pressure. Insert the catheter into the ostium of the CS without a guiding wire. After the tip of the catheter is engaged, advance the catheter into the CS. Advance the tip of the diagnostic catheter into the ostium of the CS. Use a wire to advance further into the CS to the point of the entrance of the great cardiac vein and then remove the wire. Perform cineangiography with contrast of the CS through the diagnostic catheter to evaluate size of the CS and implantation area for use with the reduction device. Advance a guidewire within the diagnostic catheter into the distal CS. Remove the diagnostic catheter. Give heparin to patient per standard. Load the CS reduction device inside a 9-Fr GC and advance the catheter over the guidewire into the CS so that the tip of the GC and the reduction device tip is slightly distal to the planned implantation target. Perform cineangiography to verify the location of the reduction device. Withdraw the GC to the most proximal marker on the reduction device balloon to expose the reduction device on its pre-mounted balloon, which is held in the landing zone previously identified. Inflate the balloon on which the reduction device was pre-mounted to a nominal pressure of 4 atm using a mixture of saline and contrast to achieve 10 to 20% oversize of the reduction device within the CS. While the balloon is fully inflated, inject a small amount of contrast through the guiding catheter to verify sufficient oversizing. To withdraw the reduction device inflation balloon, repeat a full-vacuum evacuation of contrast three times using the three-way stopcock and expelling any contrast residue from the inflation balloon. Recapture the balloon inside the 9-Fr GC and remove both. Re-insert the 6-Fr diagnostic catheter over the wire and remove the wire. Perform cineangiography one last time by manually injecting contrast through the catheter. Remove the catheter when completed.

| 0646T | Code is out of numerical sequence. See 0569T-0572T |

● **0647T**  Insertion of gastrostomy tube, percutaneous, with magnetic gastropexy, under ultrasound guidance, image documentation and report

▶(Do not report 0647T in conjunction with 76942)◀

## Rationale

Code 0647T has been established to report the insertion of a gastrostomy tube percutaneously with magnetic gastropexy under ultrasound guidance. A parenthetical note has been added to guide users on the appropriate reporting of this procedure in conjunction with other services in the CPT code set.

Code 0647T describes the placement of a percutaneous ultrasound-guided gastrostomy tube using orogastric and superficial magnets. This procedure is not currently described in the CPT code set. This new procedure differs from other procedures in the code set because it uses ultrasound guidance, guidewires, and magnets for the placement of a gastrostomy tube.

An exclusionary parenthetical note has been added following code 0647T to specify that this new procedure should not be reported with code 76942.

## Clinical Example (0647T)

A 75-year-old female presents with a massive cerebral vascular accident and inability to take oral nutrition. The patient is malnourished and needs enteral support. A swallowing evaluation is performed, confirming dysphagia. A gastrostomy tube is required to provide adequate enteral nutrition.

## Description of Procedure (0647T)

At the patient's bedside, introduce a lubricated catheter balloon with internal magnet via the mouth and esophagus into the stomach. Insufflate the stomach with air. Place a second magnet atop the abdomen, which is attracted to the catheter's magnet inside the body. Coapt the external magnet and catheter. Fill the balloon with saline or methylene blue. Use ultrasound to visualize the intervening tissue and find a safe gastrostomy tract, using the external magnet to make minor positioning adjustments. Under ultrasound guidance, advance an access needle into the stomach to form the gastrostomy tract. Feed a guidewire through the tract and capture the guidewire by deflating the balloon. Retract the balloon and guidewire out of the mouth to gain through-and-through access. Place the gastrostomy tube over the wire using the Seldinger technique.

▲ **0648T**    Quantitative magnetic resonance for analysis of tissue composition (eg, fat, iron, water content), including multiparametric data acquisition, data preparation and transmission, interpretation and report, obtained without diagnostic MRI examination of the same anatomy (eg, organ, gland, tissue, target structure) during the same session; single organ

     ▶(Do not report 0648T in conjunction with 0649T, 0697T, 0698T, when also evaluating same organ, gland, tissue, or target structure)◀

#● **0697T**       multiple organs

     ▶(Do not report 0648T, 0697T in conjunction with 70540, 70542, 70543, 70551, 70552, 70553, 71550, 71551, 71552, 72141, 72142, 72146, 72147, 72148, 72149, 72156, 72157, 72158, 72195, 72196, 72197, 73218, 73219, 73220, 73221, 73222, 73223, 73718, 73719, 73720, 73721, 73722, 73723, 74181, 74182, 74183, 75557, 75559, 75561, 75563, 76390, 76498, 77046, 77047, 77048, 77049, 0398T, when also evaluating same organ, gland, tissue, or target structure)◀

     ▶(Do not report 0697T in conjunction with 0648T, 0649T, 0698T, when also evaluating same organ, gland, tissue, or target structure)◀

+▲ **0649T**    Quantitative magnetic resonance for analysis of tissue composition (eg, fat, iron, water content), including multiparametric data acquisition, data preparation and transmission, interpretation and report, obtained with diagnostic MRI examination of the same anatomy (eg, organ, gland, tissue, target structure); single organ (List separately in addition to code for primary procedure)

     ▶(Do not report 0649T in conjunction with 0648T, 0697T, 0698T, when also evaluating same organ, gland, tissue, or target structure)◀

#+● **0698T**       multiple organs (List separately in addition to code for primary procedure)

     ▶(Use 0649T, 0698T in conjunction with 70540, 70542, 70543, 70551, 70552, 70553, 71550, 71551, 71552, 72141, 72142, 72146, 72147, 72148, 72149, 72156, 72157, 72158, 72195, 72196, 72197, 73218, 73219, 73220, 73221, 73222, 73223, 73718, 73719, 73720, 73721, 73722, 73723, 74181, 74182, 74183, 75557, 75559, 75561, 75563, 76390, 76498, 77046, 77047, 77048, 77049, 0398T, when also evaluating same organ, gland, tissue, or target structure)◀

     ▶(Do not report 0698T in conjunction with 0648T, 0649T, 0697T, when also evaluating same organ, gland, tissue, or target structure)◀

## Rationale

Two Category III codes have been revised (0648T, 0649T) and two new codes (0697T, 0698T) have been established to report quantitative multiparametric magnetic resonance

(mp-MR) for analysis of tissue composition. Additional guidance, including several parenthetical notes, have been provided for when to report and when not to report these procedures in conjunction with other services, and when performance of these services also involves evaluation of the same organ, gland, tissue, or target structure. In support of the creation of this code family, codes 0648T and 0649T have been revised to specify that the procedure is performed on a single organ.

Codes 0648T and 0649T are comprehensive codes that include quantitative magnetic resonance (MR) for analysis of tissue composition, multiparametric data acquisition, data preparation and transmission, interpretation and report, obtained with (0649T) or without (0648T) diagnostic MRI examination of the same anatomy. The language in the code descriptor specifies that analysis of the tissue composition may include fat, iron, or water content. The code descriptor also specifies that when performing the service, the same anatomy may include organ, gland, tissue, or target structure.

Code 0648T is used to report quantitative mp-MR for a single organ during the same session. Code 0649T is an add-on code and is also used to report quantitative mp-MR for a single organ. Code 0697T is used to report quantitative mp-MR for multiple organs during the same session. Code 0698T is an add-on code and is used to report quantitative mp-MR for multiple organs.

In conjunction with the revision of codes 0648T and 0649T and the establishment of codes 0697T and 0698T, one conditional and five exclusionary parenthetical notes have been created to provide instruction on the appropriate reporting of this new series of codes with other codes throughout the CPT code set. Additional instructions have also been provided to guide users on appropriate reporting when evaluation of the same organ, gland, tissue, or target structure is performed.

## Clinical Example (0648T)

A 56-year-old male presents with metabolic syndrome and abnormal liver function tests. An abdominal ultrasound showed evidence of hepatic steatosis. The patient is referred for quantitative multiparametric MRI of the liver obtained without diagnostic MRI for noninvasive assessment of steatohepatitis.

## Description of Procedure (0648T)

The physician reviews the request for service to clarify indications and determine clinical questions that need to be answered by the multiparametric MRI. Obtain scout views of the area to select the appropriate field of view and confirm adequate positioning. Obtain and review MRI sequences to check for motion or banding artifacts.

Repeat the acquisition if artifacts are identified. Process the data through an algorithm that generates parametric maps. Obtain postprocessed metrics of liver iron (T2*), proton density fat fraction (PDFF), and fibroinflammatory disease (corrected T1 [cT1]). The physician then reviews and interprets all sequences resulting from the study and multiparametric MRI data. This approach allows the physician to determine the location of the disease burden. Compare data to all pertinent available prior examinations. Prepare, dictate, and document a report in the patient's record. Communicate the study results to the referring physician to facilitate appropriate patient management.

## Clinical Example (0697T)

A 44-year-old female presents with fatigue, shortness of breath, headache, and muscle pain that have persisted for several weeks after confirmed exposure to severe acute respiratory syndrome coronavirus 2 (SARS-CoV-2) (coronavirus disease 2019 [COVID-19]). The patient is referred for quantitative multiparametric MRI of multiple organs obtained without diagnostic MRI for noninvasive assessment of suspected post-acute COVID-19 syndrome.

## Description of Procedure (0697T)

Refer the patient to an imaging center where she will be scanned with the relevant MRI protocol. Set up the patient in the scanner, acquire and use scout views of the upper body to select the appropriate field of view for the rest of the acquisitions, and confirm adequate patient positioning.

Acquire the organ-specific images using different MRI sequences to enable the radiologist to correctly set up the parameters, instruct the patient (breathing instructions), and check for specific artifacts. Repeat the acquisitions if substantial artifacts are identified.

Process the data through an algorithm that generates parametric maps. Obtain and compile manually PDFF and cT1; pancreas fat (PDF) and fibrosis (T1); cardiac function (left ventricle ejection fraction, left ventricle end diastolic volume, stroke volume, inflammation [T1] and size [left ventricle muscle mass], left ventricle muscle wall thickness); kidney size; spleen size; and lung capacity for the physician to interpret.

The physician then reviews and interprets all the metrics resulting from the study and the multiparametric MRI data. Compare the data to all pertinent available prior examinations. Prepare, dictate, and document a report in the patient's record. Communicate the study results to the referring physician and make the results available to other QHPs to facilitate appropriate patient management as needed.

## Clinical Example (0649T)

A 45-year-old male with hemochromatosis presents for evaluation of iron deposition and hepatocellular carcinoma screening. The patient is referred for quantitative multiparametric MRI for noninvasive assessment of hemochromatosis and abdominal MRI for hepatocellular carcinoma screening. [**Note:** This is an add-on service. Only consider the additional work related to quantitative multiparametric MRI of single organs.]

## Description of Procedure (0649T)

The physician reviews the request for service to clarify indications and determine clinical questions that need to be answered by the multiparametric MRI. Obtain scout views of the area to select the appropriate field of view and confirm adequate positioning. Obtain and review MRI sequences to check for motion or banding artifacts. Process the data through an algorithm that generates parametric maps. Obtain postprocessed metrics of liver iron (T2*), PDFF, and cT1. The physician then reviews and interprets all sequences resulting from the study and multiparametric magnetic resonance data.

Obtain separate abdominal MRI sequences to assess for potential lesions and organ changes. Evaluate and compare included anatomic structures of the abdomen with any available pertinent prior examinations.

Prepare, dictate, and document a report that includes quantitative multiparametric MRI data and abdominal MRI findings in the patient's record. Communicate the study results to the referring physician to facilitate appropriate patient management.

## Clinical Example (0698T)

A 47-year-old male presents with fatigue, joint pain, and palpitations that have persisted for several weeks after confirmed exposure to COVID-19. The patient is referred for quantitative multiparametric MRI of multiple organs obtained with diagnostic MRI for noninvasive assessment of suspected post-acute COVID-19 syndrome. [**Note:** This is an add-on service. Only consider the additional work related to quantitative multiparametric MRI of multiple organs.]

## Description of Procedure (0698T)

The physician reviews the request for service to clarify indications for procedure and determine the clinical questions that need to be answered by the multiparametric MRI of multiple organs.

Refer the patient to an imaging center where he will be scanned with the relevant MRI protocol. Set up the patient in the scanner, acquire and use scout views of the upper body to select appropriate field of view for the rest of the acquisitions, and confirm adequate patient positioning.

★ = Telemedicine   ✚ = Add-on code   ✐ = FDA approval pending   # = Resequenced code   ⊘ = Modifier 51 exempt

Acquire the organ-specific images using different MRI sequences to enable the radiologist to correctly set up the parameters, instruct the patient (breathing instructions), and check for specific artifacts. Repeat the acquisitions if substantial artifacts are identified.

Process the data through algorithms that generate parametric maps. Obtain and compile manually PDFF and cT1; PDF and fibrosis (T1); cardiac function (left ventricle ejection fraction, left ventricle end diastolic volume, stroke volume, inflammation [T1] and size [left ventricle muscle mass], left ventricle muscle wall thickness); kidney size; spleen size; and lung capacity.

Obtain separate MRI sequences to assess for potential lesions and organ changes. The physician then reviews and interprets all the metrics resulting from the study, the sequences, and the multiparametric MRI data. This approach allows the physician to determine the location of the disease burden. Evaluate and compare the included anatomic structures of each additional organ with any available pertinent prior examinations.

Prepare, dictate, and document a report that includes quantitative multiparametric MRI data and MRI findings in the patient's record. Communicate the study results to the referring physician and make the results available to other QHPs to facilitate appropriate patient management as needed.

## ▶Subcutaneous Cardiac Rhythm Monitor System Programming Device Evaluation (Remote)◀

▶The programming evaluation of a subcutaneous cardiac rhythm monitor system may be performed in-person or remotely. Codes 93285, 0650T are reported per procedure. Remote programming device evaluation (0650T) includes in-person device programming (93285), when performed, on the same day. Programming device evaluation includes all components of the interrogation device evaluation. Therefore, 93291 (in-person interrogation) should not be reported in conjunction with 93285, 0650T. Programming device evaluations (93285, 0650T) and remote interrogation device evaluations (93298) may both be reported during the 30-day remote interrogation device evaluation period.◀

- **0650T**  Programming device evaluation (remote) of subcutaneous cardiac rhythm monitor system, with iterative adjustment of the implantable device to test the function of the device and select optimal permanently programmed values with analysis, review and report by a physician or other qualified health care professional

    ▶(Do not report 0650T in conjunction with 33285, 93260, 93279, 93280, 93281, 93282, 93284, 93285, 93291)◀

## Rationale

A new subsection with guidelines and one new Category III code (0650T) have been established in the Category III section of the CPT code set.

Code 0650T is intended to be reported for remote programming device evaluation of a subcutaneous cardiac rhythm monitoring system. The procedure includes iterative adjustment of the implantable device to test the function of the device and select optimal permanently programmed values with analysis, review, and report.

The new guidelines clarify that programming evaluation of a subcutaneous cardiac rhythm monitor system may be performed in-person or remotely. However, remote programming device evaluation (0650T) includes in-person device programming (93285) and should not be separately reported when performed on the same day.

Subcutaneous cardiac rhythm monitors are implanted in patients to diagnose various suspected arrythmias. The subcutaneous cardiac rhythm monitor continuously records the electrocardiographic rhythm with event recordings triggered automatically by rapid and slow heart rates or by the patient during a symptomatic episode.

An exclusionary parenthetical note has been added following code 0650T to restrict users from reporting this code in conjunction with codes 33285, 93260, 93279-93282, 93284, 93285, and 93291.

## Clinical Example (0650T)

A 71-year-old female with sick sinus syndrome, who was previously treated by implanting a subcutaneous cardiac rhythm monitor system with a remote interrogation device evaluation, indicates the need for remote programming device evaluation for possible adjustment of the rhythm-detection parameters.

## Description of Procedure (0650T)

Identify and review the alert conditions. Review the patient-activated and the automatically recorded rhythm episodes for evidence of accurately identified arrythmias. Compare current data measurements to stored and trended historical data. Assess device function for underlying signal strength and battery longevity. Evaluate and adjust the sensing thresholds for detecting arrythmias until optimized. Identify the appropriate rhythm alerts, and review and adjust recording parameters. Review the total device-memory capacity and the parameters for recording capacity. Assess and adjust the amount of episode-detection recording time as needed to optimize recording function. After detailed evaluation of all parameters, make a decision about the adequacy of the current programmed parameters. Make and save any identified device programming changes to optimize device performance in the remote monitoring system.

● **0651T**   Magnetically controlled capsule endoscopy, esophagus through stomach, including intraprocedural positioning of capsule, with interpretation and report

▶(Do not report 0651T in conjunction with 91110, 91111)◀

## Rationale

Code 0651T has been established to report capsule endoscopy in the esophagus and stomach.

Code 0651T involves active control and active maneuvering while the capsule is in vivo (inside the patient). This procedure is the technical equivalent of performing an endoscopic procedure, but using the capsule as the modality. Because the capsule endoscopy is in vivo, it allows for both diagnostic and therapeutic prognostication.

Code 91110 is typically reported for the traditional wireless capsule endoscopy. For this procedure, the patient swallows a capsule and wears a recorder device. The images are captured passively, and the patient then returns the recorder device at the completion of the procedure. An exclusionary parenthetical note has been added to restrict the use of code 0651T with codes 91110 and 91111.

## Clinical Example (0651T)

A 65-year-old male presents to the emergency room with hematemesis. Wireless capsule endoscopy of the esophagus and stomach is performed.

## Description of Procedure (0651T)

Give the patient the capsule endoscope to swallow with water, which is observed by the physician. After the study is completed, staff downloads the data to the workstation. The physician reviews images. Scan the entire study and annotate key anatomic landmarks (eg, esophagogastric junction). Once the landmarks have been determined, view all images. When an abnormality is identified, create a thumbnail image. Note and record key findings or abnormalities on a localization drawing that may also be used to guide subsequent management.

● **0652T**   Esophagogastroduodenoscopy, flexible, transnasal; diagnostic, including collection of specimen(s) by brushing or washing, when performed (separate procedure)

● **0653T**       with biopsy, single or multiple

● **0654T**       with insertion of intraluminal tube or catheter

▶(For rigid transoral esophagoscopy services, see 43191, 43192, 43193, 43194, 43195)◀

▶(For diagnostic transnasal esophagoscopy, use 43197)◀

▶(For transnasal esophagoscopy with biopsy[ies], use 43198)◀

▶(For transoral esophagoscopy, esophagogastroduodenoscopy, see 43200-43232, 43235-43259, 43266, 43270)◀

▶(For other transnasal esophagogastroduodenoscopy services, see 43499, 43999, 44799)◀

## Rationale

Three new Category III codes (0652T, 0653T, 0654T) have been established to report transnasal flexible esophagogastroduodenoscopy (EGD). Code 0652T describes diagnostic transnasal EGD, code 0653T describes transnasal EGD with biopsy, and code 0654T describes transnasal EGD with insertion of intraluminal tube or catheter.

Category I codes 43210, 43233, 43235-43259, 43266, and 43270 describe flexible EGD using a transoral approach. Prior to 2022, no codes existed for flexible EGD using a transnasal approach. Transoral flexible EGD is performed using sedation. Sedation is not used in transnasal flexible EGD; topical anesthesia is used instead.

Five parenthetical notes have been added following codes 0652T, 0653T, and 0654T that clarify the appropriate reporting of other endoscopic procedures. Specifically, diagnostic transnasal esophagoscopy is reported with code 43197 and transnasal esophagoscopy with biopsy(ies) is reported with code 43198. Other transnasal EGD services not described in codes 0652T-0654T should be reported using unlisted code 43499, 43999, or 44799, as appropriate.

Transoral esophagoscopy and EGD are reported with codes 43200-43232, 43235-43259, 43266, and 43270, and rigid transoral esophagoscopy services are reported with codes 43191-43195.

## Clinical Example (0652T)

A 15-year-old male presents with the sensation that something is stuck in his throat.

★ = Telemedicine   ✚ = Add-on code   ⨏ = FDA approval pending   # = Resequenced code   ⊘ = Modifier 51 exempt

## Description of Procedure (0652T)

Spray a topical anesthetic into the patient's nose and mouth. Lubricate the distal portion of the endoscope and then pass the endoscope under direct vision into the nasal cavity. The physician is careful to avoid nasal spurs, nasal septal deviations, turbinates, nasal polyps, and other areas of constriction. Instruct the patient to breathe steadily and calmly through the nose to open the nasopharynx. Pass the endoscope into the oropharynx. Visualize the larynx and take care not to stimulate it to avoid potential laryngospasm. Ask the patient to tilt his head toward his chest and swallow; at this moment, the endoscopist advances the endoscope into the hypopharynx and through the pharyngoesophageal segment. Advance the endoscope under direct vision into the proximal stomach. Insufflate the stomach with air after suctioning liquid contents. Perform an examination of the entire stomach in the forward and retroflexed positions. Advance the endoscope through the pylorus into the duodenal bulb. Inspect the duodenum circumferentially after air insufflation and water irrigation. Withdraw the endoscope and inspect the stomach and duodenum. After suctioning air to deflate the stomach, withdraw the endoscope into the esophagus, allowing measurement of the squamocolumnar (SC) and gastroesophageal (GE) junction from the incisors. Assess for the presence of a hiatal hernia and examine the esophageal mucosa. When indicated, obtain brushings or washings of suspicious abnormalities. Obtain photo documentation of appropriate normal landmarks and abnormalities. Withdraw the endoscope at the conclusion of the procedure.

## Clinical Example (0653T)

A 13-year-old female presents with chronic abdominal pain, diarrhea, and dysphagia.

## Description of Procedure (0653T)

Spray a topical anesthetic into the patient's nose and mouth. Lubricate the distal portion of the endoscope and then pass the endoscope under direct vision into the nasal cavity. The physician is careful to avoid nasal spurs, nasal septal deviations, turbinates, nasal polyps, and other areas of constriction. Instruct the patient to breathe steadily and calmly through the nose to open the nasopharynx. Pass the endoscope is passed into the oropharynx. Visualize the larynx and take care not to stimulate it to avoid potential laryngospasm. Ask the patient to tilt her head toward her chest and swallow; at this moment, the endoscopist advances the endoscope into the hypopharynx and through the pharyngo-esophageal segment. Advance the endoscope under direct vision into the proximal stomach. Insufflate the stomach with air after suctioning liquid contents. Perform an

examination of the entire stomach in the forward and retroflexed positions. Advance the endoscope through the pylorus into the duodenal bulb. Inspect the duodenum circumferentially after air insufflation and water irrigation. Withdraw the endoscope and inspect the stomach and duodenum. Obtain endoscopically directed biopsies of abnormal tissue. After suctioning air to deflate the stomach, withdraw the endoscope into the esophagus, allowing measurement of the SC and GE junction from the incisors. Perform an assessment for the presence of a hiatal hernia and examine the esophageal mucosa. When indicated, obtain brushings or washings of suspicious abnormalities. Obtain photo documentation of appropriate normal landmarks and abnormalities. Withdraw the endoscope at the conclusion of the procedure.

## Clinical Example (0654T)

A 5-year-old female, who is unable to maintain adequate nutritional intake, is referred for endoscopic evaluation and placement of a feeding tube into the duodenum.

## Description of Procedure (0654T)

Spray a topical anesthetic into the patient's nose and mouth. Lubricate the distal portion of the endoscope and then pass the endoscope under direct vision into the nasal cavity. The physician is careful to avoid nasal spurs, nasal septal deviations, turbinates, nasal polyps, and other areas of constriction. Instruct the patient to breathe steadily and calmly through the nose to open the nasopharynx. Pass the endoscope into the oropharynx. Visualize the larynx and take care not to stimulate it to avoid potential laryngospasm. Ask the patient to tilt her head toward her chest and swallow; at this moment, the endoscopist advances the endoscope into the hypopharynx and through the pharyngoesophageal segment. Advance the endoscope under direct vision into the proximal stomach. Insufflate the stomach with air after suctioning liquid contents. Perform an examination of the entire stomach in the forward and retroflexed positions. Advance the endoscope through the pylorus into the duodenal bulb. Inspect the duodenum circumferentially after air insufflation and water irrigation. Withdraw the endoscope and inspect the stomach and duodenum. Pass a nasoenteric tube through the opposite nares into the stomach. Reinsert the endoscope through the opposite nares. Identify the tip of the nasoenteric tube, position the tube and endoscope, insert a grasping device through the endoscope biopsy channel, and grasp the tube. Advance the tube endoscopically through the pylorus into the proximal small intestine. Release the tube and withdraw the endoscope, maintaining the position of the tube. After suctioning air to deflate the stomach, withdraw the endoscope into the esophagus, allowing measurement of the SC and GE junction from the incisors. Perform an assessment for the presence of a hiatal hernia and examine the esophageal mucosa. When indicated, obtain brushings or washings of suspicious abnormalities. Obtain photo documentation of appropriate normal landmarks and abnormalities. Withdraw the endoscope at the conclusion of the procedure.

● **0655T**   Transperineal focal laser ablation of malignant prostate tissue, including transrectal imaging guidance, with MR-fused images or other enhanced ultrasound imaging

▶(Do not report 0655T in conjunction with 52000, 76376, 76377, 76872, 76940, 76942, 76998)◀

## Rationale

Code 0655T has been established to report transperineal focal laser ablation of malignant prostate tissue, including imaging guidance, with MR-fused images or other enhanced ultrasound imaging. In addition, an exclusionary parenthetical note has been added following code 0655T.

This procedure is designed to treat conditions such as prostate cancer. Ultrasound-guided or ultrasound-fusion-guided focal laser ablation of malignant prostate tissue is not currently described in the CPT code set.

An exclusionary parenthetical note following code 0655T has been included to guide users in the appropriate reporting of these procedures with other procedures within the CPT code set.

## Clinical Example (0655T)

A 67-year-old male presents with MRI-visible, biopsy-proven, prostate cancer (Gleason score 3+4) localized within the gland.

## Description of Procedure (0655T)

Induce local, regional, or general anesthesia. Place the patient in the lithotomy position. Place a transrectal ultrasound probe. After fusing the MRI scans to the real-time ultrasound, the urologist identifies the targeted tissue and plans the treatment approach to obtain the desired oncological effect. Perform the entire procedure under ultrasound guidance. Place the introducer through the perineum to access the prostate. Insert the laser applicator access device through the needle guide. Place temperature probes to monitor the temperature of important structures as needed. Using one or more laser applicators, the urologist ablates the prostate to achieve the desired margins around the targeted malignant tissue. Confirm the desired ablative effect via ultrasound.

● **0656T**   Vertebral body tethering, anterior; up to 7 vertebral segments

● **0657T**       8 or more vertebral segments

▶(Do not report 0656T, 0657T in conjunction with 22800, 22802, 22804, 22808, 22810, 22812, 22818, 22819, 22845, 22846, 22847)◀

## Rationale

Two new codes (0656T, 0657T) have been established to report anterior vertebral body tethering. Anterior vertebral body tethering is indicated for the treatment of skeletally immature patients who require surgical treatment to obtain and maintain correction of progressive idiopathic scoliosis. Prior to 2022, this service was reported with code 22899, *Unlisted procedure, spine.*

Anterior vertebral body tethering does not involve arthrodesis or fusion of the spine and thus, it is not appropriate to report codes 22800, 22802, 22804, 22808, 22810, 22812, 22818, 22819, and 22845-22847 for the new procedures. However, anterior vertebral body tethering does involve the placement of bone screws into the vertebral bodies and a tether band placed across the bone screws. Parenthetical notes have been added to provide this guidance.

In accordance with the establishment of new Category III codes 0656T and 0657T for reporting anterior vertebral body tethering, the Spine Deformity (eg, Scoliosis, Kyphosis) section guidelines have been revised and updated to provide appropriate guidance and instruction for reporting spinal deformity arthrodesis codes 22800, 22802, 22804, 22808, 22810, and 22812, and kyphectomy codes 22818 and 22819 with new codes 0656T and 0657T.

Additional exclusionary parenthetical notes have been added following codes 22804, 22812, and 22819 to support accurate reporting of these services in conjunction with codes 0656T and 0657T. A cross-reference parenthetical note has been added following code 22847, directing users to codes 0656T and 0657T for anterior vertebral body tethering.

Code 0656T is intended to describe anterior vertebral body tethering, up to seven vertebral segments. Code 0657T describes anterior vertebral body tethering for eight or more vertebral segments. As noted earlier, anterior vertebral body tethering does not involve arthrodesis or fusion of the spine; therefore, a parenthetical note has been added following the new Category III codes to provide guidance on the appropriate reporting of these new codes.

## Clinical Example (0656T)

A 12-year-old female, who has a 42° curvature due to idiopathic scoliosis, undergoes implantation of bone screws and anchors into the T6 to T11 vertebral bodies along with placement and tensioning of a tethering cord to provide initial coronal correction.

## Description of Procedure (0656T)

Position and prepare the patient. Clean the incision sites with disinfectant. Identify the scoliotic curve, the levels to be instrumented, the size and selection of the implant, and the initial target correction. Use a video-assisted thoracoscopic surgery (VATS) technique to access the anterior thoracic spine. Using an ultrasonic scalpel, incise the parietal pleura longitudinally and identify the segmental vessels along the vertebrae to be instrumented. Coagulate the segmental vessels and expose the lateral aspect of the vertebral bodies intended for instrumentation. Confirm the trajectory and placement on the vertebral body at all levels prior to anchor insertion, screw preparation, and screw insertion. Secure and segmentally tension a cord to the most cranial screw to off-load the deformity and provide growth modulation over time. Maintain compression by tightening set screws at up to six adjacent levels (ie, combining to instrument up to a total of seven vertebral segments). Following final tensioning, close the wound and place a drain as needed.

## Clinical Example (0657T)

A 12-year-old female, who has a 50° curvature due to idiopathic scoliosis, undergoes implantation of bone screws and anchors into the T6 to L2 vertebral bodies along with placement and tensioning of a tethering cord to provide initial coronal correction.

## Description of Procedure (0657T)

Position and prepare the patient. Clean the incision sites with disinfectant. Identify the scoliotic curve, the levels to be instrumented, the size and selection of the implant, and the target initial correction. Use a VATS technique to access the anterior thoracic spine and use a lateral open approach to access the anterior lumbar spine. Using an ultrasonic scalpel, incise the parietal pleura longitudinally and identify the segmental vessels along the vertebrae to be instrumented. Coagulate the segmental vessels and expose the lateral aspect of the vertebral bodies intended for instrumentation. Confirm the trajectory and placement on the vertebral body at all levels prior to anchor insertion, screw preparation, and screw insertion. Secure and segmentally tension a cord to the most cranial screw to off-load the deformity and provide growth modulation over time. Maintain compression by tightening set screws at seven or more adjacent levels (ie, combining to instrument eight or more vertebral segments). Following final tensioning, close the wound and place a drain as needed.

---

● **0658T**    Electrical impedance spectroscopy of 1 or more skin lesions for automated melanoma risk score

### Rationale

Code 0658T has been established to report electrical impedance spectroscopy for melanoma. Code 0658T describes the nonvisual detection of malignant melanoma. Currently, no codes exist in the CPT code set to describe electrical impedance spectroscopy for melanoma.

## Clinical Example (0658T)

A 65-year-old female, who has a history of extended periods of sun exposure, presents with a newly pigmented, unusual-looking growth on her skin. After an initial visual and dermoscopic examination, the physician performs electrical impedance spectroscopy (EIS) testing of this lesion to determine the risk of melanoma.

## Description of Procedure (0658T)

The physician cleans the lesion and surrounding skin with alcohol and then moistens the area with physiologic saline for 30 seconds using a compress. Remove the excess saline. Position the electrode surface on the lesion and using the device, measure the overall electrical impedance at 35 different frequencies logarithmically distributed between 1.0 kHz and 2.5 MHz at four depth settings. Analyze the measurement(s) in real time using the device's automated classifier. The device calculates an EIS score between 0 and 10, which illustrates the degree of atypia or melanoma risk for the lesion. This information is presented in the report.

---

● **0659T**    Transcatheter intracoronary infusion of supersaturated oxygen in conjunction with percutaneous coronary revascularization during acute myocardial infarction, including catheter placement, imaging guidance (eg, fluoroscopy), angiography, and radiologic supervision and interpretation

▶(Use 0659T in conjunction with 92941)◀

▶(Do not report 0659T in conjunction with 92920, 92924, 92928, 92933, 92937, 92943)◀

## Rationale

Code 0659T has been established to report intra-arterial hyperoxemic reperfusion. Code 0659T describes a new therapy involving super saturated oxygen. Two parenthetical notes have been added following code 0659T to instruct users on the appropriate reporting for intra-arterial hyperoxemic reperfusion. Prior to 2022, no codes exist in the CPT code set to describe intra-arterial hyperoxemic reperfusion.

## Clinical Example (0659T)

A 61-year-old male, who has just undergone placement of a coronary stent within the left anterior descending artery, also requires additional supersaturated oxygen ($SSO_2$) therapy to the ischemic area of the heart during revascularization of an acute total coronary artery occlusion during acute myocardial infarction, and undergoes transcatheter intracoronary hyperoxemic reperfusion.

## Description of Procedure (0659T)

Place a stent in the left descending artery (reported separately) and keep the patient in the cardiac catheterization laboratory. Obtain an angiogram of the left anterior descending coronary artery to confirm the successful reopening of the lesion with thrombolysis in myocardial infarction (TIMI) flow grade 3. Draw and analyze an arterial blood sample to ensure the systemic arterial partial pressure of oxygen ($pO_2$) status is adequate prior to beginning the intracoronary $SSO_2$ infusion. Using either percutaneous coronary intervention (PCI) access or a new femoral placement, gain arterial access. The physician advances the catheter over the wire to the ostium of the left main coronary artery under fluoroscopic guidance. Perform angiography to ensure the placement of the infusion catheter.

The physician connects the blood withdrawal tubing to the sidearm of the femoral artery sheath. Prepare the system materials. Withdraw and circulate blood from the patient's femoral artery via a roller pump through the cartridge in the console to become hyperoxemic (supersaturated). The physician connects the blood return tubing to the delivery catheter at the ostium of the left main coronary artery, creating an extracorporeal circuit. Return the supersaturated blood to the patient's left main coronary artery for distribution to the ischemic cardiac tissue. The physician operates the circuit for 60 minutes and may perform fluoroscopic imaging at 30 minutes to verify the position of the delivery catheter. Draw blood at 30 minutes to monitor anticoagulation as needed.

Perform angiography again. After supervising the discontinuation of blood flow to the extracorporeal circuit, the physician disconnects the patient's tubing, removes the catheter and the sheaths, and closes the access sites.

● **0660T** Implantation of anterior segment intraocular nonbiodegradable drug-eluting system, internal approach

▶(Report medication separately)◀

● **0661T** Removal and reimplantation of anterior segment intraocular nonbiodegradable drug-eluting implant

▶(Report medication separately)◀

## Rationale

Two Category III codes (0660T, 0661T) have been established to report the implantation of an anterior segment intraocular nonbiodegradable drug-eluting system. Medications used in conjunction with the procedures represented by codes 0660T and 0661T should be reported separately.

Code 0660T describes the internal approach for the placement of a nonbiodegradable drug implant, which is anchored through the trabecular meshwork into the sclera, that elutes drug over an extended period to lower intraocular pressure.

Code 0661T describes the removal and replacement of a new implant in order to continue therapeutic medication management.

These procedures aid in the treatment of diseases such as glaucoma. Separate instructional parenthetical notes have been added following codes 0660T and 0661T to indicate that any medication used with the procedures should be reported separately.

## Clinical Example (0660T)

A 55-year-old female, who has early open-angle glaucoma with initial response to IOP-lowering medications, is no longer meeting target pressure. Insertion of a drug-eluting device is recommended.

## Description of Procedure (0660T)

Anesthetize the eye. Create a small temporal clear corneal incision at the temporal limbus location. Use a viscoelastic solution to deepen the anterior chamber and to maintain IOP. Place a goniolens on the cornea to inspect and visualize the angle while positioning the head. Identify the trabecular meshwork, remove the

★ = Telemedicine ✚ = Add-on code ⁄⁄ = FDA approval pending # = Resequenced code ⊘ = Modifier 51 exempt

safety clip from the insertion device, and advance the tip through the incision into the anterior chamber.

The surgeon takes care to avoid the crystalline lens and iris, advancing toward the trabecular meshwork at the site opposite the incision. Slide a retractor button on the inserter backward while applying pressure so that the implant is released directly into and through the trabecular meshwork and Schlemm's canal until the barb at the tip securely penetrates the sclera. Take care to ensure the base of the cylindrical reservoir is firmly in contact with and compressing the trabecular meshwork. Backing away carefully, pull the inserter away from the seated implant and gently probe for appropriate placement.

Carefully remove the inserter. Irrigate and aspirate the anterior chamber with a BSS through the corneal wound to remove all viscoelastic solution. The surgeon presses down on the posterior edge of the incision as needed to facilitate the complete removal of the viscoelastic solution and to assure stability. Inflate the anterior chamber with saline solution as needed to achieve physiologic pressure. Apply hydration to the corneal wound to facilitate closure.

## Clinical Example (0661T)

A 55-year-old female with early open-angle glaucoma has a non-biodegradable drug-eluting implant inserted to lower IOP. Subsequently, effective drug elution has ended, with removal and reimplantation of a new device recommended.

## Description of Procedure (0661T)

Anesthetize the eye. Create a small temporal clear corneal incision at the temporal limbus location. Use a viscoelastic solution to deepen the anterior chamber and to maintain IOP. Place a goniolens on the cornea to inspect and visualize the angle while positioning the head. Identify the trabecular meshwork, remove the safety clip from the insertion device, and advance the tip through the incision into the anterior chamber.

The surgeon takes care to avoid the crystalline lens and iris, advancing toward the trabecular meshwork at the nasal site next to the existing implant. Slide a retractor button on the inserter backward while applying pressure so that the implant is released directly into and through the trabecular meshwork and Schlemm's canal until the barb at the tip securely penetrates the sclera. Take care to ensure the base of the cylindrical reservoir is firmly in contact with and compressing the trabecular meshwork. Backing away carefully, pull the inserter away from the newly seated implant and gently probe for appropriate placement. Use the inserter to grasp and remove the initial implant.

Carefully remove the inserter with the spent implant. Irrigate and aspirate the anterior chamber with a BSS through the corneal wound to remove all viscoelastic solution. The surgeon presses down on the posterior edge of the incision as needed to facilitate complete removal of the viscoelastic solution. Infiltrate the anterior chamber with saline solution as needed to achieve physiologic pressure. Apply hydration to the corneal wound to facilitate closure.

----

● **0662T**　　Scalp cooling, mechanical; initial measurement and calibration of cap

　　　　▶(Report 0662T once per chemotherapy treatment period)◀

+● **0663T**　　　placement of device, monitoring, and removal of device (List separately in addition to code for primary procedure)

　　　　▶(Use 0663T in conjunction with 96409, 96411, 96413, 96415, 96416, 96417)◀

　　　　▶(Report 0663T once per chemotherapy session)◀

　　　　▶(For selective head or total body hypothermia in the critically ill neonate, use 99184)◀

### Rationale

Category III codes 0662T and 0663T have been established to report mechanical scalp cooling. Codes 0662T and 0663T describe the use of a mechanical cooling system in conjunction with chemotherapy.

Scalp cooling methods are traditionally performed via passive devices, such as ice-filled bags or ice gel packs, to prevent chemotherapy-induced alopecia. However, the method described by codes 0662T and 0663T involves the patient wearing a special cap that circulates a liquid coolant via an active refrigeration system. This procedure is typically conducted under physician supervision in a hospital or physician office setting that provides chemotherapy. The use of this system does not involve ice or gel packs.

A parenthetical note has been added following code 0662T to instruct users to report this code once per chemotherapy treatment period. Three parenthetical notes have been added following add-on code 0663T to instruct users on how to correctly report this new code.

Prior to 2022, no codes exist in the CPT code set to describe mechanical scalp cooling.

## Clinical Example (0662T)

A 40-year-old female with breast cancer, who requires chemotherapy, engages in shared decision making in conjunction with the treating oncologist regarding the use of mechanical scalp cooling during chemotherapy sessions to reduce the likelihood of chemotherapy-induced alopecia.

## Description of Procedure (0662T)

The physician examines the scalp. The physician or a staff member under the physician's supervision measures the patient's scalp to determine the proper fit of a mechanized scalp-cooling cap. Fit the scalp-cooling cap. Instruct the patient on hair and scalp care throughout the treatment. Store the patient's cap between chemotherapy sessions according to clinician preference.

## Clinical Example (0663T)

A 40-year-old female with breast cancer requires the use of mechanical scalp cooling during chemotherapy sessions to reduce the likelihood of chemotherapy-induced alopecia. [**Note:** This is an add-on code. Only consider the additional work for the placement, monitoring, and removal of the device in conjunction with services represented by codes 96409, 96411, 96413, 96415, 96416, 96417].

## Description of Procedure (0663T)

On the day of chemotherapy infusion, direct the patient to the infusion suite. Inspect the scalp. Fit the patient's specific cooling cap, neoprene cover, and headband on the patient's head. While the patient sits, attach the cooling cap to the continuously monitored cooling system. Initiate the cooling system 30 minutes prior to chemotherapy, use it during the chemotherapy infusion(s), and continue the cooling system for 90 minutes after conclusion of the chemotherapy infusion(s). Assess the patient periodically for adverse events throughout the scalp-cooling session. At the conclusion of the scalp-cooling procedure, remove the cooling cap and inspect the scalp. Document any tolerability issues and patient assessment before, during, and after the scalp-cooling treatment in the patient's medical record.

## ▶Uterus Transplantation◀

▶Uterus allotransplantation involves three distinct components of physician work:

1. ***Cadaver donor hysterectomy,*** which includes harvesting the uterus allograft from a deceased (eg, brain-dead, cadaver) donor and cold preservation of the uterus allograft (perfusing with cold preservation solution and cold maintenance) (use 0664T). ***Living donor hysterectomy,*** which includes harvesting the uterus allograft, cold preservation of the uterus allograft (perfusing with cold preservation solution and cold maintenance), and care of the donor (see 0665T, 0666T).

2. ***Backbench work,*** which includes standard preparation of the cadaver or living uterus allograft prior to transplantation, such as dissection and removal of surrounding soft tissues to prepare uterine vein(s) and uterine artery(ies), as necessary (use 0668T). Additional reconstruction of the uterus allograft may include venous and/or arterial anastomosis(es) (see 0669T, 0670T).

3. ***Recipient uterus allotransplantation,*** which includes transplantation of the uterus allograft and care of the recipient (use 0667T).◀

● **0664T**   Donor hysterectomy (including cold preservation); open, from cadaver donor

● **0665T**   open, from living donor

● **0666T**   laparoscopic or robotic, from living donor

● **0667T**   recipient uterus allograft transplantation from cadaver or living donor

● **0668T**   Backbench standard preparation of cadaver or living donor uterine allograft prior to transplantation, including dissection and removal of surrounding soft tissues and preparation of uterine vein(s) and uterine artery(ies), as necessary

● **0669T**   Backbench reconstruction of cadaver or living donor uterus allograft prior to transplantation; venous anastomosis, each

● **0670T**   arterial anastomosis, each

## Rationale

A new subsection, new guidelines, and seven new codes (0664T-0670T) have been established in the Category III section for reporting uterus transplantation procedures.

The new subsection and code family follow coding convention for other transplantation services. Therefore, separate codes are provided to specify reporting for donor hysterectomy procedures that differentiate between the harvest of the donor organ from cadavers and from living donors, the method used to harvest the organ (open vs

★ = Telemedicine   + = Add-on code   ⇗ = FDA approval pending   # = Resequenced code   ⊘ = Modifier 51 exempt laparoscopic), where appropriate, and the transplantation procedure itself, ie, whether harvested from a living donor or a cadaver. Additional codes also allow separate reporting for backbench work performed to prepare the harvested uterus for transplant into the recipient. These codes differentiate the type of backbench work provided, whether by noting the dissection efforts necessary to prepare the transplanted uterus for implantation into the host (0668T) or by noting the reconstruction efforts necessary for venous (0669T) or arterial (0670T) anastomosis.

The new guidelines describe what is included as part of cadaver and living donor hysterectomy, backbench work, and recipient uterus allotransplantation.

## Clinical Example (0664T)

A 30-year-old multiparous brain-dead female, who has previously expressed desire to be an organ donor, is matched to a living recipient who desires uterus transplantation. Procurement of the uterus along with other life-saving organs is performed.

## Description of Procedure (0664T)

Begin surgery on the deceased donor via laparotomy using an ample midline abdominal, arrow shaped, or cruciate incision. After entry into the abdomen, identify and mobilize the uterus and ovaries. For each side, ligate the infundibulopelvic ligament. Dissect the ureter free from the iliac and ovarian vessels; transect the ovarian vessels above the pelvic brim to allow use for graft outflow; perform ureterolysis from the pelvic brim to the uterine artery. Transect the ureter at the level where it crosses the internal iliac artery. Transect the round ligament. Open the paravesical space. Dissect the bladder off the uterus and cervix and open the vesicovaginal space. For each side, dissect the internal iliac artery laterally to the external iliac artery. Ligate all branches going laterally or inferiorly toward the sacrum; take all structures medial to the obturator nerve en bloc with the uterus; ligate all vessels coursing laterally. Dissect and prepare the internal iliac vein for final removal of the graft. Open the rectovaginal space to prepare for vaginotomy. Either remove the uterus after donor heparinization and prior to cross-clamping (and flushed on the back table), or remove the uterus after donor heparinization, cross-clamping, and in-situ flush, and after the other abdominal organs have been removed.

## Clinical Example (0665T)

A 45-year-old multiparous female, who has completed childbearing, desires to donate her uterus. She meets with numerous providers to ensure that she is adequately informed of the risks of the procedure. As is standard for other solid-organ transplants, she undergoes an extensive, multidisciplinary selection process. She undergoes an abdominal hysterectomy procedure to allow donation of her organ to a matched recipient.

## Description of Procedure (0665T)

Begin surgery on the living donor via a lower midline vertical laparotomy. After entry into the abdomen, identify and mobilize the uterus and ovaries. Divide the round ligaments bilaterally. Dissect the bladder off the uterus and cervix and open the vesicovaginal space. Dissect the anterior branch of the internal iliac artery and identify all branching vessels. Perform ureterolysis bilaterally from the pelvic brim to the passage of the ureters under the uterine artery. Dissect and ligate the parametrium and deep uterine veins away, near their inlets with the internal iliac vein. Dissect and ligate the superior uterine veins to be used as alternate or accessory venous drainage of the graft. Perform vaginotomy with sufficient cuff for anastomosis. Remove the graft and immediately place it on ice. Close the vagina and incision site(s) in the standard fashion.

## Clinical Example (0666T)

A 45-year-old multiparous female, who has completed childbearing, desires to donate her uterus. As is standard for other solid-organ transplants, she undergoes an extensive, multidisciplinary selection process. She undergoes a laparoscopic hysterectomy procedure (with or without robotic assistance) to allow donation of her organ to a matched recipient.

## Description of Procedure (0666T)

Begin surgery on the living donor with laparoscopic/ robotic trocar insertion. After entry into the abdomen and insufflation, identify and mobilize the uterus and ovaries. Divide the round ligaments bilaterally. Dissect the bladder off the uterus and cervix and open the vesicovaginal space. Dissect the anterior branch of the internal iliac artery and identify all branching vessels. Perform ureterolysis bilaterally from the pelvic brim to the passage of the ureters under the uterine artery. Dissect the parametrium and deep uterine veins away, near their inlets with the internal iliac vein and ligated. Dissect and ligate the superior uterine veins to be used as alternate or accessory venous drainage of the graft. Perform vaginotomy. Remove the graft through the vagina and immediately place it on ice. Close the vagina and incision sites in the standard fashion.

## Clinical Example (0667T)

A 25-year-old nulligravida female with congenital absence of the uterus (diagnosed at age 15) has a desire to carry her genetic offspring. As is standard for other solid-organ transplants, she undergoes an extensive selection process, and a uterus transplantation is performed.

## Description of Procedure (0667T)

Begin surgery on the recipient via lower midline laparotomy after the graft is deemed satisfactory for implantation. Expose the external iliac vessels and identify the recipient vaginal apex while mobilizing the bladder anteriorly and the rectum posteriorly. Anastomose bilaterally a combination of the superior and inferior uterine veins, at least one per side, to the external iliac veins. Anastomose the uterine arteries to the external iliac arteries. Perform the vaginal anastomosis in an end-to-end fashion. Provide additional pelvic support to the uterosacral ligaments, uterine rudiment, and round ligament attachments. Confirm vascular flow with color and spectral Doppler ultrasound imaging intraoperatively and immediately postoperatively. If there are concerns regarding outflow from the graft, perform additional vascular anastomoses (eg, ovarian veins). Close the abdomen in the usual fashion.

## Clinical Example (0668T)

Following procurement of the donor uterus as part of a uterus transplantation procedure, the uterine graft is prepared prior to allotransplantation.

## Description of Procedure (0668T)

Following procurement of the uterine graft either from a cadaver or living donor, put the graft on ice and take it to a back table in the recipient operating room for thorough examination and preparation. Flush the arterial and venous pedicles with solution and assess them for vascular leakage. Tie off any vessels with evidence of leakage by suture ligation. Finally, remove all extraneous soft tissue, and mark orientation to facilitate transplantation.

## Clinical Example (0669T)

During the backbench preparation of the uterine graft, additional reconstruction of vascular grafts, including venous anastomosis, is performed prior to allotransplantation.

## Description of Procedure (0669T)

Add a venous extension graft as needed to the uterine veins.

## Clinical Example (0670T)

During the backbench preparation of the uterine graft, additional reconstruction of vascular grafts, including

arterial anastomosis, is performed prior to allotransplantation.

## Description of Procedure (0670T)

Add an arterial graft as needed to the uterine arteries.

---

**0671T** Code is out of numerical sequence. See 0175T-0200T

● **0672T** Endovaginal cryogen-cooled, monopolar radiofrequency remodeling of the tissues surrounding the female bladder neck and proximal urethra for urinary incontinence

### Rationale

Code 0672T has been established to report dual-energy tissue remodeling. Code 0672T describes remodeling of tissue at the cellular level by utilizing a cryogen-cooled, monopolar radiofrequency dual-energy approach. Prior to 2022, no codes exist in the CPT code set to describe dual-energy tissue remodeling.

## Clinical Example (0672T)

A 43-year-old female presents with a history of diagnosed urinary incontinence. The patient remains unresponsive to conservative therapies and seeks an alternative, noninvasive method of treatment.

## Description of Procedure (0672T)

Perform physical examination and prepare the patient. The physician prepares the cryogen-cooled radiofrequency device by connecting the return pad to the return cable and attaching the return pad to the patient. Prior to administering the cryogen-cooled radiofrequency, the physician administers coupling fluid into the vaginal canal. After ensuring the tissue temperature is sufficient, the physician delivers cryogen-cooled radiofrequency pulses endovaginally in a nonsurgical environment for treatment of urinary incontinence. Once sufficient rounds of treatment have been completed, the physician removes and discards the treatment tip, cleans the handpiece, and provides instructions regarding immediate postprocedural care when the patient is discharged. No prescribed pain medication is used during or after the procedure.

---

● **0673T** Ablation, benign thyroid nodule(s), percutaneous, laser, including imaging guidance

▶(Do not report 0673T in conjunction with 76940, 76942, 77013, 77022)◄

Category III 0042T-0713T

## Rationale

Code 0673T has been established to report thyroid nodule laser ablation. Code 0673T describes laser ablation of benign thyroid lesions, which is a minimally invasive outpatient procedure compared to the traditional surgical excision. In accordance with the establishment of code 0673T, an exclusionary parenthetical note has been added to instruct users on the correct use of the code. Prior to 2022, no codes exist in the CPT code set to describe thyroid nodule laser ablation.

## Clinical Example (0673T)

A 45-year-old female presents with dysphagia and a 3.0-cm palpable thyroid nodule in the lower pole of the right lobe that is solid and isoechoic by sonography and benign by fine needle aspiration cytology. The findings are consistent with a benign colloid nodule. The patient undergoes percutaneous laser ablation of the thyroid nodule.

## Description of Procedure (0673T)

Place the patient in the supine position with the neck hyperextended. Prepare and drape the surgical site. Administer local anesthesia, if required. Administer conscious sedation, if required (separately reported). Use ultrasound to localize the target lesion(s) and to position the percutaneous laser applicator. Place one or more introducer needles in the deeper portion of the target lesion(s) under real-time ultrasound guidance. Place the optical fiber(s) into the introducer needle(s). Deliver the laser energy to the target lesion(s). Monitor the ablation progress of the target lesion(s) using ultrasound imaging. Once the target lesion(s) is completely ablated, withdraw the optical fiber(s) and introducer needle(s). Apply a postoperative dressing. Provide postoperative instructions and prescriptions. Dictate an operative note.

## ▶Implantable Synchronized Diaphragmatic Stimulation System for Augmentation of Cardiac Function◀

▶An implantable synchronized diaphragmatic stimulation system for augmentation of cardiac function consists of a pulse generator and two diaphragmatic leads. The generator is placed in a subcutaneous pocket in the abdomen. The electrodes are affixed to the inferior surface of the diaphragm. The electrodes deliver synchronized diaphragmatic stimulation (SDS) pulses, causing localized contractions of the diaphragm muscle gated to the cardiac cycle, designed to augment intrathoracic pressure and improve cardiac output and left ventricular function.

For laparoscopic insertion or replacement of the complete SDS system (diaphragmatic pulse generator and lead[s]), use 0674T. For laparoscopic insertion of new or replacement of diaphragmatic lead(s), see 0675T, 0676T. For repositioning or relocation of individual components of the SDS system, see 0677T, 0678T for the diaphragmatic lead(s), or use 0681T for the diaphragmatic pulse generator. For laparoscopic removal of diaphragmatic lead(s) without replacement, use 0679T. For insertion or replacement of the diaphragmatic pulse generator only, use 0680T. For removal of the generator only, use 0682T.

Codes 0674T, 0675T, 0676T, 0677T, 0678T, 0680T, 0681T include both interrogation and programming by the implant physician, when performed. Interrogation device evaluation and programming device evaluation include parameters of pulse amplitude, pulse duration, battery status, lead and electrode selectability, impedances, and R-wave sensitivity.◀

● **0674T**    Laparoscopic insertion of new or replacement of permanent implantable synchronized diaphragmatic stimulation system for augmentation of cardiac function, including an implantable pulse generator and diaphragmatic lead(s)

▶(Do not report 0674T in conjunction with 0675T, 0676T, 0677T, 0678T, 0679T, 0680T, 0681T, 0682T, 0683T, 0684T, 0685T)◀

● **0675T**    Laparoscopic insertion of new or replacement of diaphragmatic lead(s), permanent implantable synchronized diaphragmatic stimulation system for augmentation of cardiac function, including connection to an existing pulse generator; first lead

+● **0676T**        each additional lead (List separately in addition to code for primary procedure)

▶(Use 0676T in conjunction with 0675T)◀

▶(Do not report 0675T, 0676T in conjunction with 0674T, 0677T, 0678T, 0679T, 0680T, 0681T, 0682T, 0683T, 0684T, 0685T)◀

● **0677T**    Laparoscopic repositioning of diaphragmatic lead(s), permanent implantable synchronized diaphragmatic stimulation system for augmentation of cardiac function, including connection to an existing pulse generator; first repositioned lead

+● **0678T**        each additional repositioned lead (List separately in addition to code for primary procedure)

▶(Use 0678T in conjunction with 0677T)◀

▶(Do not report 0677T, 0678T in conjunction with 0674T, 0675T, 0676T, 0679T, 0680T, 0681T, 0682T, 0683T, 0684T, 0685T)◀

● **0679T**    Laparoscopic removal of diaphragmatic lead(s), permanent implantable synchronized diaphragmatic stimulation system for augmentation of cardiac function

▲=Revised code    ●=New code    ▶◀=Contains new or revised text    ✖=Duplicate PLA test    ↕=Category I PLA    American Medical Association    **215**

Category III 0042T-0713T

▶(Use 0679T only once regardless of the number of leads removed)◀

▶(Do not report 0679T in conjunction with 0674T, 0677T, 0680T, 0681T, 0682T, 0683T, 0684T, 0685T)◀

● **0680T** Insertion or replacement of pulse generator only, permanent implantable synchronized diaphragmatic stimulation system for augmentation of cardiac function, with connection to existing lead(s)

▶(Do not report 0680T in conjunction with 0674T, 0675T, 0676T, 0677T, 0678T, 0679T, 0681T, 0682T, 0683T, 0684T, 0685T)◀

● **0681T** Relocation of pulse generator only, permanent implantable synchronized diaphragmatic stimulation system for augmentation of cardiac function, with connection to existing dual leads

▶(Do not report 0681T in conjunction with 0674T, 0675T, 0676T, 0677T, 0678T, 0679T, 0680T, 0682T, 0683T, 0684T, 0685T)◀

● **0682T** Removal of pulse generator only, permanent implantable synchronized diaphragmatic stimulation system for augmentation of cardiac function

▶(Do not report 0682T in conjunction with 0674T, 0675T, 0676T, 0677T, 0678T, 0679T, 0680T, 0681T, 0683T, 0684T, 0685T)◀

● **0683T** Programming device evaluation (in-person) with iterative adjustment of the implantable device to test the function of the device and select optimal permanent programmed values with analysis, review and report by a physician or other qualified health care professional, permanent implantable synchronized diaphragmatic stimulation system for augmentation of cardiac function

▶(Do not report 0683T in conjunction with 0674T, 0675T, 0676T, 0677T, 0678T, 0679T, 0680T, 0681T, 0682T, 0684T, 0685T, when performed by the same physician or other qualified health care professional)◀

● **0684T** Peri-procedural device evaluation (in-person) and programming of device system parameters before or after a surgery, procedure, or test with analysis, review, and report by a physician or other qualified health care professional, permanent implantable synchronized diaphragmatic stimulation system for augmentation of cardiac function

▶(Do not report 0684T in conjunction with 0674T, 0675T, 0677T, 0679T, 0680T, 0681T, 0682T, 0683T, 0685T, when performed by the same physician or other qualified health care professional)◀

● **0685T** Interrogation device evaluation (in-person) with analysis, review and report by a physician or other qualified health care professional, including connection, recording and disconnection per patient encounter, permanent implantable synchronized diaphragmatic stimulation system for augmentation of cardiac function

▶(Do not report 0685T in conjunction with 0674T, 0675T, 0677T, 0679T, 0680T, 0681T, 0682T, 0683T, 0684T, when performed by the same physician or other qualified health care professional)◀

## Rationale

A new subsection (Implantable Synchronized Diaphragmatic Stimulation System for Augmentation of Cardiac Function) and 12 new codes (0674T-0685T) have been established in the Category III section for reporting laparoscopic services using a permanent implantable synchronized diaphragmatic stimulation system for augmentation of cardiac function (0674T) and associated services. Guidelines and parenthetical notes have also been added within the new subsection and throughout the code set to provide instruction on the appropriate reporting of these services.

The new subsection, codes, guidelines, and parenthetical notes added to the Category III section, as well as the new parenthetical note added to the Surgery section, identify the services necessary to laparoscopically insert, remove, program, update, and test a system that provides stimulation of the diaphragm muscle to impact cardiac output and left ventricular function for indicated heart failure patients. The system accomplishes this by synchronizing movement of the diaphragm with the movement or beating of the heart, thereby reducing the effort necessary for the heart to pump blood throughout the body.

These changes follow CPT code convention for neurostimulator services. Therefore, all of the new codes, guidelines, and parenthetical notes reflect language and instruction commonly included for reporting these types of services (eg, placement procedures, removals, programming).

Guidelines have also been included to provide a definition and explanation regarding what the service is, what it does, and how the codes may be reported for various components identified within the codes. Parenthetical notes provide direction regarding what services may be reported together and what may not be reported together. Special restrictive circumstances are also addressed (ie, restricted reporting when performed by the same physician or QHP).

## Clinical Example (0674T)

A 60-year-old male, who has a history of New York Heart Association (NYHA) Class II heart failure, presents with an ejection fraction of 33% with fatigue. He is on optimal medical therapy and is not a candidate for cardiac resynchronization therapy.

## Description of Procedure (0674T)

After the anesthesiologist administers general anesthesia, insufflate the abdomen using a Veress needle. Establish laparoscopic access to the abdominal cavity and place two trocars, one for the laparoscopic camera and the other for the stimulation lead introduction. Under direct visualization, place two active fixation-stimulating leads on the inferior aspect of the diaphragm. A nurse or technician electrically tests these leads for impedance, stimulation, and sensing using the external programmer. If necessary, reposition the leads until acceptable performance (mapping) is obtained. Create a subcutaneous pocket in the upper-left quadrant of the abdomen to place the pulse generator and then tunnel the leads to this pocket and connect them to the generator. Desufflate the abdomen and repeat electrical testing to ensure proper performance prior to closing the wounds. Close both of the entrance points for the trocars and the subcutaneous pocket using a layered closure technique. Reverse anesthesia and transport the patient to the recovery room. In the recovery room, perform additional electrical testing with echocardiographic monitoring to confirm adequate system function.

## Clinical Example (0675T)

A 65-year-old male, who is being treated for heart failure symptoms using the diaphragmatic pacing device system that he had received 5 years ago, has been responding favorably to the therapy. One or both of the leads have lost function. Based on the patient's positive response to therapy, the physician made the decision to replace the lead(s).

## Description of Procedure (0675T)

After the anesthesiologist administers general anesthesia, the surgeon opens the subcutaneous pocket, removes the implantable pulse generator (IPG), and disconnects the leads. Insufflate the abdomen using a Veress needle. Establish laparoscopic access to the abdominal cavity and place two trocars, one for the laparoscopic camera and the other for the stimulation lead introduction. Under direct visualization, dissect any fibrosis at the lead or tissue interface and remove the previous active fixation-stimulating lead from the inferior aspect of the diaphragm. Place one new active fixation-stimulating lead on the inferior aspect of the diaphragm. Electrically test these leads for impedance, stimulation thresholds, and sensing using the external programmer. If necessary, the surgeon repositions the lead until acceptable performance (mapping) is obtained. A nurse or technician electrically tests these leads for impedance, stimulation, and sensing using the external programmer. Desufflate the abdomen and repeat electrical testing to ensure proper performance prior to closing the wounds. Close both of the entrance points for the trocars and the

subcutaneous pocket using a layered closure technique. Reverse anesthesia and transport the patient to the recovery room. In the recovery room, perform additional electrical testing with echocardiographic monitoring to confirm adequate system function.

## Clinical Example (0676T)

A 65-year-old male, who is being treated for heart failure symptoms using the diaphragmatic pacing device system that he had received 5 years ago, has been responding favorably to the therapy. Both of the leads have lost function. Based on the patient's positive response to therapy, the physician made the decision to replace the leads.

## Description of Procedure (0676T)

After the anesthesiologist administers general anesthesia, the surgeon opens the subcutaneous pocket, removes the IPG, and disconnects the leads. Insufflate the abdomen using a Veress needle. Establish laparoscopic access to the abdominal cavity and place two trocars, one for the laparoscopic camera and the other for the stimulation lead introduction. Under direct visualization, dissect any fibrosis at the lead or tissue interface and remove one of the two previous active fixation-stimulating leads from the inferior aspect of the diaphragm. Place new active fixation-stimulating leads on the inferior aspect of the diaphragm. Cardiology electrically tests these leads for impedance, stimulation thresholds, and sensing using the external programmer. If necessary, reposition the leads until acceptable performance is obtained (mapping). Desufflate the abdomen and repeat electrical testing to ensure proper performance prior to closing the wounds. Close the incision using a layered closure technique. Reverse anesthesia and transport the patient to the recovery room.

## Clinical Example (0677T)

A 65-year-old male, who is being treated for heart failure symptoms using the diaphragmatic pacing device system that he had received 5 years ago, has been responding favorably to the therapy. One of the leads has lost function. Based on the patient's positive response to therapy, the physician made the decision to reposition the lead.

## Description of Procedure (0677T)

After the anesthesiologist administers general anesthesia, the surgeon opens the subcutaneous pocket, removes the IPG, and disconnects the leads. Insufflate the abdomen using a Veress needle. Establish laparoscopic access to the abdominal cavity. Under direct visualization, dissect any fibrosis at the lead or tissue interface and reposition the lead. Electrically test both leads for impedance, stimulation thresholds, and sensing using the external programmer. Desufflate the abdomen and repeat electrical testing to ensure proper performance prior to closing the wounds. Close the incision using a layered closure technique. Reverse anesthesia and transport the patient to the recovery room.

## Clinical Example (0678T)

A 65-year-old male, who is being treated for heart failure symptoms using the diaphragmatic pacing device system that he had received 5 years ago, has been responding favorably to the therapy. Both of the leads have lost function. Based on the patient's positive response to therapy, the physician made the decision to reposition the leads.

## Description of Procedure (0678T)

After the anesthesiologist administers general anesthesia, the surgeon opens the subcutaneous pocket, removes the IPG, and disconnects the leads. Insufflate the abdomen using a Veress needle. Establish laparoscopic access to the abdominal cavity. Under direct visualization, dissect any fibrosis at the lead or tissue interface and reposition the previous two active fixation-stimulating leads. Electrically test the repositioned leads for impedance, stimulation thresholds, and sensing using the external programmer. Desufflate the abdomen and repeat electrical testing to ensure proper performance prior to closing the wounds. Close the incision using a layered closure technique. Reverse anesthesia and transport the patient to the recovery room.

## Clinical Example (0679T)

A 65-year-old male, who is being treated for heart failure symptoms using the diaphragmatic pacing device system that he had received, has developed an infection. The physician has made the decision to remove the lead(s).

## Description of Procedure (0679T)

After the anesthesiologist administers general anesthesia, the surgeon opens the subcutaneous pocket, removes the IPG, and disconnects the leads. Insufflate the abdomen using a Veress needle. Establish laparoscopic access to the abdominal cavity. Under direct visualization, dissect any fibrosis at the lead or tissue interface and remove the previous two active fixation-stimulating lead(s). Desufflate the abdomen and close the incision using a layered closure technique. Reverse anesthesia and transport the patient to the recovery room.

## Clinical Example (0680T)

A 70-year-old female, who is being treated for heart failure symptoms with a diaphragmatic pacing device system that she had received 5 years ago, has been responding favorably to the therapy. The pulse generator has reached the end of its battery life and needs to be replaced in order for the patient to continue to receive therapy.

## Description of Procedure (0680T)

Under local anesthesia, the surgeon opens the subcutaneous pocket, removes the IPG, and disconnects the leads. Electrically test these leads for impedance, stimulation thresholds, and sensing using the external programmer. Connect the existing leads to a new IPG and place them in the pocket. Close the pocket with a standard technique.

## Clinical Example (0681T)

A 70-year-old female, who is being treated for heart failure symptoms with a diaphragmatic pacing device system that she had received 3 years ago, has been responding favorably to the therapy. The pocket containing the IPG has eroded and needs to be relocated to a newly created subcutaneous pocket.

## Description of Procedure (0681T)

Under local anesthesia, the surgeon opens the subcutaneous pocket, removes the IPG, and disconnects the leads. Create a new subcutaneous pocket in another quadrant of the abdomen to place the pulse generator. Tunnel the leads to this pocket and connect them to the generator. Electrically test the leads for impedance, stimulation thresholds, and sensing using the external programmer. Connect the existing leads to an existing IPG and place them in the new subcutaneous pocket. Close the pocket with a standard technique.

## Clinical Example (0682T)

A 70-year-old female, who is being treated for heart failure symptoms with a diaphragmatic pacing device, experiences an infected subcutaneous pocket. The physician decides to remove it and discontinue therapy.

## Description of Procedure (0682T)

Under local anesthesia, the surgeon opens the subcutaneous pocket, removes the IPG, and disconnects the leads. Close the pocket with a standard technique.

## Clinical Example (0683T)

A 72-year-old male with an NYHA Class II heart failure had a diaphragmatic pacing device implanted 5 years ago. The patient calls his cardiologist because he is concerned about increasing shortness of breath and some palpitations. The cardiologist orders a programming device evaluation.

## Description of Procedure (0683T)

In the cardiologist's office, place the programming wand over the IPG to attain a communication link. Interrogate the system for diagnostic data and assess the lead system for impedance, sensing, and capture thresholds, and battery status. Reprogram the device to new parameters based on the results of the testing and physical examination.

## Clinical Example (0684T)

A 66-year-old patient with a history of NYHA Class III heart failure with an implanted synchronized diaphragmatic stimulation (SDS) system requires abdominal aortic aneurysm surgery. To avoid IPG stimuli or damage to the sensing circuitry during the surgery related to electrosurgical cautery and manipulation, the surgeon requests evaluation and programming of the IPG to prepare the patient for surgery.

## Description of Procedure (0684T)

Evaluate and deactivate the SDS system prior to the potentially hazardous procedure through the use of the external programmer. Reactivate the SDS system postoperatively and evaluate the system for any changes in function due to the indexed procedure.

## Clinical Example (0685T)

A 58-year-old female patient with a history of NYHA Class III heart failure and prior implant of an SDS system is evaluated periodically (eg, every 3 months) to monitor the function and battery status of the system as a part of her comprehensive heart failure maintenance.

## Description of Procedure (0685T)

Evaluate the SDS system for electrical performance and battery status as a part of routine patient follow-up. The physician or other QHP electrically tests the lead system and interrogates and analyzes stored diagnostic information and recordings of cardiac signals and blood pressure using the external programmer.

● **0686T**　　Histotripsy (ie, non-thermal ablation via acoustic energy delivery) of malignant hepatocellular tissue, including image guidance

### Rationale

Code 0686T has been added to report histotripsy of malignant hepatocellular tissue via use of non-thermal energy ablation. This new procedure is distinct from other methods of treatment of malignant liver tissue in that it does not ablate the tissue thermally. Instead, it destroys tissue non-thermally using acoustic energy and includes imaging guidance necessary to perform the procedure.

## Clinical Example (0686T)

A 66-year-old male, who has been diagnosed with hepatocellular carcinoma and has three ≤3-cm lesions, is not a surgical candidate and is intolerant of other therapies. The physician performs histotripsy.

## Description of Procedure (0686T)

Place the patient in the supine position. Expose the abdomen and thorax. Perform computer-assisted targeting and dosing calculations. Perform histotripsy (nonthermal tumor ablation using acoustic energy) under ultrasound guidance.

● **0687T**　　Treatment of amblyopia using an online digital program; device supply, educational set-up, and initial session

● **0688T**　　　　assessment of patient performance and program data by physician or other qualified health care professional, with report, per calendar month

▶(Do not report 0687T, 0688T in conjunction with 92065, when performed on the same day)◀

### Rationale

Codes 0687T and 0688T have been established to report the treatment of amblyopia using an online digital program. The intended use of these codes is to accurately describe treatment performed via a remote vision-training program for patients diagnosed with amblyopia.

Code 0687T is reported for an office visit during which the patient is trained on the set-up and use of the management portal, receives instruction on using the software program, and receives an initial session.

Code 0688T is reported for follow-up assessment(s) after the patient has completed at-home training sessions. The patient training activity is reviewed and interpreted, and training progress is discussed with the patient.

In accordance with the addition of codes 0687T and 0688T, a parenthetical note has been added to restrict reporting these codes with code 92065 when performed on the same day. Code 92065, *Orthoptic and/or pleoptic training, with continuing medical direction and evaluation,* is intended to report in-office training of any binocular vision disorder and would still be reported for other types of orthoptic training.

## Clinical Example (0687T)

A 20-year-old male, who was previously diagnosed with amblyopia and using best optical correction, is prescribed an online digital amblyopia vision-training program.

## Description of Procedure (0687T)

During an in-office visit, set up the patient on the management portal, instruct the patient on using the software program, and provide the patient with an initial session under the supervisory guidance of the prescribing physician or other QHP.

## Clinical Example (0688T)

A 20-year-old male, who was previously diagnosed with amblyopia and using best optical correction, is prescribed an online digital amblyopia vision-training program.

## Description of Procedure (0688T)

The prescribing physician or other QHP performs interim treatment follow-up assessment(s) after the patient has completed 20 to 40 home training sessions. Review and interpret patient-training activity and discuss training progress with the patient with respect to improvement in best corrected visual acuity (BCVA), contrast sensitivity function (CSF), and stereo and binocular functions. Document the results of the assessment in the patient's application management system.

● **0689T**  Quantitative ultrasound tissue characterization (non-elastographic), including interpretation and report, obtained without diagnostic ultrasound examination of the same anatomy (eg, organ, gland, tissue, target structure)

▶(Do not report 0689T in conjunction with 76536, 76604, 76641, 76642, 76700, 76705, 76770, 76775, 76830, 76856, 76857, 76870, 76872, 76881, 76882, 76981, 76982, 76983, 76999, 93880, 93882, 93998, 0690T)◀

+● **0690T**  Quantitative ultrasound tissue characterization (non-elastographic), including interpretation and report, obtained with diagnostic ultrasound examination of the same anatomy (eg, organ, gland, tissue, target structure) (List separately in addition to code for primary procedure)

▶(Use 0690T in conjunction with 76536, 76604, 76641, 76642, 76700, 76705, 76770, 76775, 76830, 76856, 76857, 76870, 76872, 76881, 76882, 76981, 76982, 76999, 93880, 93882, 93998)◀

▶(Do not report 0690T in conjunction with 0689T)◀

## Rationale

Codes 0689T and 0690T have been established to report non-elastographic quantitative ultrasound tissue characterization obtained without (0689T) and with (0690T) diagnostic ultrasound examination of the same anatomy. To support accurate reporting, inclusionary and exclusionary parentheticals have been added both within the code family and in the Radiology section.

Quantitative ultrasound tissue characterization (non-elastographic) is a diagnostic technology that evaluates visceral organs and other anatomic structures and does not utilize biopsy as part of the process for detection and diagnosis. This procedure uses imaging data that is analyzed for tissue characteristics. The resultant analysis may be used to determine surgical or pharmacological interventions or for quantifications, such as liver fat fraction, which is an important factor for analysis of conditions, such as hepatic steatosis (an increased build-up of fat in the liver) and nonalcoholic fatty liver disease. The procedure may be used concurrently with ultrasound visualization (0690T) or independently (0689T).

Use of add-on code 0690T differs from typical add-on codes because this code is not intended to be reported in conjunction with the code within the family that precedes it (0689T). Instead, an inclusionary parenthetical note indicates that code 0690T should be reported as an add-on code in addition to specific ultrasound procedures as listed within the parenthetical note.

To provide additional clarification regarding the intent and use of these codes, exclusionary parenthetical notes have been added following each new code, as well as following code 76983 in the Radiology section. The exclusionary parenthetical notes regarding use of code 0689T provide specific ultrasound procedures that are restricted. Additional exclusionary instruction clarifies that codes 0689T and 0690T should not be reported together.

## Clinical Example (0689T)

A 57-year-old female presents with metabolic syndrome and elevated liver enzyme tests. The patient is referred for quantitative ultrasound tissue characterization (non-elastographic) for noninvasive liver fat fraction analysis.

## Description of Procedure (0689T)

The physician reviews prior imaging studies on which the organ of interest is found and communicates to the ultrasound technologist to delineate the area to be interrogated and any structures to be avoided. Perform a measurement of liver fat fraction and report the results. The radiologist analyzes the fat-fraction measurements of the parenchyma of interest at the picture archiving and communication system (PACS) workstation and

★ = Telemedicine  ✦ = Add-on code  ✔ = FDA approval pending  # = Resequenced code  ⊘ = Modifier 51 exempt

compares the current examination to any prior examinations to evaluate for stability or interval changes. The radiologist dictates the examination report.

Review, edit, and sign a report of the quantitative ultrasound for tissue characterization (non-nelastographic) for the patient's medical record. Communicate the findings with the referring provider and/or the patient for appropriate management.

## Clinical Example (0690T)

A 63-year-old male, who has a history of diabetes, presents with elevated liver enzyme tests. The patient has suspected long-term fatty liver with elevated alanine transaminase/aspartate transaminase (ALT/AST). The patient is referred for quantitative ultrasound tissue characterization (non-elastographic) for non-invasive liver fat fraction analysis and abdominal limited ultrasound to assess for fibrosis and liver lesions. [**Note:** This is an add-on service. Only consider the additional work spent providing quantitative ultrasound tissue characterization obtained with diagnostic ultrasound examination of the same anatomy.]

## Description of Procedure (0690T)

The physician reviews prior imaging studies on which the organ of interest is found and communicates to the ultrasound technologist to delineate the area to be interrogated and any structures to be avoided. Perform a measurement of liver fat fraction and report the results. The radiologist analyzes the fat-fraction measurements of the parenchyma of interest at the PACS workstation and compares the current examination to any prior examinations to evaluate for stability or interval changes. The radiologist dictates the examination report.

Obtain a separate abdominal limited ultrasound to assess for fibrosis and liver lesions. Evaluate included anatomic structures and compare them with any available pertinent prior examinations. The radiologist dictates the examination report.

Review, edit, and sign a report of the quantitative ultrasound for tissue characterization (non-elastographic) and abdominal limited ultrasound for the patient's medical record. Communicate the findings with the referring provider and/or the patient for appropriate management.

● **0691T**     Automated analysis of an existing computed tomography study for vertebral fracture(s), including assessment of bone density when performed, data preparation, interpretation, and report

▶(Do not report 0691T in conjunction with 71250, 71260, 71270, 71271, 71275, 72125, 72126, 72127, 72128, 72129, 72130, 72131, 72132, 72133, 72191, 72192, 72193, 72194, 74150, 74160, 74170, 74174, 74175, 74176, 74177, 74178, 74261, 74262, 74263, 75571, 75572, 75573, 75574, 75635, 78814, 78815, 78816, 0554T, 0555T, 0556T, 0557T, 0558T)◀

## Rationale

Code 0691T has been established to report automated analysis of an existing CT data set for vertebral fractures, including assessment of bone density when performed, data preparation, transmission, interpretation and report.

Code 0691T enables reporting a service that uses previously acquired data, whether performed at the same institution or an outside institution, to provide information regarding bone health and detect subtle vertebral fractures, which may not have been the intent of the original study (eg, a lung cancer screening CT scan can later be used in a patient with fall risk to determine bone health and find subtle vertebral body fractures in the thoracic spine). This service would not be applied universally to every study performed but rather performed for individuals with a baseline pre-test probability (eg, elderly patients with suspected osteoporosis or patients on steroid therapy).

Typically, this service would be specifically requested by the referring clinician for this explicit purpose. This is a service that requires additional technical expertise and professional time in reviewing and interpreting outputs of this algorithm within the context of patient-specific factors. It is not inherent in the work of the existing CT code and would not be routinely part of diagnostic CT studies. This service is an entirely different service from the original CT reported, and would not have been included in the original report, even if performed by the same interpreting physician or QHP.

In accordance with the addition of code 0691T, an exclusionary parenthetical note has been added to restrict reporting this code with codes 71250, 71260, 71270, 71271, 71275, 72125-72133, 72191-72194, 74150, 74160, 74170, 74174-74178, 74261-74263, 75571-75574, 75635, 78814-78816, and 0554T-0558T. In addition, exclusionary parenthetical notes have been added following codes 0557T and 0558T to restrict the reporting of code 0691T with codes 0554T-0558T.

Category III 0042T-0713T

## Clinical Example (0691T)

A 68-year-old female with acute onset of shortness of breath was referred for computed tomographic angiogram (CTA) of the chest to rule out pulmonary embolism (PE). Weeks later, her primary care physician requested automated analysis and report of the prior CTA dataset for detection of vertebral fractures.

## Description of Procedure (0691T)

The physician or other QHP receives an order for automated analysis of vertebral fracture(s) and estimation of bone mineral density using a previously reported CT study. Prepare and send the CT data for automated analysis. The computer software interrogates the received CT data and flags vertebral bodies suspected of vertebral compression fracture. Return the flagged dataset to the physician or other QHP who then uses the flagged dataset to perform an interpretation and create a report.

● **0692T**   Therapeutic ultrafiltration

▶(Use 0692T no more than once per day)◀

▶(Do not report 0692T in conjunction with 36511, 36512, 36513, 36514, 36516, 36522, 90935, 90937, 90945, 90947)◀

▶(For therapeutic apheresis, see 36511, 36512, 36513, 36514, 36516)◀

▶(For extracorporeal photopheresis, use 36522)◀

▶(For hemodialysis procedures, see 90935, 90937)◀

▶(For dialysis procedures, see 90945, 90947)◀

### Rationale

Code 0692T has been established to report therapeutic ultrafiltration services. Parenthetical notes have been added following code 0692T, added within the Dialysis subsection of the Medicine section, and revised following code 36522 to provide instruction on the appropriate reporting of this service vs other similar services.

Therapeutic ultrafiltration is a procedure by which blood is filtered through a semipermeable membrane to remove isotonic plasma water and restore the patient's volume status. This procedure differs from others because the fluid is separated instead of the blood constituents, such as platelets or white cells.

To direct users regarding the appropriate reporting of other filtration-type services, cross-reference parenthetical notes have been added following code 0692T for therapeutic apheresis, extracorporeal photopheresis, hemodialysis, and dialysis services. Instruction has also been included to restrict reporting this service in conjunction with any of the other filtration services and to restrict use of this code more than once per day.

A cross-reference parenthetical note has also been revised within the Cardiovascular System section and added within the Dialysis subsections to direct users to the appropriate code to report therapeutic ultrafiltration.

## Clinical Example (0692T)

A 67-year-old female, who has ischemic heart disease with chronic systolic and diastolic heart failure, decompensates and develops acute congestive heart failure. Medical management with maximal doses of IV diuretics fails to improve her pulmonary edema, and it is elected to apply therapeutic ultrafiltration.

## Description of Procedure (0692T)

The physician performing the procedure determines the appropriate vascular access that will best support the extracorporeal circuit for ultrafiltration. Write specific orders for the procedure care team that include determining a specific device, treatment duration, blood flow and fluid removal rates, end-target fluid goals, anticoagulation, and hemodynamic guardrails. During the procedure, the physician or care team periodically evaluates the patient's clinical status, paying particular attention to the patient's vital signs, fluid-in and fluid-out levels, renal function status, and other relevant parameters. Based on the clinical status of the patient and the performance of the device, the physician may adjust the blood flow and/or ultrafiltration rate(s) and adjust other orders as necessary. Upon completion, document the procedure and outcomes in the patient's medical record.

● **0693T**   Comprehensive full body computer-based markerless 3D kinematic and kinetic motion analysis and report

### Rationale

New code 0693T has been established for reporting comprehensive, full body, computer-based, markerless three-dimensional (3D) kinematic and kinetic motion analysis.

The procedure involves computer calculation of 3D joint-motion data in three planes simultaneously. A computer-generated skeletal model is created based on the optical video feeds. Kinematic and kinetic information are then calculated, and a report that consists of a series of graphs and tables is generated, which physicians or other QHPs use for their report. These results are obtained without the use of a local coordinate system created from body markers.

★ =Telemedicine   ✚ =Add-on code   ✗ =FDA approval pending   # =Resequenced code   ⊘ =Modifier 51 exempt

## Clinical Example (0693T)

A 25-year-old male, who has a sprain of the anterior cruciate ligament of the left knee, is referred for markerless three-dimensional (3D) motion analysis to improve planning for physical therapy, orthotic management, and orthopedic surgery.

## Description of Procedure (0693T)

Record the patient performing various movements using frame-synced high-speed cameras located at the patient's front, back, and sides. Using computer software, calculate accurate, 3D joint-motion data in three planes simultaneously; create a computer-generated skeletal model of the subject based on the optical video feeds; calculate kinematic and kinetic information; and calculate the moments and forces acting around each of the major joints. Report the information gathered from the motion analysis conducted by the software in a series of graphs and tables showing movement data. A physician or other QHP interprets the data and issues a report of findings.

● **0694T**     3-dimensional volumetric imaging and reconstruction of breast or axillary lymph node tissue, each excised specimen, 3-dimensional automatic specimen reorientation, interpretation and report, real-time intraoperative

▶(Do not report 0694T in conjunction with 76098)◀

▶(Report 0694T once per specimen)◀

### Rationale

Code 0694T has been established to report real-time intraoperative 3D volumetric imaging and reconstruction of breast or axillary lymph node tissue. This technology is used during surgery, such as a breast lumpectomy, to assist the physician in analyzing the excised lesions (eg, tumor, mass) to determine if additional tissue should be excised from the surgical site.

Code 0694T is reported once for each excised specimen for which the procedure described by code 0694T is performed. An instructional parenthetical note has been added for clarification. An exclusionary parenthetical note has also been added, restricting the use of code 0694T with code 76098, which describes radiological examination of a surgical specimen. Interpretation and a written report must be performed to report code 0694T.

## Clinical Example (0694T)

A 70-year-old female, who is undergoing a lumpectomy to remove the lesion in her breast, requires an additional procedure in which her ex-vivo specimen is evaluated using 3D radiography and software analysis of the image data to assess the surgical margins and calcifications intraoperatively during surgery.

## Description of Procedure (0694T)

The surgeon excises the specimen during surgery (reported separately). The surgeon or operating room staff places the specimen in the cabinet of the 3D volumetric radiography machine and initiates the automated scan and 3D reconstruction algorithm. After several minutes, the surgeon or radiologist analyzes and interprets the 3D image data on the software by rotating and marking the output. The surgeon continues with the surgery knowing which additional tissue to remove. The surgeon then removes the additional tissue. The physician prepares a written report.

● **0695T**     Body surface–activation mapping of pacemaker or pacing cardioverter-defibrillator lead(s) to optimize electrical synchrony, cardiac resynchronization therapy device, including connection, recording, disconnection, review, and report; at time of implant or replacement

▶(Use 0695T in conjunction with 33224, 33225, 33226)◀

● **0696T**     at time of follow-up interrogation or programming device evaluation

▶(Use 0696T in conjunction with 93281, 93284, 93286, 93287, 93288, 93289)◀

### Rationale

Codes 0695T and 0696T have been established to report body surface–activation mapping of pacemaker or pacing cardioverter-defibrillator leads to optimize electrical synchrony, including recording and connection and disconnection of a cardiac resynchronization therapy device. Code 0695T is reported when the procedure is performed at the time of the implant or replacement of the pacemaker or pacing cardioverter-defibrillator device. Code 0696T is reported when the procedure is performed at the time of follow-up interrogation or programming device evaluation.

Body surface–activation mapping is a technology used to determine optimal placement of a cardiac resynchronization device, such as a pacemaker or cardioverter-defibrillator, to treat cardiac dyssynchrony. Cardiac dyssynchrony is a lack of harmonization of contractions in the heart ventricles. This lack of synchrony is related to heart conditions, such as congestive heart failure.

> Code 0695T is reported with codes 33224-33226. Code 0696T is reported with codes 93281, 93284, and 93286-93289. Inclusionary parenthetical notes have been added following codes 0695T and 0696T, listing the codes that may be reported with these two codes. Both codes 0695T and 0696T include review and report.

## Clinical Example (0695T)

A 70-year-old female, who has a history of heart failure, presents for the implantation of a cardiac resynchronization defibrillator.

## Description of Procedure (0695T)

Secure a 40-lead electrocardiogram (ECG) belt on the patient's chest. After the leads for the cardiac resynchronization therapy (CRT) system are placed (reported separately), obtain measurements using body-surface mapping with and without pacing. Use the readings from the ECG belt to determine if global synchrony has been achieved. If global synchrony is not achieved, the physician may adjust pacing parameter(s) or reposition the lead(s) and repeat the process. Use readings from the ECG belt to optimize the location of the pacing lead, the pacing vector, atrioventricular (A-V) timing, and interventricular (V-V) timing to create global synchrony. Repeat the process until global synchrony is achieved. Connect and place the generator in the pocket and close the pocket (reported separately).

## Clinical Example (0696T)

A 72-year-old male with a history of heart failure, who was treated with a cardiac resynchronization implantable cardioverter-defibrillator (ICD) system followed with interrogation device evaluations (in person), presents to the clinic for a follow-up to assess device function and global synchrony and to optimize device settings using body-surface mapping when necessary.

## Description of Procedure (0696T)

Perform an interrogation or programming evaluation of the CRT system (reported separately). Secure a 40-lead ECG belt on the patient's chest. Obtain measurements using body-surface mapping with and without pacing. Use the readings from the ECG belt to determine if global synchrony has been maintained. Use the readings from the ECG belt to optimize the pacing location, A-V timing, and V-V timing to create and maintain global synchrony. When the ECG belt readings indicate dyssynchrony, reprogram the CRT device to pacing settings that will achieve or optimize the global synchrony as confirmed by the ECG belt readings.

**0697T**   Code is out of numerical sequence. See 0647T-0651T

**0698T**   Code is out of numerical sequence. See 0647T-0651T

▶The anterior segment of the eye includes the cornea, lens, iris, and aqueous. The aqueous is divided into anterior and posterior chambers. The anterior chamber is by far the larger, including all of the aqueous in front of the lens and iris and behind the cornea. The posterior chamber includes the narrow area behind the iris and in front of the peripheral portion of the lens and lens zonules.◀

● **0699T**   Injection, posterior chamber of eye, medication

## Rationale

Code 0699T has been established to report injection of medication into the posterior chamber of the eye. Guidelines have been added to clarify the anatomic location of the posterior chamber.

The posterior chamber is a part of the aqueous, which is located in the anterior segment of the eye. Existing code 66030 describes injection of medication into the anterior chamber of the eye. Prior to 2022, no code was available to report a medication injection into the posterior chamber. Substances such as anti-inflammatory medication are injected into the posterior chamber to treat patients such as those with cataracts who have received an intraocular lens.

## Clinical Example (0699T)

A 73-year-old female with cataracts, who has received an intraocular lens, receives an injection of anti-inflammatory medication into the posterior chamber.

## Description of Procedure (0699T)

At the conclusion of the cataract procedure, inject dexamethasone drug-delivery suspension behind the iris in the inferior portion of the posterior chamber.

● **0700T**   Molecular fluorescent imaging of suspicious nevus; first lesion

+● **0701T**   each additional lesion (List separately in addition to code for primary procedure)

▶(Use 0701T in conjunction with 0700T)◀

## Rationale

Two new Category III codes (0700T, 0701T) have been established to report molecular fluorescent imaging of suspicious nevus, which is used to identify biological activity that may develop into melanoma. The service involves the application of a dye to the mole or lesion of interest followed by using a handheld imaging device to take photographic and fluorescent images of the suspicious nevus. The images are transferred to a computer and analyzed.

The new codes are used to report the first lesion (0700T) and each additional lesion (0701T) thereafter.

## Clinical Example (0700T)

A 56-year-old male, who has a history of atypical moles and skin cancer, presents for follow-up and evaluation when an atypical nevus is identified. Molecular fluorescent imaging of the lesion is ordered to determine the likelihood of premalignancy or malignancy.

## Description of Procedure (0700T)

Apply a molecular fluorescent dye to the mole identified. Take photographic and fluorescent images of the suspicious nevus using a handheld imaging device. Transfer the images to a computer loaded with software and analyze. Generate a written report from the computer.

## Clinical Example (0701T)

A 56-year-old male, who has a history of atypical moles and skin cancer, presents for follow-up and evaluation when atypical nevi are identified. Molecular fluorescent imaging of the lesion is ordered to determine the likelihood of premalignancy or malignancy on the additional lesions (the first lesion analysis is coded separately). [**Note:** This is an add-on service. Only consider the additional work related to the fluorescent molecular imaging test.]

## Description of Procedure (0701T)

After evaluation of the first lesion (reported separately), apply a molecular fluorescent dye to the mole identified. Take photographic and fluorescent images of the suspicious nevi using a handheld imaging device. Transfer the images to a computer loaded with software and analyze. Generate a written report from the computer.

● **0702T**    Remote therapeutic monitoring of a standardized online digital cognitive behavioral therapy program ordered by a physician or other qualified health care professional; supply and technical support, per 30 days

● **0703T**    management services by physician or other qualified health care professional, per calendar month

▶(Do not report 0702T, 0703T in conjunction with 96158, 96159, 98975, 98976, 98977, 99091, 99424, 99425, 99426, 99427, 99437, 99453, 99454, 99457, 99458, 99484, 99492, 99493, 99494)◀

## Rationale

Two new Category III codes (0702T, 0703T) have been established to report remote therapeutic monitoring of a standardized online digital cognitive behavioral therapy program.

Code 0702T is intended to be reported for the supply and technical support for each 30 days. Code 0703T is intended to be reported for management services performed by the physician or other QHP per calendar month.

These services represent online computer-based cognitive behavioral therapy that can be used for a range of disorders, including substance use. An exclusionary parenthetical note has been added to restrict the reporting of codes 0702T and 0703T with codes 96158, 96159, 98975-98977, 99091, 99424-99427, 99437, 99453, 99454, 99457, 99458, 99484, and 99492-99494.

## Clinical Example (0702T)

A 28-year-old male, who is screened at an outpatient substance-abuse facility, reports ongoing cocaine, marijuana, and alcohol use.

## Description of Procedure (0702T)

Provide the patient with secure access to the standardized online digital cognitive behavioral therapy program, which is provided based on mutually agreed upon treatment parameters.

## Clinical Example (0703T)

A 28-year-old male, who is screened at an outpatient substance-abuse facility, reports ongoing cocaine, marijuana, and alcohol use.

## Description of Procedure (0703T)

The patient uses the digital cognitive behavioral therapy program and the physician or other QHP checks in twice a month with the patient.

● **0704T**    Remote treatment of amblyopia using an eye tracking device; device supply with initial set-up and patient education on use of equipment

● **0705T**    surveillance center technical support including data transmission with analysis, with a minimum of 18 training hours, each 30 days

● **0706T**    interpretation and report by physician or other qualified health care professional, per calendar month

▶(Do not report 0704T, 0705T, 0706T in conjunction with 92065, when performed on the same day)◀

▶(Do not report 0704T, 0705T, 0706T in conjunction with 0687T, 0688T, when reported during the same period)◀

## Rationale

Three new Category III codes (0704T-0706T) have been established to report remote treatment of amblyopia using an eye-tracking device.

Code 0704T describes an office visit during which the patient is trained on the set-up of the eye-tracking device equipment and management of the amblyopia, receives instructions on using the software program, and receives an initial session.

Code 0705T describes monitoring the treatment from the surveillance center. For example, if treatment is low in frequency, the surveillance center staff may contact the patient to encourage compliance and provide technical support if needed. The surveillance center may also notify the physician of the patient's reduced treatment frequency.

Code 0706T describes the interpretation and report of the treatment. The treatment results are securely transmitted to a secured database where the data is stored and accessible for monitoring. In addition, the physician or other QHP will generate an interpretive report reflecting results of the remote monitoring and treatment for the calendar month.

Codes 0704T-0706T are intended to report remote amblyopia treatment using a dedicated device that interfaces with a remote surveillance center. Codes 0704T-0706T are different from codes 0687T and 0688T because the services described in codes 0704T-0706T are intended to report the remote treatment of amblyopia using an eye-tracking device. Codes 0687T and 0688T are intended to report the treatment of amblyopia using an online digital program.

Two exclusionary parenthetical notes have been established in this code family. The first restricts the reporting of codes 0704T-0706T with code 92065 when performed on the same day. The second restricts the reporting of codes 0704T-0706T with codes 0687T and 0688T when reported during the same period.

## Clinical Example (0704T)

A 4-year-old male is diagnosed with amblyopia following school-based visual screening. After an unsuccessful course of eye-patching treatment, the child is prescribed remote treatment using an eye-tracking device.

## Description of Procedure (0704T)

Securely transmit the treatment results to a secured database, where the data are stored and analyzed by surveillance center staff. In the event of low-treatment frequency, surveillance center staff contacts the patient to encourage compliance and provide technical support and notifies the physician of the patient's reduced treatment frequency. The surveillance center provides the physician or other QHP the treatment data generated by the device and analyzed by the surveillance center.

## Clinical Example (0705T)

A 4-year-old male is diagnosed with amblyopia following school-based visual screening. After an unsuccessful course of eye-patching treatment, the child is prescribed remote treatment using an eye-tracking device.

## Description of Procedure (0705T)

Securely transmit the treatment results to a secured database, where the data are stored and analyzed by surveillance center staff. In the event of low-treatment frequency, surveillance center staff contacts the patient to encourage compliance and provide technical support and notifies the physician of the patient's reduced treatment frequency. The surveillance center provides the physician or other QHP the treatment data generated by the device and analyzed by the surveillance center.

## Clinical Example (0706T)

A 4-year-old male is diagnosed with amblyopia following school-based visual screening. After an unsuccessful course of eye-patching treatment, the child is prescribed remote treatment using an eye-tracking device.

## Description of Procedure (0706T)

Securely transmit the treatment results to a secured database where the data are stored and accessible for monitoring by the prescribing physician. During the month, the physician updates the visual acuity and stereo acuity results through the web application, and the treatment parameters are recalculated and updated automatically as needed. For each reporting month, the physician or other QHP generates an interpretive report that reflects the results of the remote monitoring and treatment.

● **0707T**   Injection(s), bone-substitute material (eg, calcium phosphate) into subchondral bone defect (ie, bone marrow lesion, bone bruise, stress injury, microtrabecular fracture), including imaging guidance and arthroscopic assistance for joint visualization

▶(Do not report 0707T in conjunction with 29805, 29860, 29870, 77002)◀

▶(For aspiration and injection of bone cysts, use 20615)◀

★ = Telemedicine   ✛ = Add-on code   ✗ = FDA approval pending   # = Resequenced code   ⦰ = Modifier 51 exempt

## Rationale

Code 0707T has been established to report injection of bone-substitute material into a subchrondral bone defect, including imaging guidance and arthroscopic assistance for joint visualization.

An exclusionary parenthetical note restricting the reporting of code 0707T with codes 29805, 29860, 29870, and 77002 has been added. A cross-reference parenthetical note directing users to report code 20615 for aspiration and injection of bone cysts has also been added.

## Clinical Example (0707T)

A 54-year-old male presents with chronic pain associated with bone changes or joint degradation due to osteoarthritis. Upon MRI, bone marrow lesions are detected in the surrounding bony tissue.

## Description of Procedure (0707T)

Obtain anatomic anteroposterior and lateral fluoroscopic images, mark the joint plateau line and other landmarks, and approximate the entry points as desired. Make small incisions at the noted entry points. Insert an arthroscope into the joint to aid in targeting the defect and assessing the extent of the bone injury. Remove the arthroscope when finished. Drill the cannula through the cortex, just into the cancellous bone, using a drill and wire driver. Confirm the planned trajectory to the bone defect with additional fluoroscopic imaging. Continue drilling until the cannula is at the desired depth. Confirm cannula placement again with fluoroscopic imaging, and then rotate the cannula manually to direct delivery fenestrations and flow toward the defect. Mix the preferred bone-substitute material and attach the syringe to the cannula. Inject the bone-substitute material using steady manual pressure. Remove the first syringe and repeat the previous step until the desired volume has been implanted, adjusting the cannula depth to expand the area of injection. Reinsert the arthroscope into the joint to evaluate for and evacuate any extravasated material. Remove the cannula using reverse torque on the drill while pulling back. Ensure no excess bone-substitute material emerges from the insertion portal. Ensure proper placement of the bone-substitute material using fluoroscopic imaging. Seal all incisions.

| | | |
|---|---|---|
| ● **0708T** | Intradermal cancer immunotherapy; preparation and initial injection | |
| +● **0709T** | each additional injection (List separately in addition to code for primary procedure) | |

▶(Use 0709T in conjunction with 0708T)◀

▶(Do not report 0708T, 0709T in conjunction with 96372)◀

## Rationale

The CPT code set has been updated to include two new Category III codes (0708T, 0709T) to identify intradermal cancer immunotherapy services. In addition, inclusionary, exclusionary, and cross-reference parenthetical notes have been added to clarify the appropriate reporting of this new service.

Codes 0708T and 0709T are used to report cancer immunotherapy performed intradermally via injections. This procedure includes the preparation of the dosing emulsion for the intradermal cancer immunotherapy and the initial injection service used for treatment as part of a single initial service (0708T). Additional injections provided for therapy are reported using add-on code 0709T, and is reported for each additional intradermal injection as needed.

Cross-reference parenthetical notes have been added following codes 96372 and 96401 to direct users to report the appropriate codes. An additional parenthetical note has been added to restrict reporting codes 0708T and 0709T (intradermal cancer immunotherapy services) in conjunction with code 96372.

## Clinical Example (0708T)

A 58-year-old patient, who has HLA type HLA-A*02:01 and has received initial treatment with surgery and radiation with chemotherapy and has had no prior bevacizumab therapy, presents with progressive glioblastoma. The patient is scheduled to receive intradermal cancer immunotherapy.

## Description of Procedure (0708T)

The physician or other QHP prepares the dosing emulsion for the intradermal cancer immunotherapy. Preparation requires combining two active ingredients and then agitating the preparation with a third agent to create a water and oil emulsion. Filter and emulsify the solution. Following emulsification, perform a drop test to verify the emulsion was prepared accurately. If the preparation fails the drop test, discard and initiate a new preparation.

Following successful preparation of the intradermal cancer immunotherapy, fill intradermal administration syringe(s) to a 0.1-mL dose volume. The physician or other QHP performs a subdermal injection creating a small wheal or blister.

## Clinical Example (0709T)

A 62-year-old patient, who has progressive glioblastoma is receiving intradermal cancer immunotherapy and requires additional intradermal injections to achieve recommended dose. [**Note:** This is an add-on service. Only consider the additional work related to each additional intradermal injection.]

## Description of Procedure (0709T)

Following the initial injection (separately reported), the physician or other QHP prepares the next injection site and performs a subdermal injection creating a small wheal or blister.

---

● **0710T** Noninvasive arterial plaque analysis using software processing of data from non-coronary computerized tomography angiography; including data preparation and transmission, quantification of the structure and composition of the vessel wall and assessment for lipid-rich necrotic core plaque to assess atherosclerotic plaque stability, data review, interpretation and report

▶(Do not report 0710T in conjunction with 0711T, 0712T, 0713T)◀

● **0711T** data preparation and transmission

● **0712T** quantification of the structure and composition of the vessel wall and assessment for lipid-rich necrotic core plaque to assess atherosclerotic plaque stability

● **0713T** data review, interpretation and report

▶(Do not report 0710T, 0711T, 0712T, 0713T in conjunction with 0501T, 0502T, 0503T, 0504T, 0623T, 0624T, 0625T, 0626T)◀

### Rationale

Four new Category III codes (0710T-0713T) have been established to report noninvasive arterial plaque analyses. In addition, several parenthetical notes have been added in the Diagnostic Radiology (Diagnostic Imaging), Head and Neck subsection and following new codes 0710T and 0713T to provide guidance on the appropriate reporting of these new codes with other codes in the CPT code set.

A new family of codes has been created to describe a new diagnostic imaging tool, which analyzes the structural and composition biomarkers of atherosclerotic plaque stability for all arterial vessels, such as coronary, aorta, femoral, carotid, and/or intracranial artery(ies) or vessels, derived from CTA.

Code 0710T describes noninvasive arterial plaque analysis using software to analyze data from a non-coronary CTA. This comprehensive code also includes data preparation and transmission; quantification of the structure and composition of the vessel wall and assessment for lipid-rich necrotic core plaque to assess atherosclerotic plaque

stability; and data review, interpretation, and report. Code 0711T is reported when data preparation and transmission are performed for noninvasive arterial plaque analysis. Code 0712T is reported for quantification of the structure and composition of the vessel wall and assessment for lipid-rich necrotic core plaque to assess atherosclerotic plaque stability. Code 0713T is reported for data review, interpretation, and report.

To assist in the appropriate reporting of this new series of codes, two parenthetical notes have been added following codes 0710T and 0713T. The first parenthetical note restricts reporting code 0710T with codes 0711T-0713T. The second parenthetical note restricts reporting new codes 0710T-0713T in conjunction with other services in the CPT code set.

In support of the establishment of codes 0711T-0713T, several exclusionary parenthetical notes have been added following codes 70496, 70498, 72191, 73706, 74175, 75635, 76376, and 76377 to reference new codes 0711T-0713T.

## Clinical Example (0710T)

A 70-year-old male presents with recurrent episodes of left arm, face, and leg weakness. CTA of the neck demonstrated stenosis of the left carotid artery. An order is placed for the quantification of the arterial structure and an assessment of plaque composition biomarkers to include lipid-rich necrotic core to determine atherosclerotic plaque stability.

## Description of Procedure (0710T)

Select a CTA examination that was previously performed and interpreted at a different setting. The technologist extracts patient data from the medical records system and locates and transmits the images. The physician selects one or more arterial segments for analysis. The physician then selects two or more points on the artery of interest and segments the data. Review and re-edit the segmented data until the data are adequate for lumen and wall analysis. Quantify the arterial segment (wall area, stenosis, wall thickness, plaque burden, remodeling ratio). Quantify plaque composition (calcification, lipid-rich necrotic core, matrix, and intraplaque hemorrhage) biomarkers. Prepare, analyze, review, and compare the data with the relevant CTA. The physician interprets the data within the patient's clinical context. Dictate a report for the patient's record and communicate findings to the ordering physician.

## Clinical Example (0711T)

A 70-year-old male presents with recurrent episodes of left arm, face, and leg weakness. CTA of the neck demonstrated stenosis of the left carotid artery. An order is placed for the quantification of the arterial structure and an assessment of plaque composition biomarkers to include lipid-rich necrotic core to determine atherosclerotic plaque stability.

## Description of Procedure (0711T)

Select a CTA examination that was previously performed and interpreted at a different setting. The technologist extracts patient data from the medical records system and locates and transmits the images.

## Clinical Example (0712T)

A 70-year-old male presents with recurrent episodes of left arm, face, and leg weakness. CTA of the neck demonstrated stenosis of the left carotid artery. An order is placed for the quantification of the arterial structure and an assessment of plaque composition biomarkers to include lipid-rich necrotic core to determine atherosclerotic plaque stability.

## Description of Procedure (0712T)

The physician receives the extracted data and images. The physician selects one or more arterial segments for analysis. The physician then selects two or more points on the artery of interest and segments the data. Review and re-edit the segmented data until the data are adequate for lumen and wall analysis. Quantify the arterial segment (wall area, stenosis, wall thickness, plaque burden, remodeling ratio). Quantify the plaque composition (calcification, lipid rich necrotic core, matrix, and intraplaque hemorrhage) biomarkers. Perform segmentation and quantification on all selected arterial segments. Confirm the work and quantify the final output.

## Clinical Example (0713T)

A 70-year-old male presents with recurrent episodes of left arm, face, and leg weakness. CTA of the neck demonstrated stenosis of the left carotid artery. An order is placed for the quantification of the arterial structure and an assessment of plaque composition biomarkers to include lipid-rich necrotic core to determine atherosclerotic plaque stability.

## Description of Procedure (0713T)

The interpreting physician receives the segmentation and quantification data. Analyze, review, and compare this data with the relevant CTA. The physician interprets the data within the patient's clinical context. Dictate a report for the patient's record and communicate findings to the ordering physician.

▲ = Revised code   ● = New code   ▶ ◀ = Contains new or revised text   ✕ = Duplicate PLA test   ↑↓ = Category I PLA   American Medical Association   **229**

Category III  0042T-0713T

# Notes

# Appendix A

## Summary of Additions, Deletions, and Revisions

The summary of changes shows the actual changes that have been made to the code descriptors.

New codes appear with a bullet (●) and are indicated as "Code added." Revised codes are preceded with a triangle (▲). Within revised codes, or if a code symbol has been deleted, the deleted language and code symbol appear with a ~~strikethrough~~, while new text appears <u>underlined</u>.

The ✗ symbol is used to identify codes for vaccines that are pending FDA approval. The # symbol is used to identify codes that have been resequenced. CPT add-on codes are annotated by the ✚ symbol. The ⊘ symbol is used to identify codes that are exempt from the use of modifier 51. The ★ symbol is used to identify codes that may be used for reporting telemedicine services. The ✕ symbol is used to identify a proprietary laboratory analyses (PLA) test that has an identical descriptor as another PLA test. A PLA code that satisfies Category I code criteria and has been accepted by the CPT Editorial Panel is annotated with the ↑↓ symbol.

| Modifier | Modifier Descriptor |
|---|---|
| 63 | ▶**Procedure Performed on Infants less than 4 kg:** Procedures performed on neonates and infants up to a present body weight of 4 kg may involve significantly increased complexity and physician or other qualified health care professional work commonly associated with these patients. This circumstance may be reported by adding modifier 63 to the procedure number. **Note:** Unless otherwise designated, this modifier may only be appended to procedures/services listed in the 20100-69990 code series and 92920, 92928, 92953, 92960, 92986, 92987, 92990, 92997, 92998, 93312, 93313, 93314, 93315, 93316, 93317, 93318, 93452, 93505, ~~93530, 93531, 93532, 93533, 93561, 93562,~~ 93563, 93564, 93568, 93580, 93582, 93590, 93591, 93592, <u>93593, 93594, 93595, 93596, 93597, 93598,</u> 93615, 93616 from the Medicine/Cardiovascular section. Modifier 63 should not be appended to any CPT codes listed in the **Evaluation and Management Services, Anesthesia, Radiology, Pathology/Laboratory,** or **Medicine** sections (other than those identified above from the Medicine/Cardiovascular section).◀ |

# Appendix A

## Modifiers

**63** ▶**Procedure Performed on Infants less than 4 kg:**
Procedures performed on neonates and infants up to a present body weight of 4 kg may involve significantly increased complexity and physician or other qualified health care professional work commonly associated with these patients. This circumstance may be reported by adding modifier 63 to the procedure number. **Note:** Unless otherwise designated, this modifier may only be appended to procedures/services listed in the 20100-69990 code series and 92920, 92928, 92953, 92960, 92986, 92987, 92990, 92997, 92998, 93312, 93313, 93314, 93315, 93316, 93317, 93318, 93452, 93505, 93563, 93564, 93568, 93580, 93582, 93590, 93591, 93592, 93593, 93594, 93595, 93596, 93597, 93598, 93615, 93616 from the Medicine/Cardiovascular section. Modifier 63 should not be appended to any CPT codes listed in the **Evaluation and Management Services, Anesthesia, Radiology, Pathology/Laboratory,** or **Medicine** sections (other than those identified above from the Medicine/Cardiovascular section).◀

### Rationale

In accordance with the deletion of codes 93530-93533, 93561, and 93562 and the establishment of codes 93593-93598, the descriptor of modifier 63 has been revised to reflect these changes.

Refer to the codebook and the Rationale for codes 93593-93598 for a full discussion of these changes.

★=Telemedicine　✚=Add-on code　𝒩=FDA approval pending　#=Resequenced code　⊘=Modifier 51 exempt

# Appendix O

## Summary of Additions, Deletions, and Revisions

The summary of changes shows the actual changes that have been made to the code descriptors.

New codes appear with a bullet (●) and are indicated as "Code added." Revised codes are preceded with a triangle (▲). Within revised codes, or if a code symbol has been deleted, the deleted language and code symbol appear with a ~~strikethrough~~, while new text appears underlined.

The ✄ symbol is used to identify codes for vaccines that are pending FDA approval. The # symbol is used to identify codes that have been resequenced. CPT add-on codes are annotated by the ✚ symbol. The ⊘ symbol is used to identify codes that are exempt from the use of modifier 51. The ★ symbol is used to identify codes that may be used for reporting telemedicine services. The ✕ symbol is used to identify a proprietary laboratory analyses (PLA) test that has an identical descriptor as another PLA test. A PLA code that satisfies Category I code criteria and has been accepted by the CPT Editorial Panel is annotated with the ⇅ symbol.

| Proprietary Name and Clinical Laboratory or Manufacturer | Alpha-Numeric Code | Code Descriptor |
|---|---|---|
| **Administrative Codes for Multianalyte Assays with Algorithmic Analyses (MAAA)** | | |
| | ●0017M | Code added |
| | ●0018M | Code added |
| **Category I Codes for Multianalyte Assays with Algorithmic Analyses (MAAA)** | | |
| | ●81523 | Code added |
| | ●81560 | Code added |
| **Proprietary Laboratory Analyses (PLA)** | | |
| UCompliDx, Elite Medical Laboratory Solutions, LLC, Elite Medical Laboratory Solutions, LLC (LDT) | ▲0051U | Prescription drug monitoring, evaluation of drugs present by liquid chromatography tandem mass spectrometry (LC-MS/MS), urine or blood, 31 drug panel, reported as quantitative results, detected or not detected, per date of service |
| ~~BioFire® FilmArray® Respiratory Panel (RP) EZ, BioFire® Diagnostics~~ | ~~0098U~~ | ~~Respiratory pathogen, multiplex reverse transcription and multiplex amplified probe technique, multiple types or subtypes, 14 targets (adenovirus, coronavirus, human metapneumovirus, influenza A, influenza A subtype H1, influenza A subtype H3, influenza A subtype H1-2009, influenza B, parainfluenza virus, human rhinovirus/enterovirus, respiratory syncytial virus, Bordetella pertussis, Chlamydophila pneumoniae, Mycoplasma pneumoniae)~~ |

(Continued on page 234)

Appendix O

| Proprietary Name and Clinical Laboratory or Manufacturer | Alpha-Numeric Code | Code Descriptor |
|---|---|---|
| BioFire® FilmArray® Respiratory Panel (RP), BioFire® Diagnostics | 0099U | Respiratory pathogen, multiplex reverse transcription and multiplex amplified probe technique, multiple types or subtypes, 20 targets (adenovirus, coronavirus 229E, coronavirus HKU1, coronavirus, coronavirus OC43, human metapneumovirus, influenza A, influenza A subtype, influenza A subtype H3, influenza A subtype H1-2009, influenza, parainfluenza virus, parainfluenza virus 2, parainfluenza virus 3, parainfluenza virus 4, human rhinovirus/enterovirus, respiratory syncytial virus, Bordetella pertussis, Chlamydophila pneumonia, Mycoplasma pneumoniae) |
| BioFire® FilmArray® Respiratory Panel 2 (RP2), BioFire® Diagnostics | 0100U | Respiratory pathogen, multiplex reverse transcription and multiplex amplified probe technique, multiple types or subtypes, 21 targets (adenovirus, coronavirus 229E, coronavirus HKU1, coronavirus NL63, coronavirus OC43, human metapneumovirus, human rhinovirus/enterovirus, influenza A, including subtypes H1, H1-2009, and H3, influenza B, parainfluenza virus 1, parainfluenza virus 2, parainfluenza virus 3, parainfluenza virus 4, respiratory syncytial virus, Bordetella parapertussis [IS1001], Bordetella pertussis [ptxP], Chlamydia pneumoniae, Mycoplasma pneumoniae) |
| NPDX ASD Energy Metabolism, Stemina Biomarker Discovery, Inc, Stemina Biomarker Discovery, Inc | 0139U | Neurology (autism spectrum disorder [ASD]), quantitative measurements of 6 central carbon metabolites (ie, α-ketoglutarate, alanine, lactate, phenylalanine, pyruvate, and succinate), LC-MS/MS, plasma, algorithmic analysis with result reported as negative or positive (with metabolic subtypes of ASD) |
| Karius® Test, Karius Inc, Karius Inc | ▲0152U | Infectious disease (bacteria, fungi, parasites, and DNA viruses), microbial cell-free DNA, PCR and plasma, untargeted next-generation sequencing, plasma, detection of >1,000 potential microbial organismsreport for significant positive pathogens |
| Vanadis® NIPT, PerkinElmer, Inc, PerkinElmer Genomics | 0168U | Fetal aneuploidy (trisomy 21, 18, and 13) DNA sequence analysis of selected regions using maternal plasma without fetal fraction cutoff, algorithm reported as a risk score for each trisomy |
| | #●0223U | Code added |
| | ●0224U | Code added |
| | ●0225U | Code added |
| | ●0226U | Code added |
| | ●0227U | Code added |
| | ●0228U | Code added |
| | ●0229U | Code added |
| | ●0230U | Code added |
| | ●0231U | Code added |
| | ●0232U | Code added |

★ = Telemedicine   ✚ = Add-on code   ✗ = FDA approval pending   # = Resequenced code   ⊘ = Modifier 51 exempt

| Proprietary Name and Clinical Laboratory or Manufacturer | Alpha-Numeric Code | Code Descriptor |
|---|---|---|
| | ●0233U | Code added |
| | ●0234U | Code added |
| | ●0235U | Code added |
| | ●0236U | Code added |
| | ●0237U | Code added |
| | ●0238U | Code added |
| | ●0239U | Code added |
| | ●0240U | Code added |
| | ●0241U | Code added |
| | ●0242U | Code added |
| | ●0243U | Code added |
| | ●0244U | Code added |
| | ●0245U | Code added |
| | ●0246U | Code added |
| | ●0247U | Code added |
| | ●0248U | Code added |
| | ●0249U | Code added |
| | ●0250U | Code added |
| | ●0251U | Code added |
| | ●0252U | Code added |
| | ●0253U | Code added |
| | ●0254U | Code added |
| | ●0255U | Code added |
| | ●0256U | Code added |
| | ●0257U | Code added |
| | ●0258U | Code added |
| | ●0259U | Code added |
| | ӿ●0260U | Code added |
| | ●0261U | Code added |
| | ●0262U | Code added |
| | ●0263U | Code added |
| | ӿ●0264U | Code added |
| | ●0265U | Code added |
| | ●0266U | Code added |
| | ●0267U | Code added |
| | ●0268U | Code added |
| | ●0269U | Code added |
| | ●0270U | Code added |
| | ●0271U | Code added |
| | ●0272U | Code added |
| | ●0273U | Code added |

*(Continued on page 236)*

| Proprietary Name and Clinical Laboratory or Manufacturer | Alpha-Numeric Code | Code Descriptor |
|---|---|---|
| | ●0274U | Code added |
| | ●0275U | Code added |
| | ●0276U | Code added |
| | ●0277U | Code added |
| | ●0278U | Code added |
| | ●0279U | Code added |
| | ●0280U | Code added |
| | ●0281U | Code added |
| | ●0282U | Code added |
| | ●0283U | Code added |
| | ●0284U | Code added |

★ = Telemedicine   ✚ = Add-on code   ✗ = FDA approval pending   # = Resequenced code   ⊘ = Modifier 51 exempt

# Appendix O

## Multianalyte Assays with Algorithmic Analyses and Proprietary Laboratory Analyses

The following list includes three types of CPT codes:

1. Multianalyte assays with algorithmic analyses (MAAA) administrative codes
2. Category I MAAA codes
3. Proprietary laboratory analyses (PLA) codes

1. Multianalyte assays with algorithmic analyses (MAAAs) are procedures that utilize multiple results derived from assays of various types, including molecular pathology assays, fluorescent in situ hybridization assays and non-nucleic acid based assays (eg, proteins, polypeptides, lipids, carbohydrates). Algorithmic analysis using the results of these assays as well as other patient information (if used) is then performed and reported typically as a numeric score(s) or as a probability. MAAAs are typically unique to a single clinical laboratory or manufacturer. The results of individual component procedure(s) that are inputs to the MAAAs may be provided on the associated laboratory report, however these assays are not reported separately using additional codes. MAAAs, by nature, are typically unique to a single clinical laboratory or manufacturer.

The list includes a proprietary name and clinical laboratory or manufacturer in the first column, an alpha-numeric code in the second column and code descriptor in the third column. The format for the code descriptor usually includes (in order):

- Disease type (eg, oncology, autoimmune, tissue rejection),
- Chemical(s) analyzed (eg, DNA, RNA, protein, antibody),
- Number of markers (eg, number of genes, number of proteins),
- Methodology(s) (eg, microarray, real-time [RT]-PCR, in situ hybridization [ISH], enzyme linked immunosorbent assays [ELISA]),
- Number of functional domains (if indicated),
- Specimen type (eg, blood, fresh tissue, formalin-fixed paraffin-embedded),
- Algorithm result type (eg, prognostic, diagnostic),
- Report (eg, probability index, risk score).

    MAAA procedures that have been assigned a Category I code are noted in the list below and additionally listed in the Category I MAAA section (81500-81599). The Category I MAAA section introductory language and associated parenthetical instruction(s) should be used to govern the appropriate use for Category I MAAA codes. If a specific MAAA procedure has not been assigned a Category I code, it is indicated as a four-digit number followed by the letter M.

    When a specific MAAA procedure is not included in either the list below or in the Category I MAAA section, report the analysis using the Category I MAAA unlisted code (81599). The codes below are specific to the assays identified in Appendix O by proprietary name. In order to report an MAAA code, the analysis performed must fulfill the code descriptor **and**, if proprietary, must be the test represented by the proprietary name listed in Appendix O. When an analysis is performed that may potentially fall within a specific descriptor, however the proprietary name is not included in the list below, the MAAA unlisted code (81599) should be used.

    Additions in this section may be released tri-annually (or quarterly for PLA codes) via the AMA CPT website to expedite dissemination for reporting. See the Introduction section of the CPT code set for a complete list of the dates of release and implementation.

    These administrative codes encompass all analytical services required for the algorithmic analysis (eg, cell lysis, nucleic acid stabilization, extraction, digestion, amplification, hybridization and detection) in addition to the algorithmic analysis itself, when applicable. Procedures that are required prior to cell lysis (eg, microdissection, codes 88380 and 88381) should be reported separately.

The codes in this list are provided as an administrative coding set to facilitate accurate reporting of MAAA services. The minimum standard for inclusion in this list is that an analysis is generally available for patient care. The AMA has not reviewed procedures in the administrative coding set for clinical utility. The list is not a complete list of all MAAA procedures.

2. Category I MAAA codes are included below along with their proprietary names. These codes are also listed in the Pathology and Laboratory section of the CPT code set (81490-81599).

3. PLA codes created in response to the Protecting Access to Medicare Act (PAMA) of 2014 are listed along with their proprietary names. These codes are also located at the end of the Pathology and Laboratory section of the CPT code set. In some instances, the descriptor language of PLA codes may be identical, which are differentiated only by the listed propriety names.

The accuracy of a PLA code is to be maintained by the original applicant, or the current owner of the test kit or laboratory performing the proprietary test.

A new PLA code is required when:

1. Additional nucleic acid (DNA or RNA) and/or protein analysis(es) are added to the current PLA test, or

2. The name of the PLA test has changed in association with changes in test performance or test characteristics.

The addition or modification of the therapeutic applications of the test require submission of a code change application, but it may not require a new code number.

| Proprietary Name and Clinical Laboratory or Manufacturer | Alpha-Numeric Code | Code Descriptor |
|---|---|---|
| **Administrative Codes for Multianalyte Assays with Algorithmic Analyses (MAAA)** | | |
| ASH FibroSURE™, BioPredictive S.A.S | 0002M | Liver disease, ten biochemical assays (ALT, A2-macroglobulin, apolipoprotein A-1, total bilirubin, GGT, haptoglobin, AST, glucose, total cholesterol and triglycerides) utilizing serum, prognostic algorithm reported as quantitative scores for fibrosis, steatosis and alcoholic steatohepatitis (ASH) |
| NASH FibroSURE™, BioPredictive S.A.S | 0003M | Liver disease, ten biochemical assays (ALT, A2-macroglobulin, apolipoprotein A-1, total bilirubin, GGT, haptoglobin, AST, glucose, total cholesterol and triglycerides) utilizing serum, prognostic algorithm reported as quantitative scores for fibrosis, steatosis and nonalcoholic steatohepatitis (NASH) |
| ScoliScore™ Transgenomic | 0004M | Scoliosis, DNA analysis of 53 single nucleotide polymorphisms (SNPs), using saliva, prognostic algorithm reported as a risk score |
| HeproDX™, GoPath Laboratories, LLC | 0006M | Oncology (hepatic), mRNA expression levels of 161 genes, utilizing fresh hepatocellular carcinoma tumor tissue, with alpha-fetoprotein level, algorithm reported as a risk classifier |
| NETest, Wren Laboratories, LLC | 0007M | Oncology (gastrointestinal neuroendocrine tumors), real-time PCR expression analysis of 51 genes, utilizing whole peripheral blood, algorithm reported as a nomogram of tumor disease index |
| — | (0009M has been deleted) | — |
| NeoLAB™ Prostate Liquid Biopsy, NeoGenomics Laboratories | 0011M | Oncology, prostate cancer, mRNA expression assay of 12 genes (10 content and 2 housekeeping), RT-PCR test utilizing blood plasma and urine, algorithms to predict high-grade prostate cancer risk |

| Proprietary Name and Clinical Laboratory or Manufacturer | Alpha-Numeric Code | Code Descriptor |
|---|---|---|
| Cxbladder™ Detect, Pacific Edge Diagnostics USA, Ltd | 0012M | Oncology (urothelial), mRNA, gene expression profiling by real-time quantitative PCR of five genes *(MDK, HOXA13, CDC2 [CDK1], IGFBP5,* and *CXCR2)*, utilizing urine, algorithm reported as a risk score for having urothelial carcinoma |
| Cxbladder™ Monitor, Pacific Edge Diagnostics USA, Ltd | 0013M | Oncology (urothelial), mRNA, gene expression profiling by real-time quantitative PCR of five genes *(MDK, HOXA13, CDC2 [CDK1], IGFBP5,* and *CXCR2)*, utilizing urine, algorithm reported as a risk score for having recurrent urothelial carcinoma |
| Enhanced Liver Fibrosis™ (ELF™) Test, Siemens Healthcare Diagnostics Inc/Siemens Healthcare Laboratory LLC | 0014M | Liver disease, analysis of 3 biomarkers (hyaluronic acid [HA], procollagen III amino terminal peptide [PIIINP], tissue inhibitor of metalloproteinase 1 [TIMP-1]), using immunoassays, utilizing serum, prognostic algorithm reported as a risk score and risk of liver fibrosis and liver-related clinical events within 5 years |
| Adrenal Mass Panel, 24 Hour, Urine, Mayo Clinic Laboratories (MCL), Mayo Clinic | 0015M | Adrenal cortical tumor, biochemical assay of 25 steroid markers, utilizing 24-hour urine specimen and clinical parameters, prognostic algorithm reported as a clinical risk and integrated clinical steroid risk for adrenal cortical carcinoma, adenoma, or other adrenal malignancy |
| Decipher Bladder TURBT®, Decipher Biosciences, Inc | 0016M | Oncology (bladder), mRNA, microarray gene expression profiling of 209 genes, utilizing formalin-fixed paraffin-embedded tissue, algorithm reported as molecular subtype (luminal, luminal infiltrated, basal, basal claudin-low, neuroendocrine-like) |
| ▶Lymph2Cx, Mayo Clinic Arizona Molecular Diagnostics Laboratory◀ | ●0017M | ▶Oncology (diffuse large B-cell lymphoma [DLBCL]), mRNA, gene expression profiling by fluorescent probe hybridization of 20 genes, formalin-fixed paraffin-embedded tissue, algorithm reported as cell of origin◀<br><br>▶(Do not report 0017M in conjunction with 0120U)◀ |
| ▶Pleximark™, Plexision, Inc◀ | ●0018M | ▶Transplantation medicine (allograft rejection, renal), measurement of donor and third-party-induced CD154+T-cytotoxic memory cells, utilizing whole peripheral blood, algorithm reported as a rejection risk score◀<br><br>▶(Do not report 0018M in conjunction with 81560, 85032, 86353, 86821, 88184, 88185, 88187, 88230, 88240, 88241)◀ |
| **Category I Codes for Multianalyte Assays with Algorithmic Analyses (MAAA)** | | |
| Vectra® DA, Crescendo Bioscience, Inc | 81490 | Autoimmune (rheumatoid arthritis), analysis of 12 biomarkers using immunoassays, utilizing serum, prognostic algorithm reported as a disease activity score<br><br>(Do not report 81490 in conjunction with 86140) |

*(Continued on page 240)*

▲ = Revised code    ● = New code    ▶◀ = Contains new or revised text    ⋈ = Duplicate PLA test    ⇅ = Category I PLA    American Medical Association    **239**

| Proprietary Name and Clinical Laboratory or Manufacturer | Alpha-Numeric Code | Code Descriptor |
|---|---|---|
| AlloMap®, CareDx, Inc | #81595 | Cardiology (heart transplant), mRNA, gene expression profiling by real-time quantitative PCR of 20 genes (11 content and 9 housekeeping), utilizing subfraction of peripheral blood, algorithm reported as a rejection risk score |
| Corus® CAD, CardioDx, Inc | 81493 | Coronary artery disease, mRNA, gene expression profiling by real-time RT-PCR of 23 genes, utilizing whole peripheral blood, algorithm reported as a risk score |
| PreDx Diabetes Risk Score™, Tethys Clinical Laboratory | 81506 | Endocrinology (type 2 diabetes), biochemical assays of seven analytes (glucose, HbA1c, insulin, hs-CRP, adiponectin, ferritin, interleukin 2-receptor alpha), utilizing serum or plasma, algorithm reporting a risk score |
|  |  | (Do not report 81506 in conjunction with constituent components [ie, 82728, 82947, 83036, 83525, 86141], 84999 [for adopectin], and 83520 [for interleukin 2-receptor alpha]) |
| Harmony™ Prenatal Test, Ariosa Diagnostics | 81507 | Fetal aneuploidy (trisomy 21, 18, and 13) DNA sequence analysis of selected regions using maternal plasma, algorithm reported as a risk score for each trisomy |
|  |  | (Do not report 81228, 81229, 88271 when performing genomic sequencing procedures or other molecular multianalyte assays for copy number analysis) |

★ = Telemedicine   + = Add-on code   ✱ = FDA approval pending   # = Resequenced code   ⦸ = Modifier 51 exempt

Appendix O

| Proprietary Name and Clinical Laboratory or Manufacturer | Alpha-Numeric Code | Code Descriptor |
|---|---|---|
| **No proprietary name and clinical laboratory or manufacturer.** Maternal serum screening procedures are well-established procedures and are performed by many laboratories throughout the country. The concept of prenatal screens has existed and evolved for over 10 years and is not exclusive to any one facility. | 81508 | Fetal congenital abnormalities, biochemical assays of two proteins (PAPP-A, hCG [any form]), utilizing maternal serum, algorithm reported as a risk score<br><br>(Do not report 81508 in conjunction with 84163, 84702) |
| | 81509 | Fetal congenital abnormalities, biochemical assays of three proteins (PAPP-A, hCG [any form], DIA), utilizing maternal serum, algorithm reported as a risk score<br><br>(Do not report 81509 in conjunction with 84163, 84702, 86336) |
| | 81510 | Fetal congenital abnormalities, biochemical assays of three analytes (AFP, uE3, hCG [any form]), utilizing maternal serum, algorithm reported as a risk score<br><br>(Do not report 81510 in conjunction with 82105, 82677, 84702) |
| | 81511 | Fetal congenital abnormalities, biochemical assays of four analytes (AFP, uE3, hCG [any form], DIA) utilizing maternal serum, algorithm reported as a risk score (may include additional results from previous biochemical testing)<br><br>(Do not report 81511 in conjunction with 82105, 82677, 84702, 86336) |
| | 81512 | Fetal congenital abnormalities, biochemical assays of five analytes (AFP, uE3, total hCG, hyperglycosylated hCG, DIA) utilizing maternal serum, algorithm reported as a risk score<br><br>(Do not report 81512 in conjunction with 82105, 82677, 84702, 86336) |
| Aptima® BV Assay, Hologic, Inc | 81513 | Infectious disease, bacterial vaginosis, quantitative real-time amplification of RNA markers for Atopobium vaginae, Gardnerella vaginalis, and Lactobacillus species, utilizing vaginal-fluid specimens, algorithm reported as a positive or negative result for bacterial vaginosis |
| BD MAX™ Vaginal Panel, Becton Dickson and Company | 81514 | Infectious disease, bacterial vaginosis and vaginitis, quantitative real-time amplification of DNA markers for Gardnerella vaginalis, Atopobium vaginae, Megasphaera type 1, Bacterial Vaginosis Associated Bacteria-2 (BVAB-2), and Lactobacillus species (L. crispatus and L. jensenii), utilizing vaginal-fluid specimens, algorithm reported as a positive or negative for high likelihood of bacterial vaginosis, includes separate detection of Trichomonas vaginalis and/or Candida species (C. albicans, C. tropicalis, C. parapsilosis, C. dubliniensis), Candida glabrata, Candida krusei, when reported<br><br>(Do not report 81514 in conjunction with 87480, 87481, 87482, 87510, 87511, 87512, 87660, 87661) |

(*Continued on page 242*)

▲ = Revised code   ● = New code   ▶ ◀ = Contains new or revised text   ✣ = Duplicate PLA test   ↑↓ = Category I PLA

| Proprietary Name and Clinical Laboratory or Manufacturer | Alpha-Numeric Code | Code Descriptor |
|---|---|---|
| HCV FibroSURE™, FibroTest™, BioPredictive S.A.S. | #81596 | Infectious disease, chronic hepatitis C virus (HCV) infection, six biochemical assays (ALT, A2-macroglobulin, apolipoprotein A-1, total bilirubin, GGT, and haptoglobin) utilizing serum, prognostic algorithm reported as scores for fibrosis and necroinflammatory activity in liver |
| Breast Cancer Index, Biotheranostics, Inc | 81518 | Oncology (breast), mRNA, gene expression profiling by real-time RT-PCR of 11 genes (7 content and 4 housekeeping), utilizing formalin-fixed paraffin-embedded tissue, algorithms reported as percentage risk for metastatic recurrence and likelihood of benefit from extended endocrine therapy |
| EndoPredict®, Myriad Genetic Laboratories, Inc | #81522 | Oncology (breast), mRNA, gene expression profiling by RT-PCR of 12 genes (8 content and 4 housekeeping), utilizing formalin-fixed paraffin-embedded tissue, algorithm reported as recurrence risk score |
| Oncotype DX®, Genomic Health | 81519 | Oncology (breast), mRNA, gene expression profiling by real-time RT-PCR of 21 genes, utilizing formalin-fixed paraffin-embedded tissue, algorithm reported as recurrence score |
| Prosigna® Breast Cancer Assay, NanoString Technologies, Inc | 81520 | Oncology (breast), mRNA gene expression profiling by hybrid capture of 58 genes (50 content and 8 housekeeping), utilizing formalin-fixed paraffin-embedded tissue, algorithm reported as a recurrence risk score |
| MammaPrint®, Agendia, Inc | 81521 | Oncology (breast), mRNA, microarray gene expression profiling of 70 content genes and 465 housekeeping genes, utilizing fresh frozen or formalin-fixed paraffin-embedded tissue, algorithm reported as index related to risk of distant metastasis ▶(Do not report 81521 in conjunction with 81523 for the same specimen)◀ |
| ▶MammaPrint®, Agendia, Inc◀ | ●81523 | ▶Oncology (breast), mRNA, next-generation sequencing gene expression profiling of 70 content genes and 31 housekeeping genes, utilizing formalin-fixed paraffin-embedded tissue, algorithm reported as index related to risk to distant metastasis◀ ▶(Do not report 81523 in conjunction with 81521 for the same specimen)◀ |
| Oncotype DX® Colon Cancer Assay, Genomic Health | 81525 | Oncology (colon), mRNA, gene expression profiling by real-time RT-PCR of 12 genes (7 content and 5 housekeeping), utilizing formalin-fixed paraffin-embedded tissue, algorithm reported as a recurrence score |

★ = Telemedicine   ✚ = Add-on code   ✗ = FDA approval pending   # = Resequenced code   ⊘ = Modifier 51 exemp

Appendix O

| Proprietary Name and Clinical Laboratory or Manufacturer | Alpha-Numeric Code | Code Descriptor |
|---|---|---|
| Cologuard™, Exact Sciences, Inc | 81528 | Oncology (colorectal) screening, quantitative real-time target and signal amplification of 10 DNA markers (*KRAS* mutations, promoter methylation of *NDRG4* and *BMP3*) and fecal hemoglobin, utilizing stool, algorithm reported as a positive or negative result<br><br>(Do not report 81528 in conjunction with 81275, 82274) |
| DecisionDx® Melanoma, Castle Biosciences, Inc | 81529 | Oncology (cutaneous melanoma), mRNA, gene expression profiling by real-time RT-PCR of 31 genes (28 content and 3 housekeeping), utilizing formalin-fixed paraffin-embedded tissue, algorithm reported as recurrence risk, including likelihood of sentinel lymph node metastasis |
| ChemoFX®, Helomics, Corp | 81535 | Oncology (gynecologic), live tumor cell culture and chemotherapeutic response by DAPI stain and morphology, predictive algorithm reported as a drug response score; first single drug or drug combination |
| | **+**81536 | each additional single drug or drug combination (List separately in addition to code for primary procedure)<br><br>(Use 81536 in conjunction with 81535) |
| VeriStrat, Biodesix, Inc | 81538 | Oncology (lung), mass spectrometric 8-protein signature, including amyloid A, utilizing serum, prognostic and predictive algorithm reported as good versus poor overall survival |
| Risk of Ovarian Malignancy Algorithm (ROMA)™, Fujirebio Diagnostics | #81500 | Oncology (ovarian), biochemical assays of two proteins (CA-125 and HE4), utilizing serum, with menopausal status, algorithm reported as a risk score<br><br>(Do not report 81500 in conjunction with 86304, 86305) |
| OVA1™, Vermillion, Inc | #81503 | Oncology (ovarian), biochemical assays of five proteins (CA-125, apolipoprotein A1, beta-2 microglobulin, transferrin, and pre-albumin), utilizing serum, algorithm reported as a risk score<br><br>(Do not report 81503 in conjunction with 82172, 82232, 84134, 84466, 86304) |
| 4Kscore test, OPKO Health, Inc | 81539 | Oncology (high-grade prostate cancer), biochemical assay of four proteins (Total PSA, Free PSA, Intact PSA, and human kallikrein-2 [hK2]), utilizing plasma or serum, prognostic algorithm reported as a probability score |
| Prolaris®, Myriad Genetic Laboratories, Inc | 81541 | Oncology (prostate), mRNA gene expression profiling by real-time RT-PCR of 46 genes (31 content and 15 housekeeping), utilizing formalin-fixed paraffin-embedded tissue, algorithm reported as a disease-specific mortality risk score |

(*Continued on page 244*)

| Proprietary Name and Clinical Laboratory or Manufacturer | Alpha-Numeric Code | Code Descriptor |
|---|---|---|
| Decipher® Prostate, Decipher® Biosciences | 81542 | Oncology (prostate), mRNA, microarray gene expression profiling of 22 content genes, utilizing formalin-fixed paraffin-embedded tissue, algorithm reported as metastasis risk score |
| — | (81545 has been deleted) | — |
| ConfirmMDx® for Prostate Cancer, MDxHealth, Inc | 81551 | Oncology (prostate), promoter methylation profiling by real-time PCR of 3 genes (*GSTP1, APC, RASSF1*), utilizing formalin-fixed paraffin-embedded tissue, algorithm reported as a likelihood of prostate cancer detection on repeat biopsy |
| Afirma® Genomic Sequencing Classifier, Veracyte, Inc | #81546 | Oncology (thyroid), mRNA, gene expression analysis of 10,196 genes, utilizing fine needle aspirate, algorithm reported as a categorical result (eg, benign or suspicious) |
| Tissue of Origin Test Kit-FFPE, Cancer Genetics, Inc | #81504 | Oncology (tissue of origin), microarray gene expression profiling of > 2000 genes, utilizing formalin-fixed paraffin-embedded tissue, algorithm reported as tissue similarity scores |
| CancerTYPE ID, bioTheranostics, Inc | #81540 | Oncology (tumor of unknown origin), mRNA, gene expression profiling by real-time RT-PCR of 92 genes (87 content and 5 housekeeping) to classify tumor into main cancer type and subtype, utilizing formalin-fixed paraffin-embedded tissue, algorithm reported as a probability of a predicted main cancer type and subtype |
| DecisionDx®-UM test, Castle Biosciences, Inc | 81552 | Oncology (uveal melanoma), mRNA, gene expression profiling by real-time RT-PCR of 15 genes (12 content and 3 housekeeping), utilizing fine needle aspirate or formalin-fixed paraffin-embedded tissue, algorithm reported as risk of metastasis |
| Envisia® Genomic Classifier, Veracyte, Inc | 81554 | Pulmonary disease (idiopathic pulmonary fibrosis [IPF]), mRNA, gene expression analysis of 190 genes, utilizing transbronchial biopsies, diagnostic algorithm reported as categorical result (eg, positive or negative for high probability of usual interstitial pneumonia [UIP]) |
| ▶Pleximmune™, Plexision, Inc◀ | ●81560 | ▶Transplantation medicine (allograft rejection, pediatric liver and small bowel), measurement of donor and third-party-induced CD154+T-cytotoxic memory cells, utilizing whole peripheral blood, algorithm reported as a rejection risk score◀ ▶(Do not report 81560 in conjunction with 85032, 86353, 86821, 88184, 88185, 88187, 88230, 88240, 88241, 0018M)◀ |
| — | 81599 | Unlisted multianalyte assay with algorithmic analysis (Do not use 81599 for multianalyte assays with algorithmic analyses listed in Appendix O) |

★ = Telemedicine ✚ = Add-on code ✗ = FDA approval pending # = Resequenced code ⦰ = Modifier 51 exempt

| Proprietary Name and Clinical Laboratory or Manufacturer | Alpha-Numeric Code | Code Descriptor |
|---|---|---|
| | **Proprietary Laboratory Analyses (PLA)** | |
| PreciseType® HEA Test, Immucor, Inc | 0001U | Red blood cell antigen typing, DNA, human erythrocyte antigen gene analysis of 35 antigens from 11 blood groups, utilizing whole blood, common RBC alleles reported |
| PolypDX™, Atlantic Diagnostic Laboratories, LLC, Metabolomic Technologies, Inc | 0002U | Oncology (colorectal), quantitative assessment of three urine metabolites (ascorbic acid, succinic acid and carnitine) by liquid chromatography with tandem mass spectrometry (LC-MS/MS) using multiple reaction monitoring acquisition, algorithm reported as likelihood of adenomatous polyps |
| Overa (OVA1 Next Generation), Asprira Labs, Inc, Vermillion, Inc | 0003U | Oncology (ovarian) biochemical assays of five proteins (apolipoprotein A-1, CA 125 II, follicle stimulating hormone, human epididymis protein 4, transferrin), utilizing serum, algorithm reported as a likelihood score |
| ExosomeDx® Prostate (IntelliScore), Exosome Diagnostics, Inc, Exosome Diagnostics, Inc | 0005U | Oncology (prostate) gene expression profile by real-time RT-PCR of 3 genes (ERG, PCA3, and SPDEF), urine, algorithm reported as risk score |
| — | (0006U has been deleted) | — |
| ToxProtect, Genotox Laboratories LTD | 0007U | Drug test(s), presumptive, with definitive confirmation of positive results, any number of drug classes, urine, includes specimen verification including DNA authentication in comparison to buccal DNA, per date of service |
| AmHPR® H. pylori Antibiotic Resistance Panel, American Molecular Laboratories, Inc | 0008U | Helicobacter pylori detection and antibiotic resistance, DNA, 16S and 23S rRNA, gyrA, pbp1, rdxA and rpoB, next generation sequencing, formalin-fixed paraffin-embedded or fresh tissue or fecal sample, predictive, reported as positive or negative for resistance to clarithromycin, fluoroquinolones, metronidazole, amoxicillin, tetracycline, and rifabutin |
| DEPArray™ HER2, PacificDx | 0009U | Oncology (breast cancer), ERBB2 (HER2) copy number by FISH, tumor cells from formalin-fixed paraffin-embedded tissue isolated using image-based dielectrophoresis (DEP) sorting, reported as ERBB2 gene amplified or non-amplified |
| Bacterial Typing by Whole Genome Sequencing, Mayo Clinic | 0010U | Infectious disease (bacterial), strain typing by whole genome sequencing, phylogenetic-based report of strain relatedness, per submitted isolate |
| Cordant CORE™, Cordant Health Solutions | 0011U | Prescription drug monitoring, evaluation of drugs present by LC-MS/MS, using oral fluid, reported as a comparison to an estimated steady-state range, per date of service including all drug compounds and metabolites |
| MatePair Targeted Rearrangements, Congenital, Mayo Clinic | 0012U | Germline disorders, gene rearrangement detection by whole genome next-generation sequencing, DNA, whole blood, report of specific gene rearrangement(s) |

(Continued on page 246)

▲ = Revised code   ● = New code   ▶ ◀ = Contains new or revised text   ✕ = Duplicate PLA test   ↑↓ = Category I PLA   American Medical Association   **245**

| Proprietary Name and Clinical Laboratory or Manufacturer | Alpha-Numeric Code | Code Descriptor |
|---|---|---|
| MatePair Targeted Rearrangements, Oncology, Mayo Clinic | 0013U | Oncology (solid organ neoplasia), gene rearrangement detection by whole genome next-generation sequencing, DNA, fresh or frozen tissue or cells, report of specific gene rearrangement(s) |
| MatePair Targeted Rearrangements, Hematologic, Mayo Clinic | 0014U | Hematology (hematolymphoid neoplasia), gene rearrangement detection by whole genome next-generation sequencing, DNA, whole blood or bone marrow, report of specific gene rearrangement(s) |
| BCR-ABL1 major and minor breakpoint fusion transcripts, University of Iowa, Department of Pathology, Asuragen | 0016U | Oncology (hematolymphoid neoplasia), RNA, *BCR/ABL1* major and minor breakpoint fusion transcripts, quantitative PCR amplification, blood or bone marrow, report of fusion not detected or detected with quantitation |
| *JAK2* Mutation, University of Iowa, Department of Pathology | 0017U | Oncology (hematolymphoid neoplasia), *JAK2* mutation, DNA, PCR amplification of exons 12-14 and sequence analysis, blood or bone marrow, report of *JAK2* mutation not detected or detected |
| ThyraMIR™, Interpace Diagnostics | 0018U | Oncology (thyroid), microRNA profiling by RT-PCR of 10 microRNA sequences, utilizing fine needle aspirate, algorithm reported as a positive or negative result for moderate to high risk of malignancy |
| OncoTarget/OncoTreat, Columbia University Department of Pathology and Cell Biology, Darwin Health | 0019U | Oncology, RNA, gene expression by whole transcriptome sequencing, formalin-fixed paraffin-embedded tissue or fresh frozen tissue, predictive algorithm reported as potential targets for therapeutic agents |
| — | (0020U has been deleted) | — |
| Apifiny®, Armune BioScience, Inc | 0021U | Oncology (prostate), detection of 8 autoantibodies (ARF 6, NKX3-1, 5'-UTR-BMI1, CEP 164, 3'-UTR-Ropporin, Desmocollin, AURKAIP-1, CSNK2A2), multiplexed immunoassay and flow cytometry serum, algorithm reported as risk score |
| Oncomine™ Dx Target Test, Thermo Fisher Scientific | 0022U | Targeted genomic sequence analysis panel, non-small cell lung neoplasia, DNA and RNA analysis, 23 genes, interrogation for sequence variants and rearrangements, reported as presence/absence of variants and associated therapy(ies) to consider |
| LeukoStrat® CDx *FLT3* Mutation Assay, LabPMM LLC, an Invivoscribe Technologies, Inc Company, Invivoscribe Technologies, Inc | 0023U | Oncology (acute myelogenous leukemia), DNA, genotyping of internal tandem duplication, p.D835, p.I836, using mononuclear cells, reported as detection or non-detection of *FLT3* mutation and indication for or against the use of midostaurin |
| GlycA, Laboratory Corporation of America, Laboratory Corporation of America | 0024U | Glycosylated acute phase proteins (GlycA), nuclear magnetic resonance spectroscopy, quantitative |
| UrSure Tenofovir Quantification Test, Synergy Medical Laboratories, UrSure Inc | 0025U | Tenofovir, by liquid chromatography with tandem mass spectrometry (LC-MS/MS), urine, quantitative |

★ = Telemedicine    ✚ = Add-on code    ✎ = FDA approval pending    # = Resequenced code    ⃠ = Modifier 51 exemp

| Proprietary Name and Clinical Laboratory or Manufacturer | Alpha-Numeric Code | Code Descriptor |
|---|---|---|
| Thyroseq Genomic Classifier, CBLPath, Inc, University of Pittsburgh Medical Center | 0026U | Oncology (thyroid), DNA and mRNA of 112 genes, next-generation sequencing, fine needle aspirate of thyroid nodule, algorithmic analysis reported as a categorical result ("Positive, high probability of malignancy" or "Negative, low probability of malignancy") |
| *JAK2* Exons 12 to 15 Sequencing, Mayo Clinic, Mayo Clinic | 0027U | *JAK2 (Janus kinase 2)* (eg, myeloproliferative disorder) gene analysis, targeted sequence analysis exons 12-15 |
| — | (0028U has been deleted) | — |
| Focused Pharmacogenomics Panel, Mayo Clinic, Mayo Clinic | 0029U | Drug metabolism (adverse drug reactions and drug response), targeted sequence analysis (ie, *CYP1A2, CYP2C19, CYP2C9, CYP2D6, CYP3A4, CYP3A5, CYP4F2, SLCO1B1, VKORC1* and rs12777823) |
| Warfarin Response Genotype, Mayo Clinic, Mayo Clinic | 0030U | Drug metabolism (warfarin drug response), targeted sequence analysis (ie, *CYP2C9, CYP4F2, VKORC1,* rs12777823) |
| Cytochrome P450 1A2 Genotype, Mayo Clinic, Mayo Clinic | 0031U | *CYP1A2 (cytochrome P450 family 1, subfamily A, member 2)* (eg, drug metabolism) gene analysis, common variants (ie, *1F, *1K, *6, *7) |
| Catechol-O-Methyltransferase (*COMT*) Genotype, Mayo Clinic, Mayo Clinic | 0032U | *COMT (catechol-O-methyltransferase)* (eg, drug metabolism) gene analysis, c.472G>A (rs4680) variant |
| Serotonin Receptor Genotype (*HTR2A* and *HTR2C*), Mayo Clinic, Mayo Clinic | 0033U | *HTR2A (5-hydroxytryptamine receptor 2A), HTR2C (5-hydroxytryptamine receptor 2C)* (eg, citalopram metabolism) gene analysis, common variants (ie, *HTR2A* rs7997012 [c.614-2211T>C], *HTR2C* rs3813929 [c.-759C>T] and rs1414334 [c.551-3008C>G]) |
| Thiopurine Methyltransferase (*TPMT*) and Nudix Hydrolase (*NUDT15*) Genotyping, Mayo Clinic, Mayo Clinic | 0034U | *TPMT (thiopurine S-methyltransferase), NUDT15 (nudix hydroxylase 15)* (eg, thiopurine metabolism) gene analysis, common variants (ie, *TPMT* *2, *3A, *3B, *3C, *4, *5, *6, *8, *12; *NUDT15* *3, *4, *5) |
| Real-time quaking-induced conversion for prion detection (RT-QuIC), National Prion Disease Pathology Surveillance Center | 0035U | Neurology (prion disease), cerebrospinal fluid, detection of prion protein by quaking-induced conformational conversion, qualitative |
| EXaCT-1 Whole Exome Testing, Lab of Oncology-Molecular Detection, Weill Cornell Medicine-Clinical Genomics Laboratory | 0036U | Exome (ie, somatic mutations), paired formalin-fixed paraffin-embedded tumor tissue and normal specimen, sequence analyses |
| FoundationOne CDx™ (F1CDx), Foundation Medicine, Inc, Foundation Medicine, Inc | 0037U | Targeted genomic sequence analysis, solid organ neoplasm, DNA analysis of 324 genes, interrogation for sequence variants, gene copy number amplifications, gene rearrangements, microsatellite instability and tumor mutational burden |
| Sensieva™ Droplet 25OH Vitamin D2/D3 Microvolume LC/MS Assay, InSource Diagnostics, InSource Diagnostics | 0038U | Vitamin D, 25 hydroxy D2 and D3, by LC-MS/MS, serum microsample, quantitative |

*(Continued on page 248)*

▲ = Revised code   ● = New code   ▶ ◀ = Contains new or revised text   ✕ = Duplicate PLA test   ⇅ = Category I PLA     American Medical Association   **247**

| Proprietary Name and Clinical Laboratory or Manufacturer | Alpha-Numeric Code | Code Descriptor |
|---|---|---|
| Anti-dsDNA, High Salt/Avidity, University of Washington, Department of Laboratory Medicine, Bio-Rad | 0039U | Deoxyribonucleic acid (DNA) antibody, double stranded, high avidity |
| MRDx BCR-ABL Test, MolecularMD, MolecularMD | 0040U | *BCR/ABL1 (t(9;22))* (eg, chronic myelogenous leukemia) translocation analysis, major breakpoint, quantitative |
| Lyme ImmunoBlot IgM, IGeneX Inc, ID-FISH Technology Inc (ASR) (Lyme ImmunoBlot IgM Strips Only) | 0041U | Borrelia burgdorferi, antibody detection of 5 recombinant protein groups, by immunoblot, IgM |
| Lyme ImmunoBlot IgG, IGeneX Inc, ID-FISH Technology Inc (ASR) (Lyme ImmunoBlot IgG Strips Only) | 0042U | Borrelia burgdorferi, antibody detection of 12 recombinant protein groups, by immunoblot, IgG |
| Tick-Borne Relapsing Fever (TBRF) Borrelia ImmunoBlots IgM Test, IGeneX Inc, ID-FISH Technology (Provides TBRF ImmunoBlot IgM Strips) | 0043U | Tick-borne relapsing fever Borrelia group, antibody detection to 4 recombinant protein groups, by immunoblot, IgM |
| Tick-Borne Relapsing Fever (TBRF) Borrelia ImmunoBlots IgG Test, IGeneX Inc, ID-FISH Technology Inc (Provides TBRF ImmunoBlot IgG Strips) | 0044U | Tick-borne relapsing fever Borrelia group, antibody detection to 4 recombinant protein groups, by immunoblot, IgG |
| The Oncotype DX® Breast DCIS Score™ Test, Genomic Health, Inc, Genomic Health, Inc | 0045U | Oncology (breast ductal carcinoma in situ), mRNA, gene expression profiling by real-time RT-PCR of 12 genes (7 content and 5 housekeeping), utilizing formalin-fixed paraffin-embedded tissue, algorithm reported as recurrence score |
| *FLT3* ITD MRD by NGS, LabPMM LLC, an Invivoscribe Technologies, Inc Company | 0046U | *FLT3 (fms-related tyrosine kinase 3)* (eg, acute myeloid leukemia) internal tandem duplication (ITD) variants, quantitative |
| Oncotype DX Genomic Prostate Score, Genomic Health, Inc, Genomic Health, Inc | 0047U | Oncology (prostate), mRNA, gene expression profiling by real-time RT-PCR of 17 genes (12 content and 5 housekeeping), utilizing formalin-fixed paraffin-embedded tissue, algorithm reported as a risk score |
| MSK-IMPACT (Integrated Mutation Profiling of Actionable Cancer Targets), Memorial Sloan Kettering Cancer Center | 0048U | Oncology (solid organ neoplasia), DNA, targeted sequencing of protein-coding exons of 468 cancer-associated genes, including interrogation for somatic mutations and microsatellite instability, matched with normal specimens, utilizing formalin-fixed paraffin-embedded tumor tissue, report of clinically significant mutation(s) |
| NPM1 MRD by NGS, LabPMM LLC, an Invivoscribe Technologies, Inc Company | 0049U | *NPM1 (nucleophosmin)* (eg, acute myeloid leukemia) gene analysis, quantitative |
| MyAML NGS Panel, LabPMM LLC, an Invivoscribe Technologies, Inc Company | 0050U | Targeted genomic sequence analysis panel, acute myelogenous leukemia, DNA analysis, 194 genes, interrogation for sequence variants, copy number variants or rearrangements |

★ = Telemedicine   ✛ = Add-on code   ✗ = FDA approval pending   # = Resequenced code   ⊘ = Modifier 51 exempt

| Proprietary Name and Clinical Laboratory or Manufacturer | Alpha-Numeric Code | Code Descriptor |
|---|---|---|
| UCompliDx, Elite Medical Laboratory Solutions, LLC, Elite Medical Laboratory Solutions, LLC (LDT) | ▲0051U | ▶Prescription drug monitoring, evaluation of drugs present by liquid chromatography tandem mass spectrometry (LC-MS/MS), urine or blood, 31 drug panel, reported as quantitative results, detected or not detected, per date of service◀ |
| VAP Cholesterol Test, VAP Diagnostics Laboratory, Inc, VAP Diagnostics Laboratory, Inc | 0052U | Lipoprotein, blood, high resolution fractionation and quantitation of lipoproteins, including all five major lipoprotein classes and subclasses of HDL, LDL, and VLDL by vertical auto profile ultracentrifugation |
| Prostate Cancer Risk Panel, Mayo Clinic, Laboratory Developed Test | 0053U | Oncology (prostate cancer), FISH analysis of 4 genes (*ASAP1, HDAC9, CHD1* and *PTEN*), needle biopsy specimen, algorithm reported as probability of higher tumor grade |
| AssuranceRx Micro Serum, Firstox Laboratories, LLC, Firstox Laboratories, LLC | 0054U | Prescription drug monitoring, 14 or more classes of drugs and substances, definitive tandem mass spectrometry with chromatography, capillary blood, quantitative report with therapeutic and toxic ranges, including steady-state range for the prescribed dose when detected, per date of service |
| myTAIHEART, TAI Diagnostics, Inc, TAI Diagnostics, Inc | 0055U | Cardiology (heart transplant), cell-free DNA, PCR assay of 96 DNA target sequences (94 single nucleotide polymorphism targets and two control targets), plasma |
| MatePair Acute Myeloid Leukemia Panel, Mayo Clinic, Laboratory Developed Test | 0056U | Hematology (acute myelogenous leukemia), DNA, whole genome next-generation sequencing to detect gene rearrangement(s), blood or bone marrow, report of specific gene rearrangement(s) |
| — | (0057U has been deleted) | — |
| Merkel SmT Oncoprotein Antibody Titer, University of Washington, Department of Laboratory Medicine | 0058U | Oncology (Merkel cell carcinoma), detection of antibodies to the Merkel cell polyoma virus oncoprotein (small T antigen), serum, quantitative |
| Merkel Virus VP1 Capsid Antibody, University of Washington, Department of Laboratory Medicine | 0059U | Oncology (Merkel cell carcinoma), detection of antibodies to the Merkel cell polyoma virus capsid protein (VP1), serum, reported as positive or negative |
| Twins Zygosity PLA, Natera, Inc, Natera, Inc | 0060U | Twin zygosity, genomic-targeted sequence analysis of chromosome 2, using circulating cell-free fetal DNA in maternal blood |
| Transcutaneous multispectral measurement of tissue oxygenation and hemoglobin using spatial frequency domain imaging (SFDI), Modulated Imaging, Inc, Modulated Imaging, Inc | 0061U | Transcutaneous measurement of five biomarkers (tissue oxygenation [$StO_2$], oxyhemoglobin [$ctHbO_2$], deoxyhemoglobin [ctHbR], papillary and reticular dermal hemoglobin concentrations [ctHb1 and ctHb2]), using spatial frequency domain imaging (SFDI) and multi-spectral analysis |
| SLE-key® Rule Out, Veracis Inc, Veracis Inc | 0062U | Autoimmune (systemic lupus erythematosus), IgG and IgM analysis of 80 biomarkers, utilizing serum, algorithm reported with a risk score |
| NPDX ASD ADM Panel I, Stemina Biomarker Discovery, Inc, Stemina Biomarker Discovery, Inc d/b/a NeuroPointDX | 0063U | Neurology (autism), 32 amines by LC-MS/MS, using plasma, algorithm reported as metabolic signature associated with autism spectrum disorder |

(*Continued on page 250*)

▲ = Revised code   ● = New code   ▶◀ = Contains new or revised text   ✖ = Duplicate PLA test   ↑↓ = Category I PLA        American Medical Association   **249**

| Proprietary Name and Clinical Laboratory or Manufacturer | Alpha-Numeric Code | Code Descriptor |
|---|---|---|
| BioPlex 2200 Syphilis Total & RPR Assay, Bio-Rad Laboratories, Bio-Rad Laboratories | 0064U | Antibody, Treponema pallidum, total and rapid plasma reagin (RPR), immunoassay, qualitative |
| BioPlex 2200 RPR Assay, Bio-Rad Laboratories, Bio-Rad Laboratories | 0065U | Syphilis test, non-treponemal antibody, immunoassay, qualitative (RPR) |
| PartoSure™ Test, Parsagen Diagnostics, Inc, Parsagen Diagnostics, Inc, a QIAGEN Company | 0066U | Placental alpha-micro globulin-1 (PAMG-1), immunoassay with direct optical observation, cervico-vaginal fluid, each specimen |
| BBDRisk Dx™, Silbiotech, Inc, Silbiotech, Inc | 0067U | Oncology (breast), immunohistochemistry, protein expression profiling of 4 biomarkers (matrix metalloproteinase-1 [MMP-1], carcinoembryonic antigen-related cell adhesion molecule 6 [CEACAM6], hyaluronoglucosaminidase [HYAL1], highly expressed in cancer protein [HEC1]), formalin-fixed paraffin-embedded precancerous breast tissue, algorithm reported as carcinoma risk score |
| MYCODART-PCR™ Dual Amplification Real Time PCR Panel for 6 Candida species, RealTime Laboratories, Inc/MycoDART, Inc, RealTime Laboratories, Inc | 0068U | Candida species panel *(C. albicans, C. glabrata, C. parapsilosis, C. kruseii, C. tropicalis,* and *C. auris),* amplified probe technique with qualitative report of the presence or absence of each species |
| miR-31*now*™, GoPath Laboratories, GoPath Laboratories | 0069U | Oncology (colorectal), microRNA, RT-PCR expression profiling of miR-31-3p, formalin-fixed paraffin-embedded tissue, algorithm reported as an expression score |
| *CYP2D6* Common Variants and Copy Number, Mayo Clinic, Laboratory Developed Test | 0070U | *CYP2D6 (cytochrome P450, family 2, subfamily D, polypeptide 6)* (eg, drug metabolism) gene analysis, common and select rare variants (ie, *2, *3, *4, *4N, *5, *6, *7, *8, *9, *10, *11, *12, *13, *14A, *14B, *15, *17, *29, *35, *36, *41, *57, *61, *63, *68, *83, *xN) |
| *CYP2D6* Full Gene Sequencing, Mayo Clinic, Laboratory Developed Test | ✚0071U | *CYP2D6 (cytochrome P450, family 2, subfamily D, polypeptide 6)* (eg, drug metabolism) gene analysis, full gene sequence (List separately in addition to code for primary procedure) <br><br> (Use 0071U in conjunction with 0070U) |
| *CYP2D6-2D7* Hybrid Gene Targeted Sequence Analysis, Mayo Clinic, Laboratory Developed Test | ✚0072U | *CYP2D6 (cytochrome P450, family 2, subfamily D, polypeptide 6)* (eg, drug metabolism) gene analysis, targeted sequence analysis (ie, *CYP2D6-2D7* hybrid gene) (List separately in addition to code for primary procedure) <br><br> (Use 0072U in conjunction with 0070U) |
| *CYP2D7-2D6* Hybrid Gene Targeted Sequence Analysis, Mayo Clinic, Laboratory Developed Test | ✚0073U | *CYP2D6 (cytochrome P450, family 2, subfamily D, polypeptide 6)* (eg, drug metabolism) gene analysis, targeted sequence analysis (ie, *CYP2D7-2D6* hybrid gene) (List separately in addition to code for primary procedure) <br><br> (Use 0073U in conjunction with 0070U) |

★ = Telemedicine   ✚ = Add-on code   ✕ = FDA approval pending   # = Resequenced code   ⊘ = Modifier 51 exempt

Appendix O

| Proprietary Name and Clinical Laboratory or Manufacturer | Alpha-Numeric Code | Code Descriptor |
|---|---|---|
| *CYP2D6* trans-duplication/ multiplication non-duplicated gene targeted sequence analysis, Mayo Clinic, Laboratory Developed Test | ✚0074U | *CYP2D6 (cytochrome P450, family 2, subfamily D, polypeptide 6)* (eg, drug metabolism) gene analysis, targeted sequence analysis (ie, non-duplicated gene when duplication/multiplication is trans) (List separately in addition to code for primary procedure)<br><br>(Use 0074U in conjunction with 0070U) |
| *CYP2D6* 5' gene duplication/ multiplication targeted sequence analysis, Mayo Clinic, Laboratory Developed Test | ✚0075U | *CYP2D6 (cytochrome P450, family 2, subfamily D, polypeptide 6)* (eg, drug metabolism) gene analysis, targeted sequence analysis (ie, 5' gene duplication/ multiplication) (List separately in addition to code for primary procedure)<br><br>(Use 0075U in conjunction with 0070U) |
| *CYP2D6* 3' gene duplication/ multiplication targeted sequence analysis, Mayo Clinic, Laboratory Developed Test | ✚0076U | *CYP2D6 (cytochrome P450, family 2, subfamily D, polypeptide 6)* (eg, drug metabolism) gene analysis, targeted sequence analysis (ie, 3' gene duplication/ multiplication) (List separately in addition to code for primary procedure)<br><br>(Use 0076U in conjunction with 0070U) |
| M-Protein Detection and Isotyping by MALDI-TOF Mass Spectrometry, Mayo Clinic, Laboratory Developed Test | 0077U | Immunoglobulin paraprotein (M-protein), qualitative, immunoprecipitation and mass spectrometry, blood or urine, including isotype |
| INFINITI® Neural Response Panel, PersonalizeDx Labs, AutoGenomics Inc | 0078U | Pain management (opioid-use disorder) genotyping panel, 16 common variants (ie, *ABCB1, COMT, DAT1, DBH, DOR, DRD1, DRD2, DRD4, GABA, GAL, HTR2A, HTTLPR, MTHFR, MUOR, OPRK1, OPRM1),* buccal swab or other germline tissue sample, algorithm reported as positive or negative risk of opioid-use disorder |
| ToxLok™, InSource Diagnostics, InSource Diagnostics | 0079U | Comparative DNA analysis using multiple selected single-nucleotide polymorphisms (SNPs), urine and buccal DNA, for specimen identity verification |
| BDX-XL2, Biodesix®, Inc, Biodesix®, Inc | 0080U | Oncology (lung), mass spectrometric analysis of galectin-3-binding protein and scavenger receptor cysteine-rich type 1 protein M130, with five clinical risk factors (age, smoking status, nodule diameter, nodule-spiculation status and nodule location), utilizing plasma, algorithm reported as a categorical probability of malignancy |
| — | (0081U has been deleted. To report, use 81552) | — |
| NextGen Precision™ Testing, Precision Diagnostics, Precision Diagnostics LBN Precision Toxicology, LLC | 0082U | Drug test(s), definitive, 90 or more drugs or substances, definitive chromatography with mass spectrometry, and presumptive, any number of drug classes, by instrument chemistry analyzer (utilizing immunoassay), urine, report of presence or absence of each drug, drug metabolite or substance with description and severity of significant interactions per date of service |

*(Continued on page 252)*

▲ =Revised code   ● =New code   ▶ ◀ =Contains new or revised text   ✕ =Duplicate PLA test   ↑↓ =Category I PLA

| Proprietary Name and Clinical Laboratory or Manufacturer | Alpha-Numeric Code | Code Descriptor |
|---|---|---|
| Onco4D™, Animated Dynamics, Inc, Animated Dynamics, Inc | 0083U | Oncology, response to chemotherapy drugs using motility contrast tomography, fresh or frozen tissue, reported as likelihood of sensitivity or resistance to drugs or drug combinations |
| BLOODchip® ID CORE XT™, Grifols Diagnostic Solutions Inc | 0084U | Red blood cell antigen typing, DNA, genotyping of 10 blood groups with phenotype prediction of 37 red blood cell antigens |
| — | (0085U has been deleted) | — |
| Accelerate PhenoTest™ BC kit, Accelerate Diagnostics, Inc | 0086U | Infectious disease (bacterial and fungal), organism identification, blood culture, using rRNA FISH, 6 or more organism targets, reported as positive or negative with phenotypic minimum inhibitory concentration (MIC)-based antimicrobial susceptibility |
| Molecular Microscope® MMDx— Heart, Kashi Clinical Laboratories | 0087U | Cardiology (heart transplant), mRNA gene expression profiling by microarray of 1283 genes, transplant biopsy tissue, allograft rejection and injury algorithm reported as a probability score |
| Molecular Microscope® MMDx— Kidney, Kashi Clinical Laboratories | 0088U | Transplantation medicine (kidney allograft rejection), microarray gene expression profiling of 1494 genes, utilizing transplant biopsy tissue, algorithm reported as a probability score for rejection |
| Pigmented Lesion Assay (PLA), DermTech | 0089U | Oncology (melanoma), gene expression profiling by RTqPCR, *PRAME* and *LINC00518*, superficial collection using adhesive patch(es) |
| myPath® Melanoma, Myriad Genetic Laboratories | 0090U | Oncology (cutaneous melanoma), mRNA gene expression profiling by RT-PCR of 23 genes (14 content and 9 housekeeping), utilizing formalin-fixed paraffin-embedded tissue, algorithm reported as a categorical result (ie, benign, indeterminate, malignant) |
| FirstSight^CRC, CellMax Life | 0091U | Oncology (colorectal) screening, cell enumeration of circulating tumor cells, utilizing whole blood, algorithm, for the presence of adenoma or cancer, reported as a positive or negative result |
| REVEAL Lung Nodule Characterization, MagArray, Inc | 0092U | Oncology (lung), three protein biomarkers, immunoassay using magnetic nanosensor technology, plasma, algorithm reported as risk score for likelihood of malignancy |
| ComplyRX, Claro Labs | 0093U | Prescription drug monitoring, evaluation of 65 common drugs by LC-MS/MS, urine, each drug reported detected or not detected |
| RCIGM Rapid Whole Genome Sequencing, Rady Children's Institute for Genomic Medicine (RCIGM) | 0094U | Genome (eg, unexplained constitutional or heritable disorder or syndrome), rapid sequence analysis |

★ = Telemedicine ✚ = Add-on code ✎ = FDA approval pending # = Resequenced code ⊘ = Modifier 51 exempt

| Proprietary Name and Clinical Laboratory or Manufacturer | Alpha-Numeric Code | Code Descriptor |
|---|---|---|
| Esophageal String Test™ (EST), Cambridge Biomedical, Inc | 0095U | Inflammation (eosinophilic esophagitis), ELISA analysis of eotaxin-3 *(CCL26 [C-C motif chemokine ligand 26])* and major basic protein *(PRG2 [proteoglycan 2, pro eosinophil major basic protein])*, specimen obtained by swallowed nylon string, algorithm reported as predictive probability index for active eosinophilic esophagitis |
| HPV, High-Risk, Male Urine, Molecular Testing Labs | 0096U | Human papillomavirus (HPV), high-risk types (ie, 16, 18, 31, 33, 35, 39, 45, 51, 52, 56, 58, 59, 66, 68), male urine |
| BioFire® FilmArray® Gastrointestinal (GI) Panel, BioFire® Diagnostics | 0097U | Gastrointestinal pathogen, multiplex reverse transcription and multiplex amplified probe technique, multiple types or subtypes, 22 targets (Campylobacter [C. jejuni/C. coli/C. upsaliensis], Clostridium difficile [C. difficile] toxin A/B, Plesiomonas shigelloides, Salmonella, Vibrio [V. parahaemolyticus/V. vulnificus/V. cholerae], including specific identification of Vibrio cholerae, Yersinia enterocolitica, Enteroaggregative Escherichia coli [EAEC], Enteropathogenic Escherichia coli [EPEC], Enterotoxigenic Escherichia coli [ETEC] lt/st, Shiga-like toxin-producing Escherichia coli [STEC] stx1/stx2 [including specific identification of the E. coli O157 serogroup within STEC], Shigella/Enteroinvasive Escherichia coli [EIEC], Cryptosporidium, Cyclospora cayetanensis, Entamoeba histolytica, Giardia lamblia [also known as G. intestinalis and G. duodenalis], adenovirus F 40/41, astrovirus, norovirus GI/GII, rotavirus A, sapovirus [Genogroups I, II, IV, and V]) |
| — | ▶(0098U has been deleted)◀ | — |
| — | ▶(0099U has been deleted)◀ | |
| — | ▶(0100U has been deleted)◀ | — |
| ColoNext®, Ambry Genetics®, Ambry Genetics® | 0101U | Hereditary colon cancer disorders (eg, Lynch syndrome, *PTEN* hamartoma syndrome, Cowden syndrome, familial adenomatosis polyposis), genomic sequence analysis panel utilizing a combination of NGS, Sanger, MLPA, and array CGH, with mRNA analytics to resolve variants of unknown significance when indicated (15 genes [sequencing and deletion/duplication], *EPCAM* and *GREM1* [deletion/duplication only]) |

*(Continued on page 254)*

▲ = Revised code   ● = New code   ▶ ◀ = Contains new or revised text   ✕ = Duplicate PLA test   ↕ = Category I PLA   American Medical Association   **253**

**Appendix O**

| Proprietary Name and Clinical Laboratory or Manufacturer | Alpha-Numeric Code | Code Descriptor |
|---|---|---|
| BreastNext®, Ambry Genetics®, Ambry Genetics® | 0102U | Hereditary breast cancer-related disorders (eg, hereditary breast cancer, hereditary ovarian cancer, hereditary endometrial cancer), genomic sequence analysis panel utilizing a combination of NGS, Sanger, MLPA, and array CGH, with mRNA analytics to resolve variants of unknown significance when indicated (17 genes [sequencing and deletion/duplication]) |
| OvaNext®, Ambry Genetics®, Ambry Genetics® | 0103U | Hereditary ovarian cancer (eg, hereditary ovarian cancer, hereditary endometrial cancer), genomic sequence analysis panel utilizing a combination of NGS, Sanger, MLPA, and array CGH, with mRNA analytics to resolve variants of unknown significance when indicated (24 genes [sequencing and deletion/duplication], *EPCAM* [deletion/duplication only]) |
| — | (0104U has been deleted) | — |
| KidneyIntelX™, RenalytixAI, RenalytixAI | 0105U | Nephrology (chronic kidney disease), multiplex electrochemiluminescent immunoassay (ECLIA) of tumor necrosis factor receptor 1A, receptor superfamily 2 *(TNFR1, TNFR2),* and kidney injury molecule-1 (KIM-1) combined with longitudinal clinical data, including *APOL1* genotype if available, and plasma (isolated fresh or frozen), algorithm reported as probability score for rapid kidney function decline (RKFD) |
| 13C-Spirulina Gastric Emptying Breath Test (GEBT), Cairn Diagnostics d/b/a Advanced Breath Diagnostics, LLC, Cairn Diagnostics d/b/a Advanced Breath Diagnostics, LLC | 0106U | Gastric emptying, serial collection of 7 timed breath specimens, non-radioisotope carbon-13 ($^{13}$C) spirulina substrate, analysis of each specimen by gas isotope ratio mass spectrometry, reported as rate of $^{13}CO_2$ excretion |
| Singulex Clarity C. diff toxins A/B Assay, Singulex | 0107U | Clostridium difficile toxin(s) antigen detection by immunoassay technique, stool, qualitative, multiple-step method |
| TissueCypher® Barrett's Esophagus Assay, Cernostics, Cernostics | 0108U | Gastroenterology (Barrett's esophagus), whole slide–digital imaging, including morphometric analysis, computer-assisted quantitative immunolabeling of 9 protein biomarkers (p16, AMACR, p53, CD68, COX-2, CD45RO, HIF1a, HER-2, K20) and morphology, formalin-fixed paraffin-embedded tissue, algorithm reported as risk of progression to high-grade dysplasia or cancer |
| MYCODART Dual Amplification Real Time PCR Panel for 4 Aspergillus species, RealTime Laboratories, Inc/MycoDART, Inc | 0109U | Infectious disease (Aspergillus species), real-time PCR for detection of DNA from 4 species *(A. fumigatus, A. terreus, A. niger,* and *A. flavus),* blood, lavage fluid, or tissue, qualitative reporting of presence or absence of each species |

★ = Telemedicine   ✚ = Add-on code   ✎ = FDA approval pending   # = Resequenced code   ⊘ = Modifier 51 exempt

| Proprietary Name and Clinical Laboratory or Manufacturer | Alpha-Numeric Code | Code Descriptor |
|---|---|---|
| Oral OncolyticAssuranceRX, Firstox Laboratories, LLC, Firstox Laboratories, LLC | 0110U | Prescription drug monitoring, one or more oral oncology drug(s) and substances, definitive tandem mass spectrometry with chromatography, serum or plasma from capillary blood or venous blood, quantitative report with steady-state range for the prescribed drug(s) when detected) |
| Praxis™ Extended RAS Panel, Illumina, Illumina | 0111U | Oncology (colon cancer), targeted *KRAS* (codons 12, 13, and 61) and *NRAS* (codons 12, 13, and 61) gene analysis, utilizing formalin-fixed paraffin-embedded tissue |
| MicroGenDX qPCR & NGS For Infection, MicroGenDX, MicroGenDX | 0112U | Infectious agent detection and identification, targeted sequence analysis (16S and 18S rRNA genes) with drug-resistance gene |
| MiPS (Mi-Prostate Score), MLabs, MLabs | 0113U | Oncology (prostate), measurement of *PCA3* and *TMPRSS2-ERG* in urine and PSA in serum following prostatic massage, by RNA amplification and fluorescence-based detection, algorithm reported as risk score |
| EsoGuard™, Lucid Diagnostics, Lucid Diagnostics | 0114U | Gastroenterology (Barrett's esophagus), *VIM* and *CCNA1* methylation analysis, esophageal cells, algorithm reported as likelihood for Barrett's esophagus |
| ePlex Respiratory Pathogen (RP) Panel, GenMark Diagnostics, Inc, GenMark Diagnostics, Inc | 0115U | Respiratory infectious agent detection by nucleic acid (DNA and RNA), 18 viral types and subtypes and 2 bacterial targets, amplified probe technique, including multiplex reverse transcription for RNA targets, each analyte reported as detected or not detected |
| Snapshot Oral Fluid Compliance, Ethos Laboratories | 0116U | Prescription drug monitoring, enzyme immunoassay of 35 or more drugs confirmed with LC-MS/MS, oral fluid, algorithm results reported as a patient-compliance measurement with risk of drug to drug interactions for prescribed medications |
| Foundation PI℠, Ethos Laboratories | 0117U | Pain management, analysis of 11 endogenous analytes (methylmalonic acid, xanthurenic acid, homocysteine, pyroglutamic acid, vanilmandelate, 5-hydroxyindoleacetic acid, hydroxymethylglutarate, ethylmalonate, 3-hydroxypropyl mercapturic acid (3-HPMA), quinolinic acid, kynurenic acid), LC-MS/MS, urine, algorithm reported as a pain-index score with likelihood of atypical biochemical function associated with pain |
| Viracor TRAC™ dd-cfDNA, Viracor Eurofins, Viracor Eurofins | 0118U | Transplantation medicine, quantification of donor-derived cell-free DNA using whole genome next-generation sequencing, plasma, reported as percentage of donor-derived cell-free DNA in the total cell-free DNA |
| MI-HEART Ceramides, Plasma, Mayo Clinic, Laboratory Developed Test | 0119U | Cardiology, ceramides by liquid chromatography–tandem mass spectrometry, plasma, quantitative report with risk score for major cardiovascular events |

(*Continued on page 256*)

▲ = Revised code　● = New code　▶ ◀ = Contains new or revised text　✕ = Duplicate PLA test　↕ = Category I PLA　　American Medical Association　**255**

| Proprietary Name and Clinical Laboratory or Manufacturer | Alpha-Numeric Code | Code Descriptor |
|---|---|---|
| Lymph3Cx Lymphoma Molecular Subtyping Assay, Mayo Clinic, Laboratory Developed Test | 0120U | Oncology (B-cell lymphoma classification), mRNA, gene expression profiling by fluorescent probe hybridization of 58 genes (45 content and 13 housekeeping genes), formalin-fixed paraffin-embedded tissue, algorithm reported as likelihood for primary mediastinal B-cell lymphoma (PMBCL) and diffuse large B-cell lymphoma (DLBCL) with cell of origin subtyping in the latter<br><br>▶(Do not report 0120U in conjunction with 0017M)◀ |
| Flow Adhesion of Whole Blood on VCAM-1 (FAB-V), Functional Fluidics, Functional Fluidics | 0121U | Sickle cell disease, microfluidic flow adhesion (VCAM-1), whole blood |
| Flow Adhesion of Whole Blood to P-SELECTIN (WB-PSEL), Functional Fluidics, Functional Fluidics | 0122U | Sickle cell disease, microfluidic flow adhesion (P-Selectin), whole blood |
| Mechanical Fragility, RBC by shear stress profiling and spectral analysis, Functional Fluidics, Functional Fluidics | 0123U | Mechanical fragility, RBC, shear stress and spectral analysis profiling |
| — | (0124U has been deleted) | — |
| — | (0125U has been deleted) | — |
| — | (0126U has been deleted) | — |
| — | (0127U has been deleted) | — |
| — | (0128U has been deleted) | — |
| BRCAplus, Ambry Genetics | 0129U | Hereditary breast cancer–related disorders (eg, hereditary breast cancer, hereditary ovarian cancer, hereditary endometrial cancer), genomic sequence analysis and deletion/duplication analysis panel *(ATM, BRCA1, BRCA2, CDH1, CHEK2, PALB2, PTEN, and TP53)* |
| +RNAinsight™ for ColoNext®, Ambry Genetics | ✚0130U | Hereditary colon cancer disorders (eg, Lynch syndrome, PTEN hamartoma syndrome, Cowden syndrome, familial adenomatosis polyposis), targeted mRNA sequence analysis panel *(APC, CDH1, CHEK2, MLH1, MSH2, MSH6, MUTYH, PMS2, PTEN, and TP53)* (List separately in addition to code for primary procedure)<br><br>(Use 0130U in conjunction with 81435, 0101U) |
| +RNAinsight™ for BreastNext®, Ambry Genetics | ✚0131U | Hereditary breast cancer–related disorders (eg, hereditary breast cancer, hereditary ovarian cancer, hereditary endometrial cancer), targeted mRNA sequence analysis panel (13 genes) (List separately in addition to code for primary procedure)<br><br>(Use 0131U in conjunction with 81162, 81432, 0102U) |

★=Telemedicine   ✚=Add-on code   ⋆=FDA approval pending   #=Resequenced code   ⊘=Modifier 51 exempt

| Proprietary Name and Clinical Laboratory or Manufacturer | Alpha-Numeric Code | Code Descriptor |
|---|---|---|
| +RNAinsight™ for OvaNext®, Ambry Genetics | ✚0132U | Hereditary ovarian cancer–related disorders (eg, hereditary breast cancer, hereditary ovarian cancer, hereditary endometrial cancer), targeted mRNA sequence analysis panel (17 genes) (List separately in addition to code for primary procedure)<br><br>(Use 0132U in conjunction with 81162, 81432, 0103U) |
| +RNAinsight™ for ProstateNext®, Ambry Genetics | ✚0133U | Hereditary prostate cancer–related disorders, targeted mRNA sequence analysis panel (11 genes) (List separately in addition to code for primary procedure)<br><br>(Use 0133U in conjunction with 81162) |
| +RNAinsight™ for CancerNext®, Ambry Genetics | ✚0134U | Hereditary pan cancer (eg, hereditary breast and ovarian cancer, hereditary endometrial cancer, hereditary colorectal cancer), targeted mRNA sequence analysis panel (18 genes) (List separately in addition to code for primary procedure)<br><br>(Use 0134U in conjunction with 81162, 81432, 81435) |
| +RNAinsight™ for GYNPlus®, Ambry Genetics | ✚0135U | Hereditary gynecological cancer (eg, hereditary breast and ovarian cancer, hereditary endometrial cancer, hereditary colorectal cancer), targeted mRNA sequence analysis panel (12 genes) (List separately in addition to code for primary procedure)<br><br>(Use 0135U in conjunction with 81162) |
| +RNAinsight™ for *ATM*, Ambry Genetics | ✚0136U | *ATM (ataxia telangiectasia mutated)* (eg, ataxia telangiectasia) mRNA sequence analysis (List separately in addition to code for primary procedure)<br><br>(Use 0136U in conjunction with 81408) |
| +RNAinsight™ for *PALB2*, Ambry Genetics | ✚0137U | *PALB2 (partner and localizer of BRCA2)* (eg, breast and pancreatic cancer) mRNA sequence analysis (List separately in addition to code for primary procedure)<br><br>(Use 0137U in conjunction with 81307) |
| +RNAinsight™ for *BRCA1/2*, Ambry Genetics | ✚0138U | *BRCA1 (BRCA1, DNA repair associated), BRCA2 (BRCA2, DNA repair associated)* (eg, hereditary breast and ovarian cancer) mRNA sequence analysis (List separately in addition to code for primary procedure)<br><br>(Use 0138U in conjunction with 81162) |
| — | ▶(0139U has been deleted)◀ | — |
| ePlex® BCID Fungal Pathogens Panel, GenMark Diagnostics, Inc, GenMark Diagnostics, Inc | 0140U | Infectious disease (fungi), fungal pathogen identification, DNA (15 fungal targets), blood culture, amplified probe technique, each target reported as detected or not detected |

(*Continued on page 258*)

| Proprietary Name and Clinical Laboratory or Manufacturer | Alpha-Numeric Code | Code Descriptor |
|---|---|---|
| ePlex® BCID Gram-Positive Panel, GenMark Diagnostics, Inc, GenMark Diagnostics, Inc | 0141U | Infectious disease (bacteria and fungi), gram-positive organism identification and drug resistance element detection, DNA (20 gram-positive bacterial targets, 4 resistance genes, 1 pan gram-negative bacterial target, 1 pan Candida target), blood culture, amplified probe technique, each target reported as detected or not detected |
| ePlex® BCID Gram-Negative Panel, GenMark Diagnostics, Inc, GenMark Diagnostics, Inc | 0142U | Infectious disease (bacteria and fungi), gram-negative bacterial identification and drug resistance element detection, DNA (21 gram-negative bacterial targets, 6 resistance genes, 1 pan gram-positive bacterial target, 1 pan Candida target), amplified probe technique, each target reported as detected or not detected |
| CareViewRx, Newstar Medical Laboratories, LLC, Newstar Medical Laboratories, LLC | ✚0143U | Drug assay, definitive, 120 or more drugs or metabolites, urine, quantitative liquid chromatography with tandem mass spectrometry (LC-MS/MS) using multiple reaction monitoring (MRM), with drug or metabolite description, comments including sample validation, per date of service<br><br>(For additional PLA code with identical clinical descriptor, see 0150U. See Appendix O to determine appropriate code assignment) |
| CareViewRx Plus, Newstar Medical Laboratories, LLC, Newstar Medical Laboratories, LLC | 0144U | Drug assay, definitive, 160 or more drugs or metabolites, urine, quantitative liquid chromatography with tandem mass spectrometry (LC-MS/MS) using multiple reaction monitoring (MRM), with drug or metabolite description, comments including sample validation, per date of service |
| PainViewRx, Newstar Medical Laboratories, LLC, Newstar Medical Laboratories, LLC | 0145U | Drug assay, definitive, 65 or more drugs or metabolites, urine, quantitative liquid chromatography with tandem mass spectrometry (LC-MS/MS) using multiple reaction monitoring (MRM), with drug or metabolite description, comments including sample validation, per date of service |
| PainViewRx Plus, Newstar Medical Laboratories, LLC, Newstar Medical Laboratories, LLC | 0146U | Drug assay, definitive, 80 or more drugs or metabolites, urine, by quantitative liquid chromatography with tandem mass spectrometry (LC-MS/MS) using multiple reaction monitoring (MRM), with drug or metabolite description, comments including sample validation, per date of service |
| RiskViewRx, Newstar Medical Laboratories, LLC, Newstar Medical Laboratories, LLC | 0147U | Drug assay, definitive, 85 or more drugs or metabolites, urine, quantitative liquid chromatography with tandem mass spectrometry (LC-MS/MS) using multiple reaction monitoring (MRM), with drug or metabolite description, comments including sample validation, per date of service |

★ = Telemedicine   ✚ = Add-on code   ✒ = FDA approval pending   # = Resequenced code   ⊘ = Modifier 51 exempt

Appendix O

| Proprietary Name and Clinical Laboratory or Manufacturer | Alpha-Numeric Code | Code Descriptor |
|---|---|---|
| RiskViewRx Plus, Newstar Medical Laboratories, LLC, Newstar Medical Laboratories, LLC | 0148U | Drug assay, definitive, 100 or more drugs or metabolites, urine, quantitative liquid chromatography with tandem mass spectrometry (LC-MS/MS) using multiple reaction monitoring (MRM), with drug or metabolite description, comments including sample validation, per date of service |
| PsychViewRx, Newstar Medical Laboratories, LLC, Newstar Medical Laboratories, LLC | 0149U | Drug assay, definitive, 60 or more drugs or metabolites, urine, quantitative liquid chromatography with tandem mass spectrometry (LC-MS/MS) using multiple reaction monitoring (MRM), with drug or metabolite description, comments including sample validation, per date of service |
| PsychViewRx Plus, Newstar Medical Laboratories, LLC, Newstar Medical Laboratories, LLC | ⵌ0150U | Drug assay, definitive, 120 or more drugs or metabolites, urine, quantitative liquid chromatography with tandem mass spectrometry (LC-MS/MS) using multiple reaction monitoring (MRM), with drug or metabolite description, comments including sample validation, per date of service<br><br>(For additional PLA code with identical clinical descriptor, see 0143U. See Appendix O to determine appropriate code assignment) |
| BioFire® FilmArray® Pneumonia Panel, BioFire® Diagnostics, BioFire® Diagnostics | 0151U | Infectious disease (bacterial or viral respiratory tract infection), pathogen specific nucleic acid (DNA or RNA), 33 targets, real-time semi-quantitative PCR, bronchoalveolar lavage, sputum, or endotracheal aspirate, detection of 33 organismal and antibiotic resistance genes with limited semi-quantitative results |
| Karius® Test, Karius Inc, Karius Inc | ▲0152U | ▶Infectious disease (bacteria, fungi, parasites, and DNA viruses), microbial cell-free DNA, plasma, untargeted next-generation sequencing, report for significant positive pathogens◀ |
| Insight TNBCtype™, Insight Molecular Labs | 0153U | Oncology (breast), mRNA, gene expression profiling by next-generation sequencing of 101 genes, utilizing formalin-fixed paraffin-embedded tissue, algorithm reported as a triple negative breast cancer clinical subtype(s) with information on immune cell involvement |
| therascreen® *FGFR* RGQ RT-PCR Kit, QIAGEN, QIAGEN GmbH | 0154U | Oncology (urothelial cancer), RNA, analysis by real-time RT-PCR of the *FGFR3 (fibroblast growth factor receptor 3)* gene analysis (ie, p.R248C [c.742C>T], p.S249C [c.746C>G], p.G370C [c.1108G>T], p.Y373C [c.1118A>G], FGFR3-TACC3v1, and FGFR3-TACC3v3), utilizing formalin-fixed paraffin-embedded urothelial cancer tumor tissue, reported as *FGFR* gene alteration status |

(*Continued on page 260*)

| Proprietary Name and Clinical Laboratory or Manufacturer | Alpha-Numeric Code | Code Descriptor |
|---|---|---|
| therascreen *PIK3CA* RGQ PCR Kit, QIAGEN, QIAGEN GmbH | 0155U | Oncology (breast cancer), DNA, *PIK3CA (phosphatidylinositol-4,5-bisphosphate 3-kinase, catalytic subunit alpha)* (eg, breast cancer) gene analysis (ie, p.C420R, p.E542K, p.E545A, p.E545D [g.1635G>T only], p.E545G, p.E545K, p.Q546E, p.Q546R, p.H1047L, p.H1047R, p.H1047Y), utilizing formalin-fixed paraffin-embedded breast tumor tissue, reported as *PIK3CA* gene mutation status |
| SMASH™, New York Genome Center, Marvel Genomics™ | 0156U | Copy number (eg, intellectual disability, dysmorphology), sequence analysis |
| CustomNext + RNA: *APC*, Ambry Genetics®, Ambry Genetics® | ✚0157U | *APC (APC regulator of WNT signaling pathway)* (eg, familial adenomatosis polyposis [FAP]) mRNA sequence analysis (List separately in addition to code for primary procedure)<br><br>(Use 0157U in conjunction with 81201) |
| CustomNext + RNA: *MLH1*, Ambry Genetics®, Ambry Genetics® | ✚0158U | *MLH1 (mutL homolog 1)* (eg, hereditary non-polyposis colorectal cancer, Lynch syndrome) mRNA sequence analysis (List separately in addition to code for primary procedure)<br><br>(Use 0158U in conjunction with 81292) |
| CustomNext + RNA: *MSH2*, Ambry Genetics®, Ambry Genetics® | ✚0159U | *MSH2 (mutS homolog 2)* (eg, hereditary colon cancer, Lynch syndrome) mRNA sequence analysis (List separately in addition to code for primary procedure)<br><br>(Use 0159U in conjunction with 81295) |
| CustomNext + RNA: *MSH6*, Ambry Genetics®, Ambry Genetics® | ✚0160U | *MSH6 (mutS homolog 6)* (eg, hereditary colon cancer, Lynch syndrome) mRNA sequence analysis (List separately in addition to code for primary procedure)<br><br>(Use 0160U in conjunction with 81298) |
| CustomNext + RNA: *PMS2*, Ambry Genetics®, Ambry Genetics® | ✚0161U | *PMS2 (PMS1 homolog 2, mismatch repair system component)* (eg, hereditary non-polyposis colorectal cancer, Lynch syndrome) mRNA sequence analysis (List separately in addition to code for primary procedure)<br><br>(Use 0161U in conjunction with 81317) |
| CustomNext + RNA: Lynch *(MLH1, MSH2, MSH6, PMS2)*, Ambry Genetics®, Ambry Genetics® | ✚0162U | Hereditary colon cancer (Lynch syndrome), targeted mRNA sequence analysis panel *(MLH1, MSH2, MSH6, PMS2)* (List separately in addition to code for primary procedure)<br><br>(Use 0162U in conjunction with 81292, 81295, 81298, 81317, 81435) |
| BeScreened™-CRC, Beacon Biomedical Inc, Beacon Biomedical Inc | 0163U | Oncology (colorectal) screening, biochemical enzyme-linked immunosorbent assay (ELISA) of 3 plasma or serum proteins (teratocarcinoma derived growth factor-1 [TDGF-1, Cripto-1], carcinoembryonic antigen [CEA], extracellular matrix protein [ECM]), with demographic data (age, gender, CRC-screening compliance) using a proprietary algorithm and reported as likelihood of CRC or advanced adenomas |

★ = Telemedicine   ✚ = Add-on code   𝒩 = FDA approval pending   # = Resequenced code   ⊘ = Modifier 51 exempt

Appendix O

| Proprietary Name and Clinical Laboratory or Manufacturer | Alpha-Numeric Code | Code Descriptor |
|---|---|---|
| ibs-smart™, Gemelli Biotech, Gemelli Biotech | 0164U | Gastroenterology (irritable bowel syndrome [IBS]), immunoassay for anti-CdtB and anti-vinculin antibodies, utilizing plasma, algorithm for elevated or not elevated qualitative results |
| VeriMAP™ Peanut Dx – Bead-based Epitope Assay, AllerGenis™ Clinical Laboratory, AllerGenis™ LLC | 0165U | Peanut allergen-specific quantitative assessment of multiple epitopes using enzyme-linked immunosorbent assay (ELISA), blood, individual epitope results and probability of peanut allergy |
| LiverFASt™, Fibronostics, Fibronostics | 0166U | Liver disease, 10 biochemical assays (α2-macroglobulin, haptoglobin, apolipoprotein A1, bilirubin, GGT, ALT, AST, triglycerides, cholesterol, fasting glucose) and biometric and demographic data, utilizing serum, algorithm reported as scores for fibrosis, necroinflammatory activity, and steatosis with a summary interpretation |
| ADEXUSDx hCG Test, NOWDiagnostics, NOWDiagnostics | 0167U | Gonadotropin, chorionic (hCG), immunoassay with direct optical observation, blood |
| — | ▶(0168U has been deleted)◀ | — |
| NT (*NUDT15* and *TPMT*) genotyping panel, RPRD Diagnostics | 0169U | *NUDT15 (nudix hydrolase 15)* and *TPMT (thiopurine S-methyltransferase)* (eg, drug metabolism) gene analysis, common variants |
| Clarifi™, Quadrant Biosciences, Inc, Quadrant Biosciences, Inc | 0170U | Neurology (autism spectrum disorder [ASD]), RNA, next-generation sequencing, saliva, algorithmic analysis, and results reported as predictive probability of ASD diagnosis |
| MyMRD® NGS Panel, Laboratory for Personalized Molecular Medicine, Laboratory for Personalized Molecular Medicine | 0171U | Targeted genomic sequence analysis panel, acute myeloid leukemia, myelodysplastic syndrome, and myeloproliferative neoplasms, DNA analysis, 23 genes, interrogation for sequence variants, rearrangements and minimal residual disease, reported as presence/absence |
| myChoice® CDx, Myriad Genetics Laboratories, Inc, Myriad Genetics Laboratories, Inc | 0172U | Oncology (solid tumor as indicated by the label), somatic mutation analysis of *BRCA1 (BRCA1, DNA repair associated)*, *BRCA2 (BRCA2, DNA repair associated)* and analysis of homologous recombination deficiency pathways, DNA, formalin-fixed paraffin-embedded tissue, algorithm quantifying tumor genomic instability score |
| Psych HealthPGx Panel, RPRD Diagnostics, RPRD Diagnostics | 0173U | Psychiatry (ie, depression, anxiety), genomic analysis panel, includes variant analysis of 14 genes |
| LC-MS/MS Targeted Proteomic Assay, OncoOmicDx Laboratory, LDT | 0174U | Oncology (solid tumor), mass spectrometric 30 protein targets, formalin-fixed paraffin-embedded tissue, prognostic and predictive algorithm reported as likely, unlikely, or uncertain benefit of 39 chemotherapy and targeted therapeutic oncology agents |
| Genomind® Professional PGx Express™ CORE, Genomind, Inc, Genomind, Inc | 0175U | Psychiatry (eg, depression, anxiety), genomic analysis panel, variant analysis of 15 genes |

(*Continued on page 262*)

▲=Revised code　●=New code　▶◀=Contains new or revised text　✖=Duplicate PLA test　↕=Category I PLA

| Proprietary Name and Clinical Laboratory or Manufacturer | Alpha-Numeric Code | Code Descriptor |
|---|---|---|
| IB*Schek*®, Commonwealth Diagnostics International, Inc, Commonwealth Diagnostics International, Inc | 0176U | Cytolethal distending toxin B (CdtB) and vinculin IgG antibodies by immunoassay (ie, ELISA) |
| therascreen® *PIK3CA* RGQ PCR Kit, QIAGEN, QIAGEN GmbH | 0177U | Oncology (breast cancer), DNA, *PIK3CA (phosphatidylinositol-4,5-bisphosphate 3-kinase catalytic subunit alpha)* gene analysis of 11 gene variants utilizing plasma, reported as *PIK3CA* gene mutation status |
| ▶VeriMAP™ Peanut Reactivity Threshold–Bead Based Epitope Assay,◀ AllerGenis™ Clinical Laboratory, AllerGenis™ LLC | 0178U | Peanut allergen-specific quantitative assessment of multiple epitopes using enzyme-linked immunosorbent assay (ELISA), blood, report of minimum eliciting exposure for a clinical reaction |
| Resolution ctDx Lung™, Resolution Bioscience, Resolution Bioscience, Inc | 0179U | Oncology (non-small cell lung cancer), cell-free DNA, targeted sequence analysis of 23 genes (single nucleotide variations, insertions and deletions, fusions without prior knowledge of partner/breakpoint, copy number variations), with report of significant mutation(s) |
| Navigator ABO Sequencing, Grifols Immunohematology Center, Grifols Immunohematology Center | 0180U | Red cell antigen (ABO blood group) genotyping (ABO), gene analysis Sanger/chain termination/ conventional sequencing, *ABO (ABO, alpha 1-3-N-acetylgalactosaminyltransferase and alpha 1-3-galactosyltransferase)* gene, including subtyping, 7 exons |
| Navigator CO Sequencing, Grifols Immunohematology Center, Grifols Immunohematology Center | 0181U | Red cell antigen (Colton blood group) genotyping (CO), gene analysis, *AQP1 (aquaporin 1 [Colton blood group])* exon 1 |
| Navigator CROM Sequencing, Grifols Immunohematology Center, Grifols Immunohematology Center | 0182U | Red cell antigen (Cromer blood group) genotyping (CROM), gene analysis, *CD55 (CD55 molecule [Cromer blood group])* exons 1-10 |
| Navigator DI Sequencing, Grifols Immunohematology Center, Grifols Immunohematology Center | 0183U | Red cell antigen (Diego blood group) genotyping (DI), gene analysis, *SLC4A1 (solute carrier family 4 member 1 [Diego blood group])* exon 19 |
| Navigator DO Sequencing, Grifols Immunohematology Center, Grifols Immunohematology Center | 0184U | Red cell antigen (Dombrock blood group) genotyping (DO), gene analysis, *ART4 (ADP-ribosyltransferase 4 [Dombrock blood group])* exon 2 |
| Navigator FUT1 Sequencing, Grifols Immunohematology Center, Grifols Immunohematology Center | 0185U | Red cell antigen (H blood group) genotyping (FUT1), gene analysis, *FUT1 (fucosyltransferase 1 [H blood group])* exon 4 |
| Navigator FUT2 Sequencing, Grifols Immunohematology Center, Grifols Immunohematology Center | 0186U | Red cell antigen (H blood group) genotyping (FUT2), gene analysis, *FUT2 (fucosyltransferase 2)* exon 2 |
| Navigator FY Sequencing, Grifols Immunohematology Center, Grifols Immunohematology Center | 0187U | Red cell antigen (Duffy blood group) genotyping (FY), gene analysis, *ACKR1 (atypical chemokine receptor 1 [Duffy blood group])* exons 1-2 |
| Navigator GE Sequencing, Grifols Immunohematology Center, Grifols Immunohematology Center | 0188U | Red cell antigen (Gerbich blood group) genotyping (GE), gene analysis, *GYPC (glycophorin C [Gerbich blood group])* exons 1-4 |

| Proprietary Name and Clinical Laboratory or Manufacturer | Alpha-Numeric Code | Code Descriptor |
|---|---|---|
| Navigator GYPA Sequencing, Grifols Immunohematology Center, Grifols Immunohematology Center | 0189U | Red cell antigen (MNS blood group) genotyping (GYPA), gene analysis, *GYPA (glycophorin A [MNS blood group])* introns 1, 5, exon 2 |
| Navigator GYPB Sequencing, Grifols Immunohematology Center, Grifols Immunohematology Center | 0190U | Red cell antigen (MNS blood group) genotyping (GYPB), gene analysis, *GYPB (glycophorin B [MNS blood group])* introns 1, 5, pseudoexon 3 |
| Navigator IN Sequencing, Grifols Immunohematology Center, Grifols Immunohematology Center | 0191U | Red cell antigen (Indian blood group) genotyping (IN), gene analysis, *CD44 (CD44 molecule [Indian blood group])* exons 2, 3, 6 |
| Navigator JK Sequencing, Grifols Immunohematology Center, Grifols Immunohematology Center | 0192U | Red cell antigen (Kidd blood group) genotyping (JK), gene analysis, *SLC14A1 (solute carrier family 14 member 1 [Kidd blood group])* gene promoter, exon 9 |
| Navigator JR Sequencing, Grifols Immunohematology Center, Grifols Immunohematology Center | 0193U | Red cell antigen (JR blood group) genotyping (JR), gene analysis, *ABCG2 (ATP binding cassette subfamily G member 2 [Junior blood group])* exons 2-26 |
| Navigator KEL Sequencing, Grifols Immunohematology Center, Grifols Immunohematology Center | 0194U | Red cell antigen (Kell blood group) genotyping (KEL), gene analysis, *KEL (Kell metallo-endopeptidase [Kell blood group])* exon 8 |
| Navigator *KLF1* Sequencing, Grifols Immunohematology Center, Grifols Immunohematology Center | 0195U | *KLF1 (Kruppel-like factor 1)*, targeted sequencing (ie, exon 13) |
| Navigator LU Sequencing, Grifols Immunohematology Center, Grifols Immunohematology Center | 0196U | Red cell antigen (Lutheran blood group) genotyping (LU), gene analysis, *BCAM (basal cell adhesion molecule [Lutheran blood group])* exon 3 |
| Navigator LW Sequencing, Grifols Immunohematology Center, Grifols Immunohematology Center | 0197U | Red cell antigen (Landsteiner-Wiener blood group) genotyping (LW), gene analysis, *ICAM4 (intercellular adhesion molecule 4 [Landsteiner-Wiener blood group])* exon 1 |
| Navigator RHD/CE Sequencing, Grifols Immunohematology Center, Grifols Immunohematology Center | 0198U | Red cell antigen (RH blood group) genotyping (RHD and RHCE), gene analysis Sanger/chain termination/conventional sequencing, *RHD (Rh blood group D antigen)* exons 1-10 and *RHCE (Rh blood group CcEe antigens)* exon 5 |
| Navigator SC Sequencing, Grifols Immunohematology Center, Grifols Immunohematology Center | 0199U | Red cell antigen (Scianna blood group) genotyping (SC), gene analysis, *ERMAP (erythroblast membrane associated protein [Scianna blood group])* exons 4, 12 |
| Navigator XK Sequencing, Grifols Immunohematology Center, Grifols Immunohematology Center | 0200U | Red cell antigen (Kx blood group) genotyping (XK), gene analysis, *XK (X-linked Kx blood group)* exons 1-3 |
| Navigator YT Sequencing, Grifols Immunohematology Center, Grifols Immunohematology Center | 0201U | Red cell antigen (Yt blood group) genotyping (YT), gene analysis, *ACHE (acetylcholinesterase [Cartwright blood group])* exon 2 |

(Continued on page 264)

| Proprietary Name and Clinical Laboratory or Manufacturer | Alpha-Numeric Code | Code Descriptor |
|---|---|---|
| BioFire® Respiratory Panel 2.1 (RP2.1), BioFire® Diagnostics, BioFire® Diagnostics, LLC | #0202U | Infectious disease (bacterial or viral respiratory tract infection), pathogen-specific nucleic acid (DNA or RNA), 22 targets including severe acute respiratory syndrome coronavirus 2 (SARS-CoV-2), qualitative RT-PCR, nasopharyngeal swab, each pathogen reported as detected or not detected |
| | | ▶(For additional PLA code with identical clinical descriptor, see 0223U. See Appendix O or the most current listing on the AMA CPT website to determine appropriate code assignment)◀ |
| PredictSURE IBD™ Test, KSL Diagnostics, PredictImmune Ltd | 0203U | Autoimmune (inflammatory bowel disease), mRNA, gene expression profiling by quantitative RT-PCR, 17 genes (15 target and 2 reference genes), whole blood, reported as a continuous risk score and classification of inflammatory bowel disease aggressiveness |
| Afirma Xpression Atlas, Veracyte, Inc, Veracyte, Inc | 0204U | Oncology (thyroid), mRNA, gene expression analysis of 593 genes (including *BRAF, RAS, RET, PAX8,* and *NTRK*) for sequence variants and rearrangements, utilizing fine needle aspirate, reported as detected or not detected |
| Vita Risk®, Arctic Medical Laboratories, Arctic Medical Laboratories | 0205U | Ophthalmology (age-related macular degeneration), analysis of 3 gene variants (2 *CFH* gene, 1 *ARMS2* gene), using PCR and MALDI-TOF, buccal swab, reported as positive or negative for neovascular age-related macular-degeneration risk associated with zinc supplements |
| DISCERN™, NeuroDiagnostics, NeuroDiagnostics | 0206U | Neurology (Alzheimer disease); cell aggregation using morphometric imaging and protein kinase C-epsilon (PKCe) concentration in response to amylospheroid treatment by ELISA, cultured skin fibroblasts, each reported as positive or negative for Alzheimer disease |
| | +0207U | quantitative imaging of phosphorylated *ERK1* and *ERK2* in response to bradykinin treatment by in situ immunofluorescence, using cultured skin fibroblasts, reported as a probability index for Alzheimer disease (List separately in addition to code for primary procedure) |
| | | (Use 0207U in conjunction with 0206U) |
| Afirma Medullary Thyroid Carcinoma (MTC) Classifier, Veracyte, Inc, Veracyte, Inc | 0208U | Oncology (medullary thyroid carcinoma), mRNA, gene expression analysis of 108 genes, utilizing fine needle aspirate, algorithm reported as positive or negative for medullary thyroid carcinoma |
| CNGnome™, PerkinElmer Genomics, PerkinElmer Genomics | 0209U | Cytogenomic constitutional (genome-wide) analysis, interrogation of genomic regions for copy number, structural changes and areas of homozygosity for chromosomal abnormalities |
| BioPlex 2200 RPR Assay – Quantitative, Bio-Rad Laboratories, Bio-Rad Laboratories | 0210U | Syphilis test, non-treponemal antibody, immunoassay, quantitative (RPR) |

★=Telemedicine    +=Add-on code    ✗=FDA approval pending    #=Resequenced code    ⊘=Modifier 51 exempt

| Proprietary Name and Clinical Laboratory or Manufacturer | Alpha-Numeric Code | Code Descriptor |
|---|---|---|
| MI Cancer Seek™ - NGS Analysis, Caris MPI d/b/a Caris Life Sciences, Caris MPI d/b/a Caris Life Sciences | 0211U | Oncology (pan-tumor), DNA and RNA by next-generation sequencing, utilizing formalin-fixed paraffin-embedded tissue, interpretative report for single nucleotide variants, copy number alterations, tumor mutational burden, and microsatellite instability, with therapy association |
| Genomic Unity® Whole Genome Analysis – Proband, Variantyx Inc, Variantyx Inc | 0212U | Rare diseases (constitutional/heritable disorders), whole genome and mitochondrial DNA sequence analysis, including small sequence changes, deletions, duplications, short tandem repeat gene expansions, and variants in non-uniquely mappable regions, blood or saliva, identification and categorization of genetic variants, proband<br><br>(Do not report 0212U in conjunction with 81425) |
| Genomic Unity® Whole Genome Analysis – Comparator, Variantyx Inc, Variantyx Inc | 0213U | Rare diseases (constitutional/heritable disorders), whole genome and mitochondrial DNA sequence analysis, including small sequence changes, deletions, duplications, short tandem repeat gene expansions, and variants in non-uniquely mappable regions, blood or saliva, identification and categorization of genetic variants, each comparator genome (eg, parent, sibling)<br><br>(Do not report 0213U in conjunction with 81426) |
| Genomic Unity® Exome Plus Analysis – Proband, Variantyx Inc, Variantyx Inc | 0214U | Rare diseases (constitutional/heritable disorders), whole exome and mitochondrial DNA sequence analysis, including small sequence changes, deletions, duplications, short tandem repeat gene expansions, and variants in non-uniquely mappable regions, blood or saliva, identification and categorization of genetic variants, proband<br><br>(Do not report 0214U in conjunction with 81415) |
| Genomic Unity® Exome Plus Analysis – Comparator, Variantyx Inc, Variantyx Inc | 0215U | Rare diseases (constitutional/heritable disorders), whole exome and mitochondrial DNA sequence analysis, including small sequence changes, deletions, duplications, short tandem repeat gene expansions, and variants in non-uniquely mappable regions, blood or saliva, identification and categorization of genetic variants, each comparator exome (eg, parent, sibling)<br><br>(Do not report 0215U in conjunction with 81416) |
| Genomic Unity® Ataxia Repeat Expansion and Sequence Analysis, Variantyx Inc, Variantyx Inc | 0216U | Neurology (inherited ataxias), genomic DNA sequence analysis of 12 common genes including small sequence changes, deletions, duplications, short tandem repeat gene expansions, and variants in non-uniquely mappable regions, blood or saliva, identification and categorization of genetic variants |
| Genomic Unity® Comprehensive Ataxia Repeat Expansion and Sequence Analysis, Variantyx Inc, Variantyx Inc | 0217U | Neurology (inherited ataxias), genomic DNA sequence analysis of 51 genes including small sequence changes, deletions, duplications, short tandem repeat gene expansions, and variants in non-uniquely mappable regions, blood or saliva, identification and categorization of genetic variants |

(Continued on page 266)

Appendix O

| Proprietary Name and Clinical Laboratory or Manufacturer | Alpha-Numeric Code | Code Descriptor |
|---|---|---|
| Genomic Unity® DMD Analysis, Variantyx Inc, Variantyx Inc | 0218U | Neurology (muscular dystrophy), *DMD* gene sequence analysis, including small sequence changes, deletions, duplications, and variants in non-uniquely mappable regions, blood or saliva, identification and characterization of genetic variants |
| *Sentosa®* SQ HIV-1 Genotyping Assay, Vela Diagnostics USA, Inc, Vela Operations Singapore Pte Ltd | 0219U | Infectious agent (human immunodeficiency virus), targeted viral next-generation sequence analysis (ie, protease [PR], reverse transcriptase [RT], integrase [INT]), algorithm reported as prediction of antiviral drug susceptibility |
| PreciseDx™ Breast Cancer Test, PreciseDx, PreciseDx | 0220U | Oncology (breast cancer), image analysis with artificial intelligence assessment of 12 histologic and immunohistochemical features, reported as a recurrence score |
| Navigator ABO Blood Group NGS, Grifols Immunohematology Center, Grifols Immunohematology Center | 0221U | Red cell antigen (ABO blood group) genotyping (ABO), gene analysis, next-generation sequencing, *ABO (ABO, alpha 1-3-N-acetylgalactosaminyltransferase and alpha 1-3-galactosyltransferase)* gene |
| Navigator Rh Blood Group NGS, Grifols Immunohematology Center, Grifols Immunohematology Center | 0222U | Red cell antigen (RH blood group) genotyping (RHD and RHCE), gene analysis, next-generation sequencing, RH proximal promoter, exons 1-10, portions of introns 2-3 |
| ▶QIAstat-Dx Respiratory SARS CoV-2 Panel, QIAGEN Sciences, QIAGEN GmbH◀ | #●0223U | ▶Infectious disease (bacterial or viral respiratory tract infection), pathogen-specific nucleic acid (DNA or RNA), 22 targets including severe acute respiratory syndrome coronavirus 2 (SARS-CoV-2), qualitative RT-PCR, nasopharyngeal swab, each pathogen reported as detected or not detected◀ ▶(For additional PLA code with identical clinical descriptor, see 0202U. See Appendix O or the most current listing on the AMA CPT website to determine appropriate code assignment)◀ |
| ▶COVID-19 Antibody Test, Mt Sinai, Mount Sinai Laboratory◀ | ●0224U | ▶Antibody, severe acute respiratory syndrome coronavirus 2 (SARS-CoV-2) (coronavirus disease [COVID-19]), includes titer(s), when performed◀ ▶(Do not report 0224U in conjunction with 86769)◀ |
| ▶ePlex® Respiratory Pathogen Panel 2, GenMark Dx, GenMark Diagnostics, Inc◀ | ●0225U | ▶Infectious disease (bacterial or viral respiratory tract infection) pathogen-specific DNA and RNA, 21 targets, including severe acute respiratory syndrome coronavirus 2 (SARS-CoV-2), amplified probe technique, including multiplex reverse transcription for RNA targets, each analyte reported as detected or not detected◀ |
| ▶Tru-Immune™, Ethos Laboratories, GenScript® USA Inc◀ | ●0226U | ▶Surrogate viral neutralization test (sVNT), severe acute respiratory syndrome coronavirus 2 (SARS-CoV-2) (coronavirus disease [COVID-19]), ELISA, plasma, serum◀ |

★=Telemedicine  ✚=Add-on code  ✗=FDA approval pending  #=Resequenced code  ⊘=Modifier 51 exempt

| Proprietary Name and Clinical Laboratory or Manufacturer | Alpha-Numeric Code | Code Descriptor |
|---|---|---|
| ▶Comprehensive Screen, Aspenti Health◀ | ●0227U | ▶Drug assay, presumptive, 30 or more drugs or metabolites, urine, liquid chromatography with tandem mass spectrometry (LC-MS/MS) using multiple reaction monitoring (MRM), with drug or metabolite description, includes sample validation◀ |
| ▶PanGIA Prostate, Genetics Institute of America, Entopsis, LLC◀ | ●0228U | ▶Oncology (prostate), multianalyte molecular profile by photometric detection of macromolecules adsorbed on nanosponge array slides with machine learning, utilizing first morning voided urine, algorithm reported as likelihood of prostate cancer◀ |
| ▶Colvera®, Clinical Genomics Pathology Inc◀ | ●0229U | ▶*BCAT1 (Branched chain amino acid transaminase 1)* or *IKZF1 (IKAROS family zinc finger 1)* (eg, colorectal cancer) promoter methylation analysis◀ |
| ▶Genomic Unity® AR Analysis, Variantyx Inc, Variantyx Inc◀ | ●0230U | ▶*AR (androgen receptor)* (eg, spinal and bulbar muscular atrophy, Kennedy disease, X chromosome inactivation), full sequence analysis, including small sequence changes in exonic and intronic regions, deletions, duplications, short tandem repeat (STR) expansions, mobile element insertions, and variants in non-uniquely mappable regions◀ |
| ▶Genomic Unity® CACNA1A Analysis, Variantyx Inc, Variantyx Inc◀ | ●0231U | ▶*CACNA1A (calcium voltage-gated channel subunit alpha 1A)* (eg, spinocerebellar ataxia), full gene analysis, including small sequence changes in exonic and intronic regions, deletions, duplications, short tandem repeat (STR) gene expansions, mobile element insertions, and variants in non-uniquely mappable regions◀ |
| ▶Genomic Unity® CSTB Analysis, Variantyx Inc, Variantyx Inc◀ | ●0232U | ▶*CSTB (cystatin B)* (eg, progressive myoclonic epilepsy type 1A, Unverricht-Lundborg disease), full gene analysis, including small sequence changes in exonic and intronic regions, deletions, duplications, short tandem repeat (STR) expansions, mobile element insertions, and variants in non-uniquely mappable regions◀ |
| ▶Genomic Unity® FXN Analysis, Variantyx Inc, Variantyx Inc◀ | ●0233U | ▶*FXN (frataxin)* (eg, Friedreich ataxia), gene analysis, including small sequence changes in exonic and intronic regions, deletions, duplications, short tandem repeat (STR) expansions, mobile element insertions, and variants in non-uniquely mappable regions◀ |
| ▶Genomic Unity® MECP2 Analysis, Variantyx Inc, Variantyx Inc◀ | ●0234U | ▶*MECP2 (methyl CpG binding protein 2)* (eg, Rett syndrome), full gene analysis, including small sequence changes in exonic and intronic regions, deletions, duplications, mobile element insertions, and variants in non-uniquely mappable regions◀ |

(*Continued on page 268*)

| Proprietary Name and Clinical Laboratory or Manufacturer | Alpha-Numeric Code | Code Descriptor |
|---|---|---|
| ▶Genomic Unity® PTEN Analysis, Variantyx Inc, Variantyx Inc◀ | ●0235U | ▶*PTEN (phosphatase and tensin homolog)* (eg, Cowden syndrome, PTEN hamartoma tumor syndrome), full gene analysis, including small sequence changes in exonic and intronic regions, deletions, duplications, mobile element insertions, and variants in non-uniquely mappable regions◀ |
| ▶Genomic Unity® SMN1/2 Analysis, Variantyx Inc, Variantyx Inc◀ | ●0236U | ▶*SMN1 (survival of motor neuron 1, telomeric)* and *SMN2 (survival of motor neuron 2, centromeric)* (eg, spinal muscular atrophy) full gene analysis, including small sequence changes in exonic and intronic regions, duplications, deletions, and mobile element insertions◀ |
| ▶Genomic Unity® Cardiac Ion Channelopathies Analysis, Variantyx Inc, Variantyx Inc◀ | ●0237U | ▶Cardiac ion channelopathies (eg, Brugada syndrome, long QT syndrome, short QT syndrome, catecholaminergic polymorphic ventricular tachycardia), genomic sequence analysis panel including *ANK2, CASQ2, CAV3, KCNE1, KCNE2, KCNH2, KCNJ2, KCNQ1, RYR2,* and *SCN5A,* including small sequence changes in exonic and intronic regions, deletions, duplications, mobile element insertions, and variants in non-uniquely mappable regions◀ |
| ▶Genomic Unity® Lynch Syndrome Analysis, Variantyx Inc, Variantyx Inc◀ | ●0238U | ▶Oncology (Lynch syndrome), genomic DNA sequence analysis of *MLH1, MSH2, MSH6, PMS2,* and *EPCAM,* including small sequence changes in exonic and intronic regions, deletions, duplications, mobile element insertions, and variants in non-uniquely mappable regions◀ |
| ▶FoundationOne® Liquid CDx, Foundation Medicine Inc, Foundation Medicine Inc◀ | ●0239U | ▶Targeted genomic sequence analysis panel, solid organ neoplasm, cell-free DNA, analysis of 311 or more genes, interrogation for sequence variants, including substitutions, insertions, deletions, select rearrangements, and copy number variations◀ |
| ▶Xpert® Xpress SARS-CoV-2/Flu/RSV (SARS-CoV-2 & Flu targets only), Cepheid◀ | ●0240U | ▶Infectious disease (viral respiratory tract infection), pathogen-specific RNA, 3 targets (severe acute respiratory syndrome coronavirus 2 [SARS-CoV-2], influenza A, influenza B), upper respiratory specimen, each pathogen reported as detected or not detected◀ |
| ▶Xpert® Xpress SARS-CoV-2/Flu/RSV (all targets), Cepheid◀ | ●0241U | ▶Infectious disease (viral respiratory tract infection), pathogen-specific RNA, 4 targets (severe acute respiratory syndrome coronavirus 2 [SARS-CoV-2], influenza A, influenza B, respiratory syncytial virus [RSV]), upper respiratory specimen, each pathogen reported as detected or not detected◀ |
| ▶Guardant360® CDx, Guardant Health Inc, Guardant Health Inc◀ | ●0242U | ▶Targeted genomic sequence analysis panel, solid organ neoplasm, cell-free circulating DNA analysis of 55-74 genes, interrogation for sequence variants, gene copy number amplifications, and gene rearrangements◀ |

★=Telemedicine   ✛=Add-on code   ✗=FDA approval pending   #=Resequenced code   ⊘=Modifier 51 exempt

| Proprietary Name and Clinical Laboratory or Manufacturer | Alpha-Numeric Code | Code Descriptor |
|---|---|---|
| ▶PlGF Preeclampsia Screen, PerkinElmer Genetics, PerkinElmer Genetics, Inc◀ | ●0243U | ▶Obstetrics (preeclampsia), biochemical assay of placental-growth factor, time-resolved fluorescence immunoassay, maternal serum, predictive algorithm reported as a risk score for preeclampsia◀ |
| ▶Oncotype MAP™ Pan-Cancer Tissue Test, Paradigm Diagnostics, Inc, Paradigm Diagnostics, Inc◀ | ●0244U | ▶Oncology (solid organ), DNA, comprehensive genomic profiling, 257 genes, interrogation for single-nucleotide variants, insertions/deletions, copy number alterations, gene rearrangements, tumor-mutational burden and microsatellite instability, utilizing formalin-fixed paraffin-embedded tumor tissue◀ |
| ▶ThyGeNEXT® Thyroid Oncogene Panel, Interpace Diagnostics, Interpace Diagnostics◀ | ●0245U | ▶Oncology (thyroid), mutation analysis of 10 genes and 37 RNA fusions and expression of 4 mRNA markers using next-generation sequencing, fine needle aspirate, report includes associated risk of malignancy expressed as a percentage◀ |
| ▶PrecisionBlood™, San Diego Blood Bank, San Diego Blood Bank◀ | ●0246U | ▶Red blood cell antigen typing, DNA, genotyping of at least 16 blood groups with phenotype prediction of at least 51 red blood cell antigens◀ |
| ▶PreTRM®, Sera Prognostics, Sera Prognostics, Inc®◀ | ●0247U | ▶Obstetrics (preterm birth), insulin-like growth factor–binding protein 4 (IBP4), sex hormone–binding globulin (SHBG), quantitative measurement by LC-MS/MS, utilizing maternal serum, combined with clinical data, reported as predictive-risk stratification for spontaneous preterm birth◀ |
| ▶3D Predict Glioma, KIYATEC®, Inc◀ | ●0248U | ▶Oncology (brain), spheroid cell culture in a 3D microenvironment, 12 drug panel, tumor-response prediction for each drug◀ |
| ▶Theralink® Reverse Phase Protein Array (RPPA), Theralink® Technologies, Inc, Theralink® Technologies, Inc◀ | ●0249U | ▶Oncology (breast), semiquantitative analysis of 32 phosphoproteins and protein analytes, includes laser capture microdissection, with algorithmic analysis and interpretative report◀ |
| ▶PGDx elio™ tissue complete, Personal Genome Diagnostics, Inc, Personal Genome Diagnostics, Inc◀ | ●0250U | ▶Oncology (solid organ neoplasm), targeted genomic sequence DNA analysis of 505 genes, interrogation for somatic alterations (SNVs [single nucleotide variant], small insertions and deletions, one amplification, and four translocations), microsatellite instability and tumor-mutation burden◀ |
| ▶Intrinsic Hepcidin IDx™ Test, IntrinsicDx, Intrinsic LifeSciences™ LLC◀ | ●0251U | ▶Hepcidin-25, enzyme-linked immunosorbent assay (ELISA), serum or plasma◀ |
| ▶POC (Products of Conception), Igenomix®, Igenomix® USA◀ | ●0252U | ▶Fetal aneuploidy short tandem–repeat comparative analysis, fetal DNA from products of conception, reported as normal (euploidy), monosomy, trisomy, or partial deletion/duplication, mosaicism, and segmental aneuploidy◀ |

(Continued on page 270)

▲=Revised code   ●=New code   ▶◀=Contains new or revised text   ✕=Duplicate PLA test   ↿⇂=Category I PLA

| Proprietary Name and Clinical Laboratory or Manufacturer | Alpha-Numeric Code | Code Descriptor |
|---|---|---|
| ▶ERA® (Endometrial Receptivity Analysis), Igenomix®, Igenomix® USA◀ | ●0253U | ▶Reproductive medicine (endometrial receptivity analysis), RNA gene expression profile, 238 genes by next-generation sequencing, endometrial tissue, predictive algorithm reported as endometrial window of implantation (eg, pre-receptive, receptive, post-receptive)◀ |
| ▶SMART PGT-A (Pre-implantation Genetic Testing - Aneuploidy), Igenomix®, Igenomix® USA◀ | ●0254U | ▶Reproductive medicine (preimplantation genetic assessment), analysis of 24 chromosomes using embryonic DNA genomic sequence analysis for aneuploidy, and a mitochondrial DNA score in euploid embryos, results reported as normal (euploidy), monosomy, trisomy, or partial deletion/duplication, mosaicism, and segmental aneuploidy, per embryo tested◀ |
| ▶Cap-Score™ Test, Androvia LifeSciences, Avantor Clinical Services (previously known as Therapak)◀ | ●0255U | ▶Andrology (infertility), sperm-capacitation assessment of ganglioside GM1 distribution patterns, fluorescence microscopy, fresh or frozen specimen, reported as percentage of capacitated sperm and probability of generating a pregnancy score◀ |
| ▶Trimethylamine (TMA) and TMA N-Oxide, Children's Hospital Colorado Laboratory◀ | ●0256U | ▶Trimethylamine/trimethylamine N-oxide (TMA/TMAO) profile, tandem mass spectrometry (MS/MS), urine, with algorithmic analysis and interpretive report◀ |
| ▶Very-Long Chain Acyl-CoA Dehydrogenase (VLCAD) Enzyme Activity, Children's Hospital Colorado Laboratory◀ | ●0257U | ▶Very long chain acyl-coenzyme A (CoA) dehydrogenase (VLCAD), leukocyte enzyme activity, whole blood◀ |
| ▶Mind.Px, Mindera, Mindera Corporation◀ | ●0258U | ▶Autoimmune (psoriasis), mRNA, next-generation sequencing, gene expression profiling of 50-100 genes, skin-surface collection using adhesive patch, algorithm reported as likelihood of response to psoriasis biologics◀ |
| ▶GFR by NMR, Labtech™ Diagnostics◀ | ●0259U | ▶Nephrology (chronic kidney disease), nuclear magnetic resonance spectroscopy measurement of myo-inositol, valine, and creatinine, algorithmically combined with cystatin C (by immunoassay) and demographic data to determine estimated glomerular filtration rate (GFR), serum, quantitative◀ |
| ▶Augusta Optical Genome Mapping, Georgia Esoteric and Molecular (GEM) Laboratory, LLC, Bionano Genomics Inc◀ | ✕●0260U | ▶Rare diseases (constitutional/heritable disorders), identification of copy number variations, inversions, insertions, translocations, and other structural variants by optical genome mapping◀<br><br>▶(For additional PLA code with identical clinical descriptor, see 0264U. See Appendix O or the most current listing on the AMA CPT website to determine appropriate code assignment)◀ |

Appendix O

| Proprietary Name and Clinical Laboratory or Manufacturer | Alpha-Numeric Code | Code Descriptor |
|---|---|---|
| ▶Immunoscore®, HalioDx, HalioDx◀ | ●0261U | ▶Oncology (colorectal cancer), image analysis with artificial intelligence assessment of 4 histologic and immunohistochemical features (CD3 and CD8 within tumor-stroma border and tumor core), tissue, reported as immune response and recurrence-risk score◀ |
| ▶OncoSignal 7 Pathway Signal, Protean BioDiagnostics, Philips Electronics Nederland BV◀ | ●0262U | ▶Oncology (solid tumor), gene expression profiling by real-time RT-PCR of 7 gene pathways (ER, AR, PI3K, MAPK, HH, TGFB, Notch), formalin-fixed paraffin-embedded (FFPE), algorithm reported as gene pathway activity score◀ |
| ▶NPDX ASD and Central Carbon Energy Metabolism, Stemina Biomarker Discovery, Inc, Stemina Biomarker Discovery, Inc◀ | ●0263U | ▶Neurology (autism spectrum disorder [ASD]), quantitative measurements of 16 central carbon metabolites (ie, α-ketoglutarate, alanine, lactate, phenylalanine, pyruvate, succinate, carnitine, citrate, fumarate, hypoxanthine, inosine, malate, S-sulfocysteine, taurine, urate, and xanthine), liquid chromatography tandem mass spectrometry (LC-MS/MS), plasma, algorithmic analysis with result reported as negative or positive (with metabolic subtypes of ASD)◀ |
| ▶Praxis Optical Genome Mapping, Praxis Genomics LLC◀ | ✂●0264U | ▶Rare diseases (constitutional/heritable disorders), identification of copy number variations, inversions, insertions, translocations, and other structural variants by optical genome mapping◀ ▶(For additional PLA code with identical clinical descriptor, see 0260U. See Appendix O or the most current listing on the AMA CPT website to determine appropriate code assignment)◀ |
| ▶Praxis Whole Genome Sequencing, Praxis Genomics LLC◀ | ●0265U | ▶Rare constitutional and other heritable disorders, whole genome and mitochondrial DNA sequence analysis, blood, frozen and formalin-fixed paraffin-embedded (FFPE) tissue, saliva, buccal swabs or cell lines, identification of single nucleotide and copy number variants◀ |
| ▶Praxis Transcriptome, Praxis Genomics LLC◀ | ●0266U | ▶Unexplained constitutional or other heritable disorders or syndromes, tissue-specific gene expression by whole-transcriptome and next-generation sequencing, blood, formalin-fixed paraffin-embedded (FFPE) tissue or fresh frozen tissue, reported as presence or absence of splicing or expression changes◀ |
| ▶Praxis Combined Whole Genome Sequencing and Optical Genome Mapping, Praxis Genomics LLC◀ | ●0267U | ▶Rare constitutional and other heritable disorders, identification of copy number variations, inversions, insertions, translocations, and other structural variants by optical genome mapping and whole genome sequencing◀ |
| ▶Versiti™ aHUS Genetic Evaluation, Versiti™ Diagnostic Laboratories, Versiti™◀ | ●0268U | ▶Hematology (atypical hemolytic uremic syndrome [aHUS]), genomic sequence analysis of 15 genes, blood, buccal swab, or amniotic fluid◀ |

(Continued on page 272)

| Proprietary Name and Clinical Laboratory or Manufacturer | Alpha-Numeric Code | Code Descriptor |
|---|---|---|
| ▶Versiti™ Autosomal Dominant Thrombocytopenia Panel, Versiti™ Diagnostic Laboratories, Versiti™◀ | ●0269U | ▶Hematology (autosomal dominant congenital thrombocytopenia), genomic sequence analysis of 14 genes, blood, buccal swab, or amniotic fluid◀ |
| ▶Versiti™ Coagulation Disorder Panel, Versiti™ Diagnostic Laboratories, Versiti™◀ | ●0270U | ▶Hematology (congenital coagulation disorders), genomic sequence analysis of 20 genes, blood, buccal swab, or amniotic fluid◀ |
| ▶Versiti™ Congenital Neutropenia Panel, Versiti™ Diagnostic Laboratories, Versiti™◀ | ●0271U | ▶Hematology (congenital neutropenia), genomic sequence analysis of 23 genes, blood, buccal swab, or amniotic fluid◀ |
| ▶Versiti™ Comprehensive Bleeding Disorder Panel, Versiti™ Diagnostic Laboratories, Versiti™◀ | ●0272U | ▶Hematology (genetic bleeding disorders), genomic sequence analysis of 51 genes, blood, buccal swab, or amniotic fluid, comprehensive◀ |
| ▶Versiti™ Fibrinolytic Disorder Panel, Versiti™ Diagnostic Laboratories, Versiti™◀ | ●0273U | ▶Hematology (genetic hyperfibrinolysis, delayed bleeding), genomic sequence analysis of 8 genes *(F13A1, F13B, FGA, FGB, FGG, SERPINA1, SERPINE1, SERPINF2, PLAU),* blood, buccal swab, or amniotic fluid◀ |
| ▶Versiti™ Comprehensive Platelet Disorder Panel, Versiti™ Diagnostic Laboratories, Versiti™◀ | ●0274U | ▶Hematology (genetic platelet disorders), genomic sequence analysis of 43 genes, blood, buccal swab, or amniotic fluid◀ |
| ▶Versiti™ Heparin-Induced Thrombocytopenia Evaluation – PEA, Versiti™ Diagnostic Laboratories, Versiti™◀ | ●0275U | ▶Hematology (heparin-induced thrombocytopenia), platelet antibody reactivity by flow cytometry, serum◀ |
| ▶Versiti™ Inherited Thrombocytopenia Panel, Versiti™ Diagnostic Laboratories, Versiti™◀ | ●0276U | ▶Hematology (inherited thrombocytopenia), genomic sequence analysis of 23 genes, blood, buccal swab, or amniotic fluid◀ |
| ▶Versiti™ Platelet Function Disorder Panel, Versiti™ Diagnostic Laboratories, Versiti™◀ | ●0277U | ▶Hematology (genetic platelet function disorder), genomic sequence analysis of 31 genes, blood, buccal swab, or amniotic fluid◀ |
| ▶Versiti™ Thrombosis Panel, Versiti™ Diagnostic Laboratories, Versiti™◀ | ●0278U | ▶Hematology (genetic thrombosis), genomic sequence analysis of 12 genes, blood, buccal swab, or amniotic fluid◀ |
| ▶Versiti™ VWF Collagen III Binding, Versiti™ Diagnostic Laboratories, Versiti™◀ | ●0279U | ▶Hematology (von Willebrand disease [VWD]), von Willebrand factor (VWF) and collagen III binding by enzyme-linked immunosorbent assays (ELISA), plasma, report of collagen III binding◀ |
| ▶Versiti™ VWF Collagen IV Binding, Versiti™ Diagnostic Laboratories, Versiti™◀ | ●0280U | ▶Hematology (von Willebrand disease [VWD]), von Willebrand factor (VWF) and collagen IV binding by enzyme-linked immunosorbent assays (ELISA), plasma, report of collagen IV binding◀ |

★=Telemedicine     ✚=Add-on code     ✎=FDA approval pending     #=Resequenced code     ⊘=Modifier 51 exempt

| Proprietary Name and Clinical Laboratory or Manufacturer | Alpha-Numeric Code | Code Descriptor |
|---|---|---|
| ▶Versiti™ VWF Propeptide Antigen, Versiti™ Diagnostic Laboratories, Versiti™◀ | ●0281U | ▶Hematology (von Willebrand disease [VWD]), von Willebrand propeptide, enzyme-linked immunosorbent assays (ELISA), plasma, diagnostic report of von Willebrand factor (VWF) propeptide antigen level◀ |
| ▶Versiti™ Red Cell Genotyping Panel, Versiti™ Diagnostic Laboratories, Versiti™◀ | ●0282U | ▶Red blood cell antigen typing, DNA, genotyping of 12 blood group system genes to predict 44 red blood cell antigen phenotypes◀ |
| ▶Versiti™ VWD Type 2B Evaluation, Versiti™ Diagnostic Laboratories, Versiti™◀ | ●0283U | ▶von Willebrand factor (VWF), type 2B, platelet-binding evaluation, radioimmunoassay, plasma◀ |
| ▶Versiti™ VWD Type 2N Binding, Versiti™ Diagnostic Laboratories, Versiti™◀ | ●0284U | ▶von Willebrand factor (VWF), type 2N, factor VIII and VWF binding evaluation, enzyme-linked immunosorbent assays (ELISA), plasma◀ |

# Rationale

In accordance with the changes made in the Pathology and Laboratory section, including the addition of new codes and code revisions and deletions, Appendix O has been revised. Two new administrative multianalyte assays with algorithmic analysis (MAAA) codes (0017M, 0018M), two new Category I MAAA codes (81523, 81560), and 62 new Proprietary Laboratory Analyses (PLA) codes (0223U-0284U) have been added.

New administrative MAAA code 0017M has been established to report oncology (diffuse large B-cell lymphoma [DLBCL]), mRNA, gene expression profiling by fluorescent probe hybridization of 20 genes, formalin-fixed paraffin-embedded tissue, algorithm reported as cell of origin. In addition, a parenthetical note has been added following code 0017M to restrict reporting this code with PLA code 0120U.

Code 0017M is intended to identify diffuse large B-cell lymphoma (DLBCL). It specifies the type of testing being performed. The procedure decribed in code 0017M uses the same methodology as the procedure described in code 0120U, but the purpose of the procedure is different in that it provides the likelihood of the type of lymphoma diagnostic category (primary large B-cell thymic lymphoma or diffuse large B-cell lymphoma). The test described in code 0017M is used within the diffuse large B-cell lymphoma diagnostic category to provide the "cell-of-origin" subtyping.

New administrative MAAA code 0018M has been established to report transplantation medicine (allograft rejection, renal), measurement of donor and third party–induced CD154+T-cytotoxic memory cells, utilizing whole peripheral blood, algorithm reported as a rejection risk score. In addition, a parenthetical note has been added following code 0018M to restrict reporting this code with codes that include components of this service, such as blood counting for lymphocytes (85032) or HLA typing for mixed lymphocyte culture (MLC).

PLA test codes are released and posted online on a quarterly basis (Fall, Winter, Spring, and Summer) at https://www.ama-assn. org/practice-management/cpt/cpt-pla-codes. They are effective the quarter following their publication online. Other PLA changes include the deletion of five codes (0098U, 0099U, 0100U, 0139U, 0168U), the revision of two codes (0051U, 0152U), the addition of parenthetical notes to instruct on the proper use of the codes (0120U, 0224U), the revision of a test name (0178U), and the addition of parenthetical notes to inform users of PLA codes that have identical clinical descriptors (0202U, 0223U, 0260U, 0264U).

Also, in support of the addition of Molecular Pathology Tier 1 code 81349, which is used to report cytogenomic (genome-wide) analysis for constitutional chromosomal abnormalities using low-pass sequencing, a cross-reference parenthetical note has been added to Appendix O following code 81507 to direct users to the new code.

Refer to the codebook and the Rationale for codes 81349, 81523, 81560, and 0223U-0284U for a full discussion of these changes.

### Clinical Example (0017M)

A 66-year-old male, who has confirmed diffuse large B-cell lymphoma (DLBCL), has formalin-fixed, paraffin-embedded tumor tissue submitted for gene expression profiling.

### Clinical Example (0017M)

Microdissect the tumor tissue and extract total RNA from the unstained sections. Quantify the RNA and hybridize it overnight with specific probes. Analyze the RNA via single molecule imaging. Process the recorded counts using an algorithm for determining the DLBCL cell-of-origin. Report the results.

### Clinical Example (0018M)

A 35-year-old male requires regular surveillance clinical visits to assess the status of his renal transplant (allograft). In addition to other clinical assessments (eg, kidney function tests), the patient's physician orders the test to predict whether he is at increased or decreased risk of acute cellular rejection (ACR).

### Clinical Example (0018M)

Isolate, count, and assess the viability of peripheral blood leukocytes (PBLs) from the patient's blood sample. Use patient human leukocyte antigen (HLA) information supplied with the sample to identify the appropriate cryopreserved PBL stimulators that resemble the donor (donor) or are different (reference). Thaw, count, and assess the viability of these stimulators. Pre-label the recipient PBLs and stimulator PBLs. Separately mix the recipient PBLs with each type of stimulator PBL (donor and reference, respectively), add antibodies to CD154, and culture separately overnight. Enumerate the number of CD154+T-cytotoxic memory cells induced in the donor and reference cultures. Report the test results as a binary risk score for ACR, which is calculated algorithmically by expressing the ratio of donor-induced CD154+CD8-memory cells and those induced by reference. Send the patient report to the ordering physician.

# Appendix P

## Summary of Additions, Deletions, and Revisions

The summary of changes shows the actual changes that have been made to the code descriptors.

New codes appear with a bullet (●) and are indicated as "Code added." Revised codes are preceded with a triangle (▲). Within revised codes, or if a code symbol has been deleted, the deleted language and code symbol appear with a ~~strikethrough~~, while new text appears <u>underlined</u>.

The ⚕ symbol is used to identify codes for vaccines that are pending FDA approval. The # symbol is used to identify codes that have been resequenced. CPT add-on codes are annotated by the + symbol. The ⊘ symbol is used to identify codes that are exempt from the use of modifier 51. The ★ symbol is used to identify codes that may be used for reporting telemedicine services. The ✖ symbol is used to identify a proprietary laboratory analyses (PLA) test that has an identical descriptor as another PLA test. A PLA code that satisfies Category I code criteria and has been accepted by the CPT Editorial Panel is annotated with the ↑↓ symbol.

| Code |
|------|
| <u>90785</u> |
| <u>90839</u> |
| <u>90840</u> |
| <u>90963</u> |
| <u>90964</u> |
| <u>90965</u> |
| <u>90966</u> |
| <u>90967</u> |
| <u>90968</u> |
| <u>90969</u> |
| <u>90970</u> |
| <u>96160</u> |
| <u>96161</u> |
| <u>97110</u> |
| <u>97112</u> |
| <u>97116</u> |
| <u>97161</u> |
| <u>97162</u> |
| <u>97165</u> |
| <u>97166</u> |

| Code |
|------|
| __97530__ |
| __97535__ |
| __97750__ |
| __97755__ |
| __97760__ |
| __97761__ |
| __99211__ |
| __99356__ |
| __99357__ |
| __99497__ |
| __99498__ |

★=Telemedicine   ✚=Add-on code   ✎=FDA approval pending   #=Resequenced code   ⊘=Modifier 51 exempt

# Appendix P

## CPT Codes That May Be Used For Synchronous Telemedicine Services

This listing is a summary of CPT codes that may be used for reporting synchronous (real-time) telemedicine services when appended by modifier 95. Procedures on this list involve electronic communication using interactive telecommunications equipment that includes, at a minimum, audio and video. The codes listed below are identified in CPT 2022 with the ★ symbol.

| | | | |
|---|---|---|---|
| 90785 | 90966 | 97750 | 99245 |
| 90791 | 90967 | 97755 | 99251 |
| 90792 | 90968 | 97760 | 99252 |
| 90832 | 90969 | 97761 | 99253 |
| 90833 | 90970 | 97802 | 99254 |
| 90834 | 92227 | 97803 | 99255 |
| 90836 | 92228 | 97804 | 99307 |
| 90837 | 93228 | 98960 | 99308 |
| 90838 | 93229 | 98961 | 99309 |
| 90839 | 93268 | 98962 | 99310 |
| 90840 | 93270 | 99202 | 99354 |
| 90845 | 93271 | 99203 | 99355 |
| 90846 | 93272 | 99204 | 99356 |
| 90847 | 96040 | 99205 | 99357 |
| 90863 | 96116 | 99211 | 99406 |
| 90951 | 96160 | 99212 | 99407 |
| 90952 | 96161 | 99213 | 99408 |
| 90954 | 97110 | 99214 | 99409 |
| 90955 | 97112 | 99215 | 99417 |
| 90957 | 97116 | 99231 | 99495 |
| 90958 | 97161 | 99232 | 99496 |
| 90960 | 97162 | 99233 | 99497 |
| 90961 | 97165 | 99241 | 99498 |
| 90963 | 97166 | 99242 | |
| 90964 | 97530 | 99243 | |
| 90965 | 97535 | 99244 | |

### Rationale

The listing in Appendix P has been revised to include codes 90785, 90839, 90840, 90963-90970, 96160, 96161, 97110, 97112, 97116, 97161, 97162, 97165, 97166, 97530, 97535, 97750, 97755, 97760, 97761, 99211, 99356, 99357, 99497, and 99498. These codes have been identified throughout the code set with the telemedicine (★) symbol.

To enable the reporting of additional telemedicine services, commercial and public payers continue to add CPT codes to their list of covered services that may be provided as telemedicine services. Note that the codes added this year were services that have been included in telemedicine coverage policies of at least one payer. As stated in the descriptor of modifier 95, Appendix P includes a list of CPT codes that describe services that are typically performed face-to-face but may be rendered via a real-time (synchronous) interactive audio and video telecommunications system.

# Notes

# ▶Appendix Q◀

## ▶Severe Acute Respiratory Syndrome Coronavirus 2 (SARS-CoV-2) (coronavirus disease [COVID-19]) Vaccines◀

▶This table links the individual severe acute respiratory syndrome coronavirus 2 (SARS-CoV-2) (coronavirus disease [COVID-19]) vaccine product codes (91300, 91301, 91302, 91303, 91304) to their associated immunization administration codes (0001A, 0002A, 0011A, 0012A, 0021A, 0022A, 0031A, 0041A, 0042A), manufacturer name, vaccine name(s), 10- and 11-digit National Drug Code (NDC) Labeler Product ID, and interval between doses. These codes are also located in the **Medicine** section of the CPT code set.

Additional introductory and instructional information for codes 0001A, 0002A, 0011A, 0012A, 0021A, 0022A, 0031A, 0041A, 0042A and 91300, 91301, 91302, 91303, 91304 can be found in the **Immunization Administration for Vaccines/Toxoids** and **Vaccines, Toxoids** guidelines in the **Medicine** section of the CPT code set.◀

| ▶Vaccine Code | Vaccine Administration Code(s) | Vaccine Manufacturer | Vaccine Name(s) | NDC 10/NDC 11 Labeler Product ID (Vial) | Dosing Interval |
|---|---|---|---|---|---|
| #●91300 Severe acute respiratory syndrome coronavirus 2 (SARS-CoV-2) (coronavirus disease [COVID-19]) vaccine, mRNA-LNP, spike protein, preservative free, 30 mcg/0.3 mL dosage, diluent reconstituted, for intramuscular use | ●0001A (1st Dose) ●0002A (2nd Dose) | Pfizer, Inc | Pfizer-BioNTech COVID-19 Vaccine | 59267-1000-1 59267-1000-01 | 21 Days |
| #●91301 Severe acute respiratory syndrome coronavirus 2 (SARS-CoV-2) (coronavirus disease [COVID-19]) vaccine, mRNA-LNP, spike protein, preservative free, 100 mcg/0.5 mL dosage, for intramuscular use | ●0011A (1st Dose) ●0012A (2nd Dose) | Moderna, Inc | Moderna COVID-19 Vaccine | 80777-273-10 80777-0273-10 | 28 Days |
| #✔●91302 Severe acute respiratory syndrome coronavirus 2 (SARS-CoV-2) (coronavirus disease [COVID-19]) vaccine, DNA, spike protein, chimpanzee adenovirus Oxford 1 (ChAdOx1) vector, preservative free, $5\times10^{10}$ viral particles/0.5 mL dosage, for intramuscular use | ●0021A (1st Dose) ●0022A (2nd Dose) | AstraZeneca, Plc | AstraZeneca COVID-19 Vaccine | 0310-1222-10 00310-1222-10 | 28 Days |
| #●91303 Severe acute respiratory syndrome coronavirus 2 (SARS-CoV-2) (coronavirus disease [COVID-19]) vaccine, DNA, spike protein, adenovirus type 26 (Ad26) vector, preservative free, $5\times10^{10}$ viral particles/0.5 mL dosage, for intramuscular use | ●0031A (Single Dose) | Janssen | Janssen COVID-19 Vaccine | 59676-580-05 59676-0580-05 | Not Applicable |
| #✔●91304 Severe acute respiratory syndrome coronavirus 2 (SARS-CoV-2) (coronavirus disease [COVID-19]) vaccine, recombinant spike protein nanoparticle, saponin-based adjuvant, preservative free, 5 mcg/0.5 mL dosage, for intramuscular use | ●0041A (1st Dose) ●0042A (2nd Dose) | Novavax, Inc | Novavax COVID-19 Vaccine | 80631-100-01 80631-1000-01 | 21 Days◀ |

▲=Revised code   ●=New code   ▶◀=Contains new or revised text   ✖=Duplicate PLA test   ↑↓=Category I PLA          American Medical Association   **279**

## Rationale

To accommodate the addition of new codes for reporting severe acute respiratory syndrome coronavirus 2 (SARS-CoV-2) (coronavirus disease [COVID-19]) vaccine products and their administration, Appendix Q has been added to the CPT code set.

Appendix Q includes a table that links the individual COVID-19 vaccine product codes (91300-91304) to their associated immunization administration codes (0001A, 0002A, 0011A, 0012A, 0021A, 0022A, 0031A, 0041A, 0042A), manufacturer name, vaccine name(s), 10- and 11-digit National Drug Code (NDC) Labeler Product ID, and interval between doses. This table allows easy visualization of all information related to a particular COVID vaccine product and its administration code. Guidelines have also been included for direction regarding what the table does and how it is used.

Refer to the codebook and the Rationale for codes 0001A-0042A for a full discussion of these changes.

# ►Appendix R◄

## ►Digital Medicine–Services Taxonomy◄

►Appendix R is a listing of digital medicine services described in the CPT code set. The digital medicine–services taxonomy table in this appendix classifies CPT codes that are related to digital medicine services into discrete categories of clinician-to-patient services (eg, visit), clinician-to-clinician services (eg, consultation), patient-monitoring services, and digital diagnostic services. The clinician-to-patient services and clinician-to-clinician services categories are differentiated by the nature of their services, ie, synchronous and asynchronous communication. The patient-monitoring services represent ongoing, extended monitoring that produces data that require physician assessment and interpretation and are further categorized into device/software set-up and education, data transfer, and data-interpretation services. The digital diagnostic services differentiate automated/autonomous, algorithmically enabled diagnostic-support services into patient-directed and image/specimen-directed services. The term "clinician" in the table represents a physician or other qualified health care professional (QHP) who may use the specific code(s).

This taxonomy is intended to support increased awareness and understanding of approaches to patient care through the multifaceted digital medicine services available for reporting in the CPT code set. The taxonomy is not intended to be a complete representation of all applicable digital medicine service codes in the CPT code set and does not supersede specific coding guidance listed in specific sections of the CPT code set. Furthermore, the table does not denote services that are currently payable through coverage policies by either public or commercial payers.

For purposes of this appendix, the following terms should be understood as:

- Digital medicine services represent the use of technologies for measurement and intervention in the service of patient health.

- Synchronous services represent real-time interactions between a distant-site physician or other QHP and a patient and/or family located at a remote originating site.

- Asynchronous services represent store-and-forward transmissions of health information over periods of time using a secure Web server, encrypted email, specially designed store-and-forward software, or electronic health record. Asynchronous services enable a patient to share health information for later review by the physician or other QHP. These services also allow a physician or other QHP to share a patient's medical history, images, physiologic/non-physiologic clinical data and/or pathology and laboratory reports with a specialist physician for diagnostic and treatment expertise.◄

▲ Digital Medicine–Services Taxonomy ▼

| | Clinician*-to-Patient Services (Eg, visit) | | Clinician-to-Clinician Services (Eg, consultation) | | Patient Monitoring and/or Therapeutic Services | | | Digital Diagnostic Services | |
| --- | --- | --- | --- | --- | --- | --- | --- | --- | --- |
| | Synchronous | Asynchronous | Synchronous | Asynchronous | Device/Software Set-Up and Education | Data Transfer | Data Interpretation | Patient Directed | Image/Specimen Directed |
| **Encounter Activity** | Real-time audiovisual interaction | Store-and-forward digital communication | Real-time consultative communication between requesting and consulting clinicians | Store-and-forward consultative digital exchange of clinical information between requesting and consulting clinicians | In-person, virtual face-to-face, telephone, or other modalities of communication with patient to support device set-up education/supply | Acquisition of patient data with transfer to managing or inter-preting physician/other QHP/clinical staff | Data review, interpretation, and patient management by clinical staff/physician/other QHP with associated patient communication | Automated and autonomous algorithmically enabled diagnostic support | |
| **CPT Service** | E/M performed as virtual face-to-face visit (*Use modifier 95*); Telephone services (Audio only) (99441-99443) | Online digital evaluation & management (99421-99423) (98970-98972) | Interprofessional telephone/Internet/EHR consultation (Typically via telephone) (99446-99449, 99451); If patient is present at originating site → transition to virtual face-to-face E/M consultation (*Use modifier 95*) | Interprofessional telephone/Internet/EHR consultation (99446-99449, 99451, 99452) | Remote physiologic monitoring initial set-up/education (99453) | Remote physiologic monitoring device supply (99454) | Physiologic data collection/interpretation by physician/other QHP (99091); Remote physiologic monitoring treatment management by clinical staff/physician/other QHP (99457, 99458) | Automated retinopathy screening (92229) | Multianalyte assays with algorithmic analyses (MAAA) |

**▶ Digital Medicine—Services Taxonomy ◀ (cont'd)**

| CPT Service | Clinician*-to-Patient Services (Eg. visit) Synchronous | Asynchronous | Clinician-to-Clinician Services (Eg. consultation) Synchronous | Asynchronous | Patient Monitoring and/or Therapeutic Services — Device/Software Set-Up and Education | Data Transfer | Data Interpretation | Digital Diagnostic Services — Patient Directed | Image/Specimen Directed |
|---|---|---|---|---|---|---|---|---|---|
| | | | | | Remote therapeutic monitoring initial set-up/education (98975) | Remote therapeutic monitoring device supply (98976 for respiratory system; 98977 for musculoskeletal system) | Remote therapeutic monitoring treatment management by physician/other QHP (98980, 98981) | | Computer-aided detection (CAD) imaging (77048, 77049, 77065-77067, 0042T, 0174T, 0175T) |
| | | | | | Remote pulmonary artery pressure sensor monitoring treatment management by physician/other QHP (93264) | | | | |
| | | | | | | Ambulatory continuous glucose monitoring hook-up, education, recording print-out (95250 for office-equipped; 95249 for patient-equipped) | Ambulatory continuous glucose monitoring analysis (95251) | | |
| | | | | | External electrocardiographic recording (Recording, scanning analysis with report, review and interpretation) (93224, 93241, 93245) | | | | |
| | | | | | External electrocardiographic recording (Recording) (93224, 93225, 93241, 93242, 93245, 93246) | External electrocardiographic recording (Scanning analysis with report only) (93226, 93241, 93243, 93247) | External electrocardiographic recording (Review and interpretation) (93224, 93227, 93241, 93244, 93245, 93248) | External electrocardiographic recording (Autonomous algorithms used to analyze/create report) (93241-93243, 93245-93247) | |

(Continued on page 284)

**Appendix R**

**Appendix R**

### ▶ Digital Medicine—Services Taxonomy ◀ (cont'd)

| CPT Service | ▶ Clinician*-to-Patient Services (Eg. visit) | | Clinician-to-Clinician Services (Eg. consultation) | | Patient Monitoring and/or Therapeutic Services | | | Digital Diagnostic Services | |
|---|---|---|---|---|---|---|---|---|---|
| | Synchronous | Asynchronous | Synchronous | Asynchronous | Device/Software Set-Up and Education | Data Transfer | Data Interpretation | Patient Directed | Image/Specimen Directed |
| | | | | | | External mobile cardiovascular telemetry technical support (93229) | External mobile cardiovascular telemetry review and interpretation (93228) | | |
| | | | | | Remote monitoring of digital cognitive behavioral therapy program (Supply and technical support) (0702T) | | Remote monitoring treatment management by physician/other QHP (0703T) | | |
| | | | | | Digital amblyopia services (0704T for initial set-up/education; 0705T for surveillance center technical support, including data transmission) | | Digital amblyopia services (Assessment of patient performance, program data) (0706T) | | |
| | | | | | | Automated analysis of CT study (Data preparation, interpretation and report) (0691T) ◢▼ | | | |

*The term "clinician" in the table represents a physician or other qualified health care professional (QHP) by whom the specific code may be used.

★ = Telemedicine   ✦ = Add-on code   ✒ = FDA approval pending   # = Resequenced code   ⊘ = Modifier 51 exempt

# Rationale

Appendix R has been added to the CPT code set to provide a taxonomy of digital medicine services currently described in the CPT code set. Appendix R classifies existing CPT codes that describe digital medicine into discrete categories that are organized by the provider of the services and the activities involved in the clinician work.

Digital medicine services are a rapidly growing area of medicine and thus, within the CPT code set. As digital medicine services become more and more ubiquitous, accurately understanding and categorizing these services in the CPT code set will be increasingly important. The intent is for Appendix R to be used to support increased awareness and understanding of digital medicine services; it is not intended to have any implications on payer-coverage policy.

While Appendix R is not meant to be a comprehensive list of every digital medicine service currently in the CPT code set, it is anticipated that it will be updated regularly to reflect newly described services.

Refer to the codebook for a full list of definitions and descriptions of the individual categories.

# Notes

# Indexes

## Instructions for the Use of the Changes Indexes

The Changes Indexes are not a substitute for the main text of *CPT Changes 2022* or the main text of the CPT codebook. The changes indexes consist of two types of content—coding changes and modifiers—all of which are intended to assist users in searching and locating information quickly within *CPT Changes 2022*.

## Index of Coding Changes

The Index of Coding Changes list new, revised, and deleted codes, and/or some codes that may be affected by revised and/or new guidelines and parenthetical notes. This index enables users to quickly search and locate the codes within a page(s), in addition to discerning the status of a code (new, revised, deleted, or textually changed) because the status of each new, revised, or deleted code is noted in parentheses next to the code number:

0099U (deleted)..............................................................94, 123, 126, 234, 253, 273
64629 (new) ..............................................................................29, 35, 74–75

## Index of Modifiers

The Index of Modifiers does not list all modifiers unless they are new, revised, or deleted, and/or if the modifier may be affected by revised and/or new codes, guidelines, and parenthetical notes. A limited Index of Modifiers, ie, limited to only those modifiers that appear in the Rationales and new or revised guidelines and/or parenthetical notes, is provided to help users quickly locate these modifiers and to know where in the book these modifiers are listed or mentioned.

50, Bilateral Procedure............................................................................51, 60
51, Multiple Procedures ...................................................................51, 60, 145

★ = Telemedicine   ✚ = Add-on code   ✗ = FDA approval pending   # = Resequenced code   ⊘ = Modifier 51 exempt

# Index of Coding Changes

Codes in this index are in numerical order, with the four-digit alphanumeric codes first:

Category II changes (a four-digit code followed by the letter "F"); Category III changes (a four-digit code followed by the letter "T"); changes to administrative codes for multianalyte assays with algorithmic analyses (MAAA) (a four-digit code followed by the letter "M"); and changes to proprietary laboratory analysis (PLA) codes (a four-digit code followed by the letter "U"). Five-digit CPT codes follow.

★ = Telemedicine    ✚ = Add-on code    𝗡 = FDA approval pending    # = Resequenced code    ⊘ = Modifier 51 exempt

Indexes

Indexes

Indexes

★ = Telemedicine    ✚ = Add-on code    ✖ = FDA approval pending    # = Resequenced code    ⊘ = Modifier 51 exempt

# Index of Modifiers

The modifiers in this Index of Modifiers is limited to only the modifiers that appear in the Rationales and in the new or revised guidelines and/or parenthetical notes.

## Modifier, Descriptor             **Page Numbers**

# NOTES

# NOTES

# NOTES

# NOTES

# NOTES

# NOTES

# NOTES

# NOTES

# NOTES

# NOTES

# NOTES

# NOTES

# NOTES

# NOTES

# NOTES